The Handbook of
SURGICAL
INTENSIVE CARE

The Handbook of
SURGICAL
INTENSIVE CARE

**Practices of the Surgical Residents
at Duke University Medical Center**

FOURTH EDITION

Edited by

Thomas A. D'Amico, M.D.
Fellow in Cardiothoracic Surgery
Duke University Medical Center
Durham, North Carolina

Scott K. Pruitt, M.D., Ph.D.
Senior Resident
Duke University Medical Center
Durham, North Carolina

with 34 illustrations

M Mosby

St. Louis Baltimore Boston Carlsbad Chicago Naples New York
Philadelphia Portland London Madrid Mexico City Singapore
Sydney Tokyo Toronto Wiesbaden

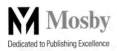

M Mosby

Dedicated to Publishing Excellence

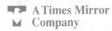

A Times Mirror Company

Editor: *Susie Baxter*
Developmental Editor: *Anne Gunter*
Project Manager: *Linda McKinley*
Production Editor: *Catherine Bricker*
Designer: *Elizabeth Fett*

FOURTH EDITION

Printed in the United States of America

Composition by Graphic World, Inc.

Printing/binding by Malloy Lithography, Inc.

Mosby-Year Book, Inc.
11830 Westline Industrial Drive, St. Louis, Missouri 63146

International Standard Book Number 0-8151-2249-7

96   97   98   99   /   9   8   7   6   5   4   3   2

CONTRIBUTORS

All contributors are from the Department of Surgery, Duke University Medical Center, Durham, North Carolina.

Paul M. Ahearne, M.D.
Chief Resident

Ravi S. Chari, M.D.
Senior Resident

Bradley H. Collins, M.D.
Senior Resident

Thomas A. D'Amico, M.D.
Fellow in Cardiothoracic
Surgery

Andrew M. Davidoff, M.D.
Chief Resident

Stanley A. Gall, Jr., M.D.
Fellow in Cardiothoracic
Surgery

Jeffrey S. Heinle, M.D.
Fellow in Cardiothoracic
Surgery

Allan D. Kirk, M.D., Ph.D.
Chief Resident

James R. Mault, M.D.
Chief Resident

Cary H. Meyers, M.D.
Senior Resident

Carmelo A. Milano, M.D.
Senior Resident

Clarence H. Owen, M.D.
Senior Resident

David S. Peterseim, M.D.
Chief Resident

**William N. Peugh, M.D.,
Ph.D.**
Chief Resident

Scott K. Pruitt, M.D., Ph.D.
Senior Resident

Cemil M. Purut, M.D.
Chief Resident

Lewis B. Schwartz, M.D.
Chief Resident

Mark W. Sebastian, M.D.
Fellow in Cardiothoracic
Surgery

Mark Tedder, M.D.
Chief Resident

FOREWORD

As the field of surgery continues to expand, the complexity of many surgical procedures becomes greater each year. With these advances, increasing emphasis has been placed on intensive care. Since this specialty constitutes one of the most important factors determining the clinical outcome of these patients, previous editions of *The Handbook of Surgical Intensive Care* have had a wide impact and have served as valuable resources in the management of a variety of difficult clinical problems.

The last edition was edited by Drs. H. Kim Lyerly and J. William Gaynor, both of whom now have academic surgical appointments at Duke University Medical Center and at the University of Pennsylvania—Philadelphia Children's Hospital, respectively. Previous editions of the *Handbook* reached impressive heights with translations into both Spanish and German, which made certain that the texts had an expanded impact in Europe as well as in South America. It is astonishing that over forty thousand copies have been printed in three languages, assuring worldwide use of this very important text.

In this fourth edition the new editors, Dr. Thomas A. D'Amico, Fellow in Cardiothoracic Surgery, and Dr. Scott K. Pruitt, Senior Resident in Surgery, and 17 of their colleagues have continued the tradition of this manual. They have meticulously updated each chapter in a most commendable manner and have simultaneously maintained the standard of excellence set by the previous editions. It is important to emphasize that this handbook, written by surgical residents, is primarily designed for use by surgical residents. In addition, it will also be quite useful for all surgeons, nurses, physicians assistants, and medical students in managing patients in intensive care units. The surgical residents obtain their training in this field by individually caring for acutely ill patients, through discussions on teaching rounds and conferences, and by remaining abreast of the surgical literature. There are currently 56 beds in the surgical intensive care units at Duke University Medical Center, where the residents gain an extensive knowledge of many surgical problems, including those that occur in general and cardiothoracic surgery as well as in the surgical subspecialties of neurosurgery, orthopedics, otolaryngology, pediatric surgery, plastic and maxillo-facial surgery, and urology.

Through the years my greatest pleasure has been derived from close association with surgical residents in their clinical work, research, publishing, and assisting in their career plans. It is a special privilege to acknowledge the scholarly talents to the current editors, Drs. Thomas A. D'Amico and Scott K. Pruitt and their colleagues in preparing this *masterwork*. It is easy to predict that they will become leaders in academic surgery and much will be heard from them and their contributions in the future. Just as in the last edition, this fourth edition can be expected to follow the same upward path of its predecessors.

Finally, *The Handbook of Surgical Intensive Care* can be highly recommended to surgeons everywhere as the standard reference in the field. Patients managed by these principles will predictably have the best possible clinical outcomes. The authors are deserving of much praise for their attention to detail in updating this splendid text, which is highly recommended with both confidence and enthusiasm.

David C. Sabiston, Jr., M.D.
James B. Duke Professor of Surgery and Chief of Staff
Distinguished Physician of the Veterans Administration
Duke University Medical Center

PREFACE

Previous editions of *The Handbook of Surgical Intensive Care: Practices of the Surgical Residents at Duke University Medical Center* have succeeded in providing an established standard for the management of the critically ill surgical patient. We are indebted to the preceding editors for their stamina and attention to detail in making this text a premier guide for surgical intensive care. The third edition, edited by H. Kim Lyerly and J. William Gaynor, was particularly successful in presenting a thorough description of the pathophysiology of the critically ill patient.

Rapid advances in the understanding of critical care and the management of the critically ill surgical patient have brought forth a new edition of the *Handbook*. This volume, which continues to represent the practices of the surgical residents at Duke University Medical Center, is a reflection of the outstanding education provided by our faculty. Each chapter has been revised to represent the current understanding of a dynamic field. We are indebted to our contributors for their outstanding efforts in presenting a discipline with such a wide scope in a concise and cogent format.

The goal of the fourth edition is to uphold the standard set by the foregoing editions, provide current understanding of the pathophysiology of critical illness, establish a framework for the study of intensive care, and convey the essential aspects of the management of complex problems in the surgical intensive care unit.

Thomas A. D'Amico
Scott K. Pruitt

LIST OF ABBREVIATIONS

AAA	abdominal aortic aneurysm
ABI	ankle-brachial index
ABG	arterial blood gas
ACE	angiotensin-converting enzyme
ACLS	advanced cardiac life support
ACT	activated clotting time
ACTH	adrenocorticotropic hormone
ADH	antidiuretic hormone
AHA	American Heart Association
AIOD	aortoiliac occlusive disease
APTT	activated partial thromboplastin time
ARF	acute renal failure; acute respiratory failure
ARDS	adult respiratory distress syndrome
ATN	acute tubular necrosis
AVo$_2$	arteriovenous O_2 content difference
BLS	basic life support
BP	blood pressure
BSA	body surface area
BUN	blood urea nitrogen
CABG	coronary artery bypass graft
CAD	coronary artery disease
CAVHD	continuous arteriovenous hemodialysis
Cao$_2$	arterial oxygen content
CBC	complete blood count
C$_{CR}$	creatinine clearance
CDH	congenital diaphragmatic hernia

CHF	congestive heart failure
CI	cardiac index
CK	creatine kinase
CMV	cytomegalovirus; controlled mechanical ventilation
CNS	central nervous system
CO	cardiac output
COPD	chronic obstructive pulmonary disease
CPAP	continuous positive airway pressure
CPB	cardiopulmonary bypass
CPK	creatine phosphokinase
CSF	cerebrospinal fluid
CT	computed tomography
CVA	cerebrovascular accident
Cvo_2	mixed venous oxygen content
CVP	central venous pressure
CXR	chest x-ray
DIC	disseminated intravascular coagulation
Do_2	oxygen delivery
DVT	deep vein thrombosis
EBV	Epstein-Barr virus
ECG	electrocardiogram
ECMO	extracorporeal membrane oxygenation
EEG	electroencephalogram
EMD	electromechanical dissociation
ERCP	endoscopic retrograde cholangiopancreatography
ERV	expiratory reserve volume
FDP	fibrin degradation product
FE_{NA}	fractional excretion of sodium
FEV	forced expiratory volume
FFP	fresh frozen plasma
Fio_2	fractional concentration of oxygen in inspired gas
FRC	functional residual capacity
GABA	γ-aminobutyric acid
GE	gastroesophageal

GFR	glomerular filtration rate
GH	growth hormone
GHIF	growth hormone inhibiting factor
GHRF	growth hormone releasing factor
GI	gastrointestinal
HATT	heparin-associated thrombotic thrombocytopenia
Hct	hematocrit
HPLC	high performance liquid chromatography
HR	heart rate
HRS	hepatorenal syndrome
HSV	herpes simplex virus
IABP	intraaortic balloon pump
IC	inspiratory capacity
ICP	intracranial pressure
I:E	inspiration to expiration ratio
IFR	inspiratory flow rate
IL	interleukin
IMA	inferior mesenteric artery
IMV	intermittent mandatory ventilation
IPPB	intermittent positive pressure breathing
IRV	inspiratory reserve volume
ITP	immune thrombocytopenia purpura
JVD	jugular venous distention
KUB	kidney, ureter, bladder
LA	left atrium/atrial
LAP	left atrial pressure
LDH	lactate dehydrogenase
LDL	low density lipoprotein
LFT	liver function test
LUQ	left upper quadrant
LV	left ventricle
LVEDP	left ventricular end-diastolic pressure
MAP	mean systemic arterial pressure
MAS	meconium aspiration syndrome

MAST	medical antishock trousers
MB	muscle-brain
MI	myocardial infarction
MIBG	metaiodobenzylguanidine
MOF	multiple organ failure
MUGA	multigated
MVo$_2$	myocardial oxygen consumption
NG	nasogastric
NS	normal saline
NSAID	nonsteroidal antiinflammatory drug
NTG	nitroglycerin
O$_2$ER	oxygen extraction ratio
OI	oxygen index
PA	pulmonary artery
Pao$_2$	arterial oxygen partial pressure
Paco$_2$	arterial carbon dioxide partial pressure
PCWP	pulmonary capillary wedge pressure
PE	pulmonary embolism
PEEP	positive end-expiratory pressure
PIP	peak inspiratory pressure
PPHN	persistent pulmonary hypertension of the newborn
P$_{osm}$	plasma osmolality
PRBCs	packed red blood cells
PSVT	paroxysmal supraventricular tachycardia
PT	prothrombin time
PTCA	percutaneous transluminal angioplasty
PTHC	percutaneous transhepatic cholangiography
PTT	partial thromboplastin time
PVC	premature ventricular contraction
RA	right atrium/atrial
RATG	rabbit antithymocyte globulin
RBC	red blood cell
RIA	radioimmunoassay
RIND	reversible ischemic neurologic deficit

rt-PA	recombinant tissue plasminogen activator
RV	right ventricle/ventricular; residual volume
Sao$_2$	arterial oxygen saturation
SGOT	serum glutamic-oxaloacetic transaminase
SIADH	syndrome of inappropriate secretion of antidiuretic hormone
SIMV	synchronized intermittent mandatory ventilation
SLE	systemic lupus erythematosus
SNP	sodium nitroprusside
SV	stroke volume
Svo$_2$	mixed venous oxygen saturation
SVR	systemic vascular resistance
T$_3$	triiodothyronine
T$_4$	thyroxine
TCT	thrombin clotting time
TE	tracheoesophageal
TIA	transient ischemic attack
TLC	total lung capacity
TNF	tumor necrosis factor
TPN	total parenteral nutrition
TSH	thyroid stimulating hormone
TTP	thrombotic thrombocytopenia purpura
UGI	upper gastrointestinal series
U$_{osm}$	urine osmolality
UPJ	ureteropelvic junction
URI	upper respiratory infection
VC	vital capacity
V$_d$	ventilatory dead space
V$_E$	minute volume ventilation
VMA	vanillylmendelic acid
V/Q	ventilation/perfusion
Vo$_2$	oxygen consumption
VSD	ventricular septal defect
V$_T$	tidal volume

vWD	von Willebrand's disease
vWF	von Willebrand's factor
VZV	varicella zoster virus
WBC	white blood cell
WDHA	watery diarrhea hypophosphatemia acidosis

CONTENTS

The Handbook of
SURGICAL
INTENSIVE CARE

PART ONE

Fundamental Principles of Surgical Intensive Care

HEMODYNAMIC MANAGEMENT 1

Thomas A. D'Amico

I. **RATIONALE FOR HEMODYNAMIC MONITORING**
A. **Basic Hemodynamic Monitoring**
   1. In the SICU, some patients may be noninvasively monitored with continuous ECG, automatic BP cuff systems, and pulse oximetry to provide continuous (or nearly continuous) recording of BP, HR, cardiac rhythm, and Sao_2.
   2. Invasive monitoring is reserved for high-risk or critically ill patients.
B. **High-Risk Populations**
   1. Patients with known CAD undergoing major procedures
   2. Patients undergoing major vascular procedures; 40% to 70% have significant CAD
   3. Patients with other significant cardiac risk factors
      a. Arrhythmia on preoperative ECG
      b. Left ventricular hypertrophy
      c. Age > 65 years
   4. Patients with significant pulmonary risk factors
      a. COPD
      b. Heavy tobacco use
      c. Asthma
   5. Patients with previous stroke
   6. Patients with other organ system failure, such as hepatic insufficiency (cirrhosis), renal insufficiency, coagulation disorders, or immunodeficiency
C. **Criteria for Critical Illness**
   1. Extensive ablative procedure for carcinoma (>5 hours), such as esophagogastrectomy, pancreaticoduodenectomy
   2. Severe multisystem trauma
   3. Massive blood loss (>8 units)
   4. Shock on presentation

5. Sepsis
6. Nutritional insufficiency associated with surgical illness (≥10 kg weight loss; albumin < 3 mg/dl)
7. Respiratory failure, prolonged mechanical ventilation
8. Acute abdominal catastrophe
9. Acute renal failure
10. Acute hepatic failure
11. Acute decompensation in mental status
12. Acute MI, cardiac failure
13. PE
14. Sustained postoperative hemorrhage
15. Sustained fluid and electrolyte or acid-base abnormality

II. CONTINUOUS ECG
A. Purpose
1. Facilitates detection of rhythm and conduction abnormalities
2. Continuous determination of HR
B. Indications
1. Used in all critically ill patients
2. Particularly useful in patients with high risk for postoperative arrhythmias
   a. Cardiac surgery
   b. Pulmonary resection
   c. Patients with known CAD
   d. Patients receiving inotropic support

III. SYSTEMIC ARTERIAL CATHETER
A. Purpose
1. Continuous determination of systolic, diastolic, and mean arterial pressures
2. Facilitation of frequent ABG analysis
B. Indications
1. Hemodynamic monitoring in patients receiving inotropic or vasoactive agents
2. Hemodynamically unstable patients
3. Patients who require prolonged mechanical ventilation as a consequence of either acute or chronic pulmonary processes

IV. CENTRAL VENOUS CATHETER
A. Purpose
1. Determination of central venous (RA) pressures and, indirectly, volume status in patients with normal RV function

   2. Delivery of inotropes or other medications that require central access
B. Indications
   1. Estimation of cardiac filling pressures in patients without preexisting cardiac or pulmonary disease who are subject to rapid changes in volume status
      a. Procedures in which major blood loss is common, such as hepatic resection
      b. Procedures anticipated to last longer than 3 hours or during which estimation of third space fluid loss is judged to be inadequate
      c. GI bleeding or other hemorrhagic conditions
      d. Pancreatitis or other conditions with extensive third-space fluid sequestration
   2. Useful in the diagnosis of cardiac tamponade
   3. Not accurate in the estimation of left-sided cardiac filling pressures in patients with cardiac valvular disease, pulmonary hypertension, or low ejection fraction

V. PULMONARY ARTERY CATHETER
A. Purpose
   1. Measurement of right ventricular filling pressures: CVP, RA pressure, RV pressure
   2. Measurement of PA pressures: PA systolic, diastolic, mean pressures; PCWP
   3. Measurement of cardiac output
   4. Estimation of perfusion: Svo_2
   5. Assessment of Do_2 and Vo_2
   6. Cardiac pacing
B. Indications
   1. Direct determination of CVP, RA pressure, RV pressure, PA pressures (systolic, diastolic, mean), and PCWP in high-risk or critically ill patients
   2. Indirect assessment of LAP and LVEDP; determination of volume status
      a. When the balloon is properly advanced into the pulmonary vasculature and wedged, the distal pulmonary circulation is isolated from the proximal pulmonary pressure.
      b. An unbroken fluid column exists between the tip of the catheter and the pulmonary veins. The PCWP is the best estimate of the LAP.

      c. In patients with normal hearts, the LAP is a good estimate of the LVEDP.

      d. Conditions in which the relationship between PCWP and LVEDP fails:

         (1) Pulmonary veno-occlusive disease, atrial tumors

         (2) Mitral valve disease

         (3) Aortic insufficiency

         (4) Diminished LV compliance

3. Determination of cardiac output by the thermodilution technique

4. Assessment of Svo_2

      a. Available continuously with oximetric PA catheters

      b. May alternatively be obtained serially by aspirating mixed venous blood from the distal port and performing blood gas analysis

5. Calculation of Do_2 and Vo_2

6. Intracardiac pacing in patients with acute heart block

VI. USE OF HEMODYNAMIC PARAMETERS IN PATIENT MANAGEMENT

A. Systemic Blood Pressure

1. Arterial catheters and continuous BP monitoring are useful in patients with hypotension or hypertension to guide therapy.

      a. Patients receiving inotropic or chronotropic support with β-adrenergic agonists

      b. Patient receiving vasopressor therapy with α-adrenergic agonists

      c. Patients receiving intravenous vasodilator therapy

2. In addition to the determination and maintenance of systolic, diastolic, and mean arterial pressures, continuous arterial pressure monitoring is essential in the optimization of afterload.

3. Systemic vascular resistance (SVR) is an index of afterload. The SVR index (SVRI) is a normalized value (normal range is 900 to 1400 dynes/sec/cm^{-5}):

$$SVRI = [(MAP - MRAP) \times 80]/CI$$

where MAP is mean systemic arterial pressure, MRAP is mean RA pressure, and CI is cardiac index

4. SVR may be manipulated to optimize cardiac output with afterload-reducing agents
   a. Nitrates: Sodium nitroprusside, nitroglycerin
   b. Phosphodiesterase inhibitors: Milrinone, amrinone
   c. ACE inhibitors: Captopril, enalapril
   d. Calcium channel blockade: Nifedipine, diltiazem
   e. α-Adrenergic antagonists: Prazosin, labetolol
   f. IABP

B. Ventricular Filling Pressures
   1. Critically ill patients should be aggressively resuscitated with crystalloid solution, colloids, or blood products as appropriate.
   2. The best index of complete fluid resuscitation is the determination of ventricular filling pressures.
   3. In patients with normal cardiac function, CVP is adequate.
   4. In patients with cardiopulmonary disease or patients requiring cardiac or pulmonary support, determination of left ventricular filling pressures with a PA catheter is required.

C. Mixed Venous Oxygen Saturation
   1. Svo_2 is an estimate of the oxygen extracted by the systemic circulation and is used as an index of perfusion. The Svo_2 in a normal individual is 75%.
   2. In critically ill patients Svo_2 is used to monitor trends in overall perfusion to detect periods of inadequate perfusion and to intervene in order to prevent organ system failure.
      a. An increase in Svo_2 is considered to represent an improvement in perfusion (an increase in Do_2 with no significant change in Vo_2); alternatively, an increase in Svo_2 may represent stable Do_2 and a decrease in Vo_2 (metabolic uncoupling) secondary to changes in a single organ system (such as hepatic failure) or systemic processes (such as sepsis).
      b. A decrease in Svo_2 is considered to represent a deterioration in perfusion (a decrease in Do_2 with no significant change in Vo_2); alternatively, a decrease in Svo_2 may represent stable Do_2 and an increase in Vo_2.
   3. Svo_2 may be used to monitor the effect of interventions intended to improve perfusion (inotropes, afterload-reducing agents, blood transfusions).
   4. Svo_2 may be used to monitor the systemic manifestations of ventilator weaning.

5. Evaluation of a patient with a sustained decrease in Svo_2 requires the consideration of several variables:
   a. Increased oxygen consumption?
      (1) Movement, incomplete relaxation during mechanical ventilation, shivering
      (2) Pain
      (3) Fever
   b. Decreased oxygenation?
      (1) Ventilator disconnection
      (2) Endotracheal tube malposition
      (3) Pneumothorax
      (4) Other pulmonary pathophysiology: ARDS, pneumonia
   c. Decreased cardiac output?
      (1) Preload
      (2) Afterload
      (3) HR
      (4) Contractility
   d. Decreased oxygen-carrying capacity?
      (1) Acidosis
      (2) Hb concentration

D. **Oxygen Delivery and Consumption**
   1. *Oxygen content* (Cao_2) is the sum of oxygen bound to hemoglobin (Hb) and the oxygen dissolved in blood (Sao_2):

   $$Cao_2 = (Hb \times 1.36 \times Sao_2) + (Pao_2 \times 0.03)$$

   Oxygen bound by 1 g Hb at full saturation (Sao_2) = 1.36 ml O_2
   Solubility coefficient of O_2 = 0.03 ml O_2/L blood/mm Hg

   2. *Oxygen delivery* (Do_2) depends on arterial oxygen content (Cao_2) and cardiac output (CO) (normal value is 800 to 1200 ml/min at rest):

   $$Do_2 = Cao_2 \times CO$$

   3. *Oxygen consumption* (Vo_2) is the rate at which the body takes up oxygen. It depends on the difference among arterial oxygen content (Cao_2) and venous oxygen content (Cvo_2) and cardiac output (CO) (normal value is 225 to 275 ml/min at rest):

$$Vo_2 = (Cao_2 \times CO) - (Cvo_2 \times CO) = (Cao_2 - Cvo_2) \times CO$$

4. *Oxygen utilization ratio* is the relationship of oxygen consumption to delivery (normal value is 15% to 25%):

$$Vo_2/Do_2$$

E. Therapeutic Goals

1. The relationship between Do_2 and Vo_2 is determined by five factors:
   a. Hb content of blood
   b. Affinity of Hb for oxygen (oxyhemoglobin dissociation curve)
   c. Hb oxygen saturation
   d. Cardiac output
   e. Oxygen consumption

2. Oxygen debt (inadequate Vo_2) appears to be a major determinant of organ failure and outcome in critically injured patients. Avoidance of oxygen debt may be achieved by optimizing the factors that determine Do_2:
   a. Hb content of blood: RBC transfusion to keep Hb at 10 to 15 g/dl
   b. Affinity of Hb for oxygen: Optimizing temperature and pH
   c. Hb oxygen saturation: Adequate oxygen administration
   d. Cardiac output: Aggressive fluid resuscitation and inotropic support as needed; dobutamine is the inotropic agent of choice

3. The achievement of a set of therapeutic hemodynamic goals in critically ill patients is associated with improved survival.
   a. Supranormal cardiac output: CI > 4.5 L/min/m^2
   b. Do_2 > 600 ml/min/m^2
   c. Vo_2 > 170 ml/min/m^2

4. Optimization of Do_2 and Vo_2 is considered complete when an incremental increase in Do_2 is not associated with an increase in Vo_2.

SUGGESTED READING

Reid KR, Leasa DJ, Sibbald WJ: Postoperative monitoring of the thoracic surgical patient, *Chest Surg Clin North Am* 2:317–335, 1991.

Shoemaker WC, Appel PL, Kram HB: Tissue oxygen debt as a determinant of lethal and nonlethal postoperative organ failure, *Crit Care Med* 16:1117–1120, 1988.

Shoemaker WC, Bland RD, Appel PL: Therapy of critically ill postoperative patients based on outcome prediction and prospective clinical trials, *Surg Clin North Am* 65:811–833, 1985.

Shoemaker WC et al: Prospective trial of supranormal values of survivors as therapeutic goals in high-risk surgical patients, *Chest* 94:1176–1186, 1988.

Snyder JV: *Oxygen transport: the model and reality.* In Snyder JV, Pinsky MR, eds: *Oxygen transport in the critically ill,* Chicago, Year Book, 1987.

SHOCK 2

Mark Tedder

I. INTRODUCTION

A. Definition

Shock defines a physiologic state in which tissue perfusion is inadequate to maintain normal organ function.

B. Pathophysiology

Although for over a century the clinical assessment of shock was based on BP and cardiac output, currently it is best described by the relationship between Do_2 and Vo_2. In shock, Vo_2 decreases at the "critical Do_2" (or "anaerobic threshold") (Fig. 2-1), signifying inadequate Do_2 to meet the metabolic demand.

C. Diagnosis

Early diagnosis remains difficult as early symptoms and physical findings are frequently nonspecific (Table 2-1).

1. Symptoms
   a. Shortness of breath
   b. Altered mental status (from minimal agitation or anxiety to obtundation or coma)
2. Signs
   a. Hypotension
   b. Tachycardia
   c. Tachypnea/respiratory distress
   d. Decreased urine output

D. Treatment

After diagnosis, therapy is immediately instituted with the specific treatment dependent on the etiology.

E. Results

Despite aggressive therapy and recent advances in provided care in the SICU, the mortality rate remains unacceptably high.

F. Complications

Persistent shock will result in MOF and ultimately death.

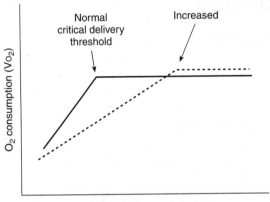

FIG 2-1.

The Do_2-Vo_2 relationship is biphasic. Patients are normally in the oxygen supply–independent phase; however, various stresses including shock can result in a progression to the oxygen supply–dependent phase where cellular metabolic requirements are not being met. (From Shumaker PT, Samsel RW: Oxygen delivery and uptake by peripheral tissues, *Crit Care Clin* 5:259, 1989.)

TABLE 2-1.
Clinical Presentation of the Various Types of Shock

Etiology	Skin	Urine Output	JVD	Cardiac Index	PCWP	SVR	Cvo_2
Hypovolemic	Cool, pale	↓	↓	↓	↓	↑	↓
Traumatic	Cool, pale	↓	↓	↓	↓	↑	↓
Cardiogenic	Cool, pale	↓	↑	↓	↑	↑	↓
Early septic	Warm, pink	↓↑	↓↑	↑	↓↑	↓	↑
Late septic	Cool, pale	↓	↓	↓	↓	↑	↓↑
Neurogenic	Warm, pink	↓	↓	↓	↓	↓	↓
Anaphylactic	Cool, pale	↓	↓	↓	↓	↑	↓

TABLE 2-2.

Normal Values for Oxygen Delivery and Consumption Variables

Variable	Value
Do_2	640-1400 ml O_2/min (500-600 ml O_2/min/m^2)
Cao_2	18-24 ml O_2/dl
Vo_2	180-280 ml O_2/min (110-160 ml O_2/min/m^2)
Cvo_2	14-20 ml O_2/dl
O_2ER	22%-30%
AVo_2	3.5-5.5 ml O_2/dl

II. BACKGROUND

A. Definition

1. Do_2 is dependent on arterial oxygen content (Cao_2) and cardiac output (CO):

$$Do_2 \text{ (ml } O_2\text{/min)} = CaO_2 \text{ (ml } O_2\text{/dl blood)} \times CO \text{ (L/min)} \times 10 \text{ dl/L}$$

(Normal values are listed in Table 2-2.)

2. Cao_2 is determined by the hemoglobin concentration ([Hb]), ther arterial hemoglobin oxygen saturation (Sao_2), and the partial pressure of oxygen in arterial blood (Pao_2):

$$Cao_2 \text{ (ml } O_2\text{/dl)} = [Hb] \text{ (g Hb/dl)} \times Sao_2\% \times 1.36 \text{ ml } O_2\text{/g Hb} + 0.003 \text{ ml } O_2\text{/mm Hg/dl} \times Pao_2 \text{ (mm Hg)}$$

At normal physiologic states, the latter contribution is insignificant, and Cao_2 may be approximated as the following:

$$Cao_2 = [Hb] \times Sao_2 \times 1.36$$

3. Vo_2 is dependent on the oxygen content of mixed venous blood (Cvo_2), Cao_2, and CO:

$$Vo_2 \text{ (ml } O_2\text{/min)} = (Cao_2 - Cvo_2) \text{ (ml } O_2\text{/dl)} \times CO \text{ (L blood/min)} \times 10 \text{ dl/L}$$

4. Cvo_2 is determined by the [Hb], the mixed venous

hemoglobin oxygen saturation (Svo_2), and the partial pressure of oxygen in mixed venous blood (Pvo_2):

$$Cvo_2 \text{ (ml } O_2/dl) = [Hb] \text{ (g Hb/dl)} \times Svo_2\%$$
$$\times 1.36 \text{ ml } O_2/g \text{ Hb} + 0.003 \text{ ml } O_2/mm \text{ Hg/dl}$$
$$\times Pvo_2 \text{ (mm Hg)}$$

At normal physiologic states, the last factor is insignificant, and Cvo_2 may be approximated as follows:

$$Cvo_2 = [Hb] \times Svo_2 \times 1.36$$

5. The relationship between Vo_2 and Do_2 can be expressed in terms of the oxygen extraction ratio (O_2ER):

$$O_2ER\% = Vo_2/Do_2 \times 100\%$$

6. The arteriovenous oxygen content difference (AVo_2) is the difference between Cao_2 and Cvo_2:

$$AVo_2 \text{ (ml } o_2/dl) = (Cao_2 - Cvo_2) \text{ (ml } O_2/dl)$$

B. Normal Physiology
The Biphasic Vo_2-Do_2 Model (Fig. 2-1) represents both adequate perfusion, where Vo_2 remains constant with decreasing Do_2 (oxygen supply–independent phase), and inadequate perfusion, where Vo_2 decreases with decreasing Do_2 (oxygen supply–dependent phase).

III. CLASSIFICATION
Shock may be classified as one or more of the following (it must be emphasized that patients may have any *combination* of shock etiologies, which may make the diagnosis more difficult to make):
A. Hypovolemic Shock
  1. Subtypes
    a. Pure hypovolemic
      (1) Hemorrhagic
      (2) Other fluid loss
    b. Traumatic
      (1) Associated tissue edema
      (2) Significant burn injuries

2. Pathophysiology: Decreased preload secondary to plasma volume losses
   a. External (e.g., near amputation)
   b. Internal (e.g., gastrointestinal)
   c. Interstitial (e.g., increased vascular permeability)
3. Diagnosis (Table 2-3)
   a. The symptoms are dependent on the degree of hypovolemia
   b. Patients who have lost up to 15% of their blood volume may have normal or mildly abnormal vital signs.
   c. Patients who have lost more than 40% of their blood volume have symptoms including hypotension, tachycardia, tachypnea, anuria, and altered mental status.
4. Treatment: Volume resuscitation
   a. Noninvasive assessment of volume replacement: No single variable can be used to determine the adequacy of fluid resuscitation, but several of the variables utilized include the following:
      (1) Creatinine clearance and urine output
      (2) HR
      (3) Arterial pH
      (4) Serum lactic acid
      (5) Capillary refill
      (6) Mental status
   b. Invasive evaluation of volume replacement includes the following:
      (1) CVP provides valuable data in patients with a normal cardiovascular system and early in the course of shock.
      (2) PA catheter monitoring is helpful in patients with impaired cardiac function. This allows for determination of many variables, including PCWP, CI, Svo_2, and the Vo_2-Do_2 relationship.
5. Clinical conditions
   a. Hemorrhage
   b. Vomiting
   c. Diarrhea
   d. Bowel obstruction
   e. Trauma
   f. Burns

TABLE 2-3.

Classification of Degrees of Hypovolemic Shock

	Class I	Class II	Class III	Class IV
Blood loss (ml)	<750	750-1500	1500-2000	>2000
Blood loss (%)	<15%	15%-30%	30%-40%	>40%
HR (beats/min)	<100	100-120	120-140	>140
BP	Normal	Normal	Decreased	Decreased
Pulse pressure	Normal	Decreased	Decreased	Decreased
Capillary refill	Normal	Delayed	Delayed	Delayed
Respiratory rate (breaths/min)	14-20	20-30	30-40	>40
Urine output (ml/hr)	>30	20-30	5-15	Negligible
Mental status	Slight anxiety	Mild anxiety	Confusion	Lethargy
Fluid replacement	Crystalloid	Crystalloid	Crystalloid and PRBCs	Crystalloid and PRBCs

TABLE 2-4.
Properties of Frequently Used Cardioactive Agents

Agent	Inotropy (β_1)	Chronotropy (β_1)	Vasodilatation (β_2)	Vasoconstriction (α_1)	Cardiac output	SVR	BP
Dobutamine	+++	+++	++	0	↑	→↑	0 - ↑
Dopamine	+++	++	+	0 - +++*	0 - ↑	→↑	0 - ↑
Ephedrine	++	++	0	+	0 - ↑	←	←
Epinephrine	+++	+++	++	+++	↑	→	←
Isoproterenol	+++	+++	+++	0	↑	←	←
Norepinephrine	++	++	0	+++	0 - →	←	←
Phenylephrine	0	0	0	+++	→	→	→↑
Milrinone	−	−	−	−	↑	←	→
Nitroprusside	−	−	−	−	↑	→	→

*Dose dependent.

B. Cardiogenic Shock
1. Subtypes include the following:
   a. Primary (pump failure)
   b. Secondary
      (1) Compressive
      (2) Obstructive
2. Pathophysiology: Cardiogenic shock is the failure of the heart to provide adequate Do_2 to maintain normal cellular metabolism and organ function.
3. Diagnosis (See Table 2-1.): A combination of the clinical, laboratory, radiographic, and electrocardiographic findings assists in determining the etiology of cardiogenic shock. A PA catheter echocardiography, coronary angiogram, ventilation/perfusion scans, and aortography may be of further assistance in specific circumstances.
4. Treatment (Tables 2-4 and 2-5): The goal is to optimize cardiac output so that further increases in Do_2 do not lead to an increase in Vo_2 (oxygen supply–independent phase).
   a. HR
      (1) Tachyarrhythmias preclude adequate ventricular filling and diastolic coronary flow, thereby resulting in cardiogenic shock.
      (2) Bradyarrhythmias lead to cardiogenic shock because there is not a proportional *increase* in SV to maintain adequate cardiac output (cardiac output = SV × HR).

TABLE 2-5.

Commonly Used Cardioactive Agents and Appropriate Dosages

Agent	Starting Dose (µg/kg/min)	Usual Dose (µg/kg/min)	Moderate Dose (µg/kg/min)	High Dose (µg/kg/min)
Dopamine	2-4	6-10	15	25
Dobutamine	2-4	6-10	15	25
Epinephrine	0.03-0.05	0.05-0.1	0.2	0.4
Isoproterenol	0.01	0.025	0.05	0.2
Milrinone	0.375	0.375	0.5	0.75
Norepinephrine	0.05	0.1	0.2	0.4
Nitroglycerin	0.2	1	2	3
Nitroprusside	0.5-1	1-3	3-5	5-7
Phenylephrine	0.6	0.6-1	1-2	3

b. Preload
    (1) SV (and therefore cardiac output) may be improved by increasing preload.
    (2) PCWP is the invasive parameter used most frequently to estimate left ventricular filling. It may be increased to 16 to 20 mm Hg under normal conditions; however, it is less useful in the presence of mitral valve abnormalities, substantial ventilator support, and chronic lung disease.
c. Afterload
    (1) Preload must be optimized before decreasing afterload; otherwise severe hypotension may ensue.
    (2) Sodium nitroprusside is effective in decreasing afterload and is the agent of choice in the ICU. Rarely, and only following prolonged use of high doses, can cyanide or thiocyanate toxicity occur. This may be suggested by a high Svo_2 and lactic acidosis.
    (3) Captopril, hydralazine, and prazosin are other less frequently used agents.
    (4) IABP can increase myocardial Do_2 (and functional cardiac output) and is usually employed following a cardiac event (e.g., MI, cardiac surgery). This is *not* a first line therapy and should be considered only after other less invasive interventions have been utilized.
d. Contractility
    (1) Should Do_2 need to be further increased, inotropic agents may be indicated after optimization of heart rate, preload, and afterload.
    (2) Tables 2-4 and 2-5 provide general information and recommended dosing of the commonly used agents.
5. Additional therapy
    a. Ventricular assist devices: If cardiogenic shock is not reversed by the aforementioned methods, ventricular assist devices may be considered as an alternative therapy.
    b. Primary: The correction of structural defects (e.g., repair of congenital heart defects, valve replacement) is frequently therapeutic.
    c. Secondary: The evacuation of a pericardial effusion or tension pneumothorax may be lifesaving. In addition,

appropriate ventilator management and aggressive therapy of associated conditions (e.g., polycythemia vera, ascites) may also be helpful.
6. Clinical conditions
   a. Primary
      (1) Congenital heart defects
      (2) Dysrhythmias
      (3) Myocardial ischemia
      (4) Acquired heart defects
         (a) Valvular abnormalities
         (b) Postinfarction VSD
      (5) Cardiomyopathy
      (6) Coronary air embolism
   b. Secondary
      (1) Compressive (compression of the heart and/or the great vessels)
         (a) Pericardial tamponade
         (b) Tension pneumothorax
         (c) Ascites
         (d) Diaphragmatic rupture
         (e) Mechanical ventilation
      (2) Obstructive (impairment of flow to the pulmonary and/or systemic circulation)
         (a) PE
         (b) Increased systemic arteriolar resistance
         (c) Pulmonary hypertension
         (d) Mechanical ventilation
         (e) Polycythemia
         (f) Aortic dissection

C. Septic Shock
1. Subtypes
   a. Gram-positive organisms
   b. Gram-negative organisms
2. Pathophysiology
   a. The increased cardiac output associated with sepsis is *not* a result of arteriovenous shunting; it is a compensatory response to increase Do_2 to tissues that are inadequately processing oxygen. Since tissue perfusion is often *enhanced* in various phases of sepsis, the *decrease* in Vo_2 may be explained by a cellular metabolic component.
   b. Numerous mediators of inflammation are released

Mediators of the Response to Shock

Prostaglandins	Leukotrienes
Bradykinin	Histamine
Endotoxin	Endogenous catecholamines
Oxygen free radicals	Interleukin-1
Tumor necrosis factor	Interleukin-6
Complement	Endothelin
Nitric oxide	β-Endorphins
Platelet activating factor	

during sepsis, which may contribute to the cellular dysfunction (See box above.)

3. Additional symptoms and signs
   a. Fever and chills are frequently seen in septic shock.
   b. Gram-positive sepsis is associated with normal urine output, sensorium, and serum lactic acid and has a significantly better prognosis than does gram-negative sepsis.
   c. The earliest manifestations of gram-negative sepsis are hyperventilation, respiratory alkalosis, and altered sensorium. A high index of suspicion must be present to make the diagnosis at this stage.
4. Diagnosis (See Table 2-1.)
   a. An early diagnosis is rarely made. Frequently, fever, hypotension, and cutaneous flushing are present, as is a significant fluid requirement.
   b. Low SVR, high CO, and high Svo_2 help to distinguish sepsis from other types of shock.
5. Treatment
   a. Treatment of the underlying infection is the most important aspect of therapy.
   b. Abscesses must be adequately drained, and infections must be treated with appropriate antimicrobial agents.
6. Associated clinical conditions: Include any infectious diseases because they may progress to sepsis.

D. Neurogenic Shock
   1. Subtypes include the following:
      a. Spinal cord injury
      b. Regional anesthesia
      c. Autonomic blocking agents

2. Pathophysiology: Venous pooling of blood follows the loss of sympathetic tone in neurogenic shock.
3. Additional symptoms and signs include the following:
   a. Cutaneous flush
   b. Decreased SVR
4. Diagnosis (Table 2-1): Diagnosis is usually obvious since it is iatrogenic (anesthetic) or associated with trauma to the spinal cord.
5. Treatment: In the absence of significant cardiovascular disease, volume resuscitation is usually effective in correcting the acute impairment in Do_2.

E. **Anaphylactic Shock**
1. Pathophysiology: The exposure of a sensitized individual (i.e., one with IgE-bound mast cells and basophils) to a foreign antigen releases large quantities of histamine and other vasoactive substances.
2. Additional symptoms and signs include the following:
   a. Laryngeal edema
   b. Bronchospasm
   c. Pulmonary hypertension and edema
   d. Hemolysis
   e. Urticaria
   f. Flushing
   g. Vascular collapse
3. Diagnosis (See Table 2-1.): The history and physical examination are sufficient.
4. Therapy for anaphylactic shock includes the following:
   a. Stop the allergen.
   b. Consider endotracheal intubation.
   c. Administer intravenous fluids (isotonic).
   d. Administer medications.
      (1) Epinephrine 0.1 to 0.2 mg IV and titrate as needed
      (2) Diphenhydramine 50 mg IV
      (3) H_2 antagonist: Cimetidine 300 mg IV or ranitidine 50 mg IV
      (4) Glucocorticoid: Methylprednisolone 100 to 250 mg IV

IV. **MULTIPLE ORGAN FAILURE**
A. **General**
1. Responsible for 50% to 80% of all SICU deaths
2. Costs over $150,000 per patient

TABLE 2-6.

Organ System Response to Multiple Organ Failure

Organ System	Dysfunction (Early)	Impending Failure (Late)
Pulmonary	Hypoxia and ventilator dependence for 3–5 days	Progressive ARDS
Hepatic	Serum bilirubin > 2 mg/dl or LFTs > 2× normal	Serum bilirubin > 8 mg/dl
Renal	Oliguria or ↑ creatinine (>2 mg/dl)	Dialysis
Intestinal	Ileus and feeding intolerance > 5 days	Stress ulcers requiring transfusion or acalculous cholecystitis
Hematologic	PT/PTT ↑ > 25% or platelets < 50,000	DIC
CNS	Confusion or mild disorientation	Progressive coma
Cardiovascular	↓ Ejection fraction or capillary-leak syndrome	Hemodynamic collapse refractory to inotropes

Modified from Deitch EA: *Crit Care* 14:134, 1993.

     3. No change in mortality rates since its original description approximately 20 years ago

     4. Makes up 7% to 8% of multiple trauma patients and 11% of patients undergoing emergency surgery

B. Clinical Syndrome

Major inflammatory response

     1. Uncontrolled infection (two thirds of patients)

     2. Shock

     3. Mechanical/thermal trauma

     4. Pancreatitis

C. Degree of Organ System Injury (Table 2-6)

D. Etiology

Although the etiology is unknown, mechanisms by which MOF occur include the following:

     1. Macrophage hypothesis and associated mediators (See Table 2-6.)

     2. Microcirculatory hypothesis (circulatory shock, DIC, increased vascular permeability)

     3. Gut hypothesis (bacterial translocation)

     4. Integrated hypothesis (any or combination of above)

E. Therapy

     1. Treat the underlying pathology.

     2. Provide supportive care for each involved organ.

SUGGESTED READING

Astiz ME, Rackow EC, Weil MH: Pathophysiology and treatment of circulatory shock, *Crit Care Clin* 9:183, 1993.

Carrico CJ et al: Multiple-organ-failure syndrome, *Arch Surg* 121:196, 1986.

Dantzker D: Oxygen delivery and utilization in sepsis, *Crit Care Clin* 5:83, 1989.

Fiddian-Green RG et al: Goals for the resuscitation of shock, *Crit Care Med* 18:S25, 1993.

Fleming A et al: Prospective trial of supranormal values as goals of resuscitation in severe trauma, *Arch Surg* 127:1175, 1992.

Moore FA et al: Incommensurate oxygen consumption in response to maximal oxygen availability predicts postinjury multiple organ failure, *J Trauma* 33:58, 1992.

Reed II RL: Oxygen consumption and delivery, *Curr Opin Anaesth* 6:329, 1993.

Shoemaker WC: Relation of oxygen transport patterns to the pathophysiology and therapy of shock states; *Intensive Care Med* 13:230, 1987.

Shoemaker WC, Kram HB, Appel PL: Therapy of shock based on pathophysiology, monitoring, and outcome prediction, *Crit Care Med* 18:S19, 1990.

Shumaker PT, Samsel RW: Oxygen delivery and uptake by peripheral tissues, *Crit Care Clin* 5:259, 1989.

Teich S, Chernow B: Specific cardiovascular drugs utilized in the critically ill, *Crit Care Clin* 1:491, 1985.

FLUIDS, ELECTROLYTES, AND ACID-BASE MANAGEMENT

3

David S. Peterseim

I. BODY FLUIDS
A. Total Body Water
1. 60% of the kilogram body mass in males
2. 50% of the kilogram body mass in females
3. 75% to 80% of the kilogram body mass in infants
4. Decreases with age so that by one year of age total body water approximately equals that of an adult; less water in fat than in muscle

B. Compartment Distribution
1. Intracellular fluid compartment: 40% of the kilogram mass
2. Extracellular fluid compartment: 20% of the kilogram mass
   a. Interstitial fluid compartment: 15% of the kilogram mass
   b. Intravascular fluid compartment: 5% of the kilgram mass

C. Regulation of Plasma Volume
Plasma volume is primarily a function of the total amount of sodium in the body; positive sodium balance will increase plasma volume. Plasma volume is most directly sensed by atrial receptors and is regulated by the renin-angiotensin-aldosterone axis.
1. Volume deficit is the most common volume disorder encountered in surgery. Typical causes include emesis, blood loss, and third space fluid losses due to any inflammatory process.
2. The signs and symptoms of acute water loss include the following:

a. CNS signs (lethargy and apathy progressing to stupor and coma) are the first to occur. Cardiovascular signs include orthostasis, tachycardia, and diminished pulses.
b. Tissue signs (decreased turgor, soft tongue with longitudinal wrinkles) and muscle atony usually do not appear before 24 hours.
c. Body temperature decreases.

3. Acute volume overload is almost always iatrogenic.
   a. Young patients can compensate for moderate to severe overload.
   b. The signs include distended veins, a bounding pulse, functional murmurs, edema, and basilar rales.

II. ELECTROLYTES
A. Electrolyte Composition
1. Intracellular
   a. Principal intracellular anions: Proteins and phosphates
   b. Principal intracellular cations: Potassium and magnesium
2. Extracellular
   a. Principal extracellular anions: Chloride and bicarbonate
   b. Principal extracellular cation: Sodium

B. Osmolarity
1. Osmolarity refers to the number of osmotically active particles in solution.
2. Normal osmolarity is 290 to 310 mOsm/L. Plasma osmolarity is calculated as follows:

$$P_{osm} = 2[Na^+] + glucose/18 + (BUN)/2.8$$

3. Nonpermeable plasma proteins are responsible for the effective oncotic pressure between the plasma compartment and the interstitial fluid compartment (the colloid oncotic pressure).
4. The effective oncotic pressure between extracellular and intracellular compartments is regulated primarily by sodium, which does not freely cross the cell membrane.
5. Since water diffuses freely between compartments, the effective oncotic pressures within the fluid compartments are equal.

C. Regulation of Serum Sodium
Serum sodium concentration reflects the water balance of the body and is an index of how much sodium is diluted by water.

Serum sodium concentration is a reliable index of serum osmolarity. Osmoreceptors in the brain are stimulated by a rise in serum osmolarity, stimulate the thirst mechanism to increase water intake, and release ADH, which increases free water resorption in the collecting duct of the kidney.

III. INTRAVENOUS FLUID THERAPY

IV fluids are necessary when adequate oral intake is not possible. The fluids delivered should fulfill the maintenance requirements of the patient, replace previous losses, and replace ongoing losses.

A. Electrolyte Content of Intravenous Fluids (Table 3-1)

B. Maintenance Fluid Requirement (Table 3-2)
1. Daily fluid requirements (per 24 hours)
   a. 100 ml/kg for the first 10 kg
   b. 50 ml/kg for the second 10 kg
   c. 20 ml/kg for each kilogram thereafter
2. Daily maintenance requirements: Can usually be met with D_5W ½ NS plus 20 mEq KCl/L at the above rate for adults.

TABLE 3-1.

Electrolyte Content of Intravenous Fluids (mEq/L)

Fluid	Na^+	K^+	Ca^{++}	Cl^-	HCO_3^-
Lactated Ringer's	130	4	2.7	109	28
Normal saline (0.9%)	154	—	—	154	—
½ Normal saline (0.45%)	77	—	—	77	—
¼ Normal saline (0.21%)	34	—	—	34	—
Hypertonic saline (3%)	513	—	—	513	—

TABLE 3-2.

Daily Fluid and Electrolyte Losses

Losses	H_2O (ml/day)	Na^+ (mEq/day)	K^+ (mEq/day)
Sensible losses			
Urine	800-1500	10-150	50-80
Stool	0-250	0-20	Trace
Sweat	0-100	10-60	0-10
Insensible losses			
Lungs	250-450	—	—
Skin	250-450	—	—
TOTAL OUTPUT	1300-2750	20-230	50-90

C. Replacement of Previous Fluid Losses

1. If the patient is hemodynamically unstable, 2 L of lactated Ringer's solution should be given, but if the patient has evidence of metabolic alkalosis, normal saline should be given.
2. Dextrose should only be given with the replacement if there is hypoglycemia.
3. Risks of large infusions of crystalloid include the development of peripheral and pulmonary edema. Patients should receive colloids if (1) they have CHF, liver failure and ascites, and (2) if following CPB they already have evidence of peripheral edema but have low intravascular volumes from fluid losses.
4. Patients should receive colloids after they receive the initial 2 L of crystalloid if hemodynamic stability is not attained. One hundred ml of 25% albumin increases plasma volume by 450 ml, whereas 1000 ml of lactated Ringer's solution increases plasma volume by 200 ml.
5. The primary risk of receiving colloids is pulmonary edema, especially when coupled with any process that increases capillary permeability.
6. After hemodynamic stability is achieved, replace half the remaining volume deficit (based on weight loss, history, and physical exam) within the first 8 hours. The remainder can be replaced over a 16 to 24 hour period.
7. Follow the patient's hemodynamics, urine output, electrolytes, and plasma osmolarity and adjust as indicated.

D. Replacement of Ongoing Fluid Losses (Tables 3-3 and 3-4)

1. Fever: Add 2 to 2.5 ml/kg/d of insensible losses for each degree above 37°C.
2. Third space losses: Fluids of extracellular composition shift into a pathologic space which cannot be regulated (inter-

TABLE 3-3.

Electrolyte Content of Body Fluids (mEq/L)

Fluid	Na$^+$	K$^+$	H$^+$	Cl$^-$	HCO$_3^-$
Sweat	30-50	5	—	45-55	—
Gastric secretions	40-65	10	90	100-140	—
Pancreatic fistula	135-155	5	—	55-75	70-90
Biliary fistula	135-155	5	—	80-110	35-50
Ileostomy fluid	120-130	10	—	50-60	50-70
Diarrhea fluid	25-50	35-60	—	20-40	30-45

stitium, retroperitoneum, and visceral parenchyma). Therefore this fluid is lost for the physiologic compartments which
can be regulated. In adults, 1 L of fluid is lost to the third
space for each quadrant of the abdomen explored, traumatized, or inflamed. (See Chapter 19.)

3. Osmotic diuresis: This is secondary to urea, mannitol, glucose,
myoglobin, hemoglobin, or dextran.
4. Tubes and drains: Measure electrolyte composition and replace
as needed.

E. **Assessment of Adequacy of Intravenous Therapy**
1. History: Thirst with minimal clinical signs indicates a 2%
body weight water deficit. Marked thirst, dry mouth,
oliguria, and previous poor oral intake indicates a 6% body
weight water deficit. All of the above, in addition to
weakness and changes in mental status, indicates a 7 to 14%
body weight water deficit.
a. Adults: Adequate urine output is 0.5 to 1.0 ml/kg/hr
b. Children older than 1 year of age: Adequate urine output
is 1.0 ml/kg/hr
c. Children less than 1 year of age: Adequate urine output
is 2.0 ml/kg/hr
2. Vital signs: Tachycardia, orthostatic blood pressure, and
hypotension indicate hypovolemia.
3. Examination includes the following considerations:
a. Flat neck veins when the patient is horizontal indicates
hypovolemia.
b. Dry mucous membranes suggest hypovolemia.
c. Skin tenting suggests hypovolemia; pitting edema suggests CHF or hypervolemia
d. Rales on pulmonary auscultation indicate hypervolemia

TABLE 3-4.
Replacement of Body Fluids

Fluid	Replacement Fluid
Sweat	D_5W ¼ NS + 5 mEq KCl/L
Gastric	D_5W ½ NS + 30-40 mEq KCl/L
Biliary or pancreatic	Lactated Ringer's
Small bowel	Lactated Ringer's
Colon	Lactated Ringer's or ½ NS + 20 mEq KCl/L + 25 mEq Na HCO_3^-/L
Third space losses	Lactated Ringer's

    e. If the patient is over 40 years of age, a dull, low-pitched, early diastolic murmur heard most clearly at the apex with the patient in the left lateral decubitus position (S_3) may indicate hypervolemia and heart failure.

4. Laboratory assessment includes the following:
   a. Serial serum electrolytes are important until stability is achieved.
   b. Urine electrolytes and osmolarity need to be drawn either before diuretics are given or no less than 12 hours after the last diuretic.

5. Central venous monitoring: This is especially helpful in patients with multisystem disease, elderly patients with limited cardiopulmonary reserve, and patients with a prior history of moderate to severe heart failure or COPD.

IV. ELECTROLYTE ABNORMALITIES

A. Sodium

The daily requirements are 1 to 2 mEq/kg/day, and the normal serum sodium is 136 to 144 mEq/L.

1. Hyponatremia
   a. Hyponatremia with overhydration
      (1) Nephrotic syndrome
      (2) CHF
      (3) Cirrhosis
      (4) Iatrogenic overadministration of free water
      (5) Severe hypovolemia: Increase in ADH secretion because volume regulation takes priority over osmolarity regulation
   b. Hyponatremia with euhydration
      (1) Diuretics
      (2) SIADH
      (3) Tumors (especially small cell carcinoma of the lung)
      (4) CNS disease (meningitis and encephalitis may affect the osmoreceptors which regulate ADH secretion)
      (5) Pulmonary infections
      (6) Drugs: Clofibrate, cyclophosphamide, or chlorpropamide (increase ADH secretion or renal sensitivity to ADH)
   c. Hyponatremia with dehydration
      (1) Have signs and symptoms of hypovolemia
      (2) More renal or nonrenal sodium loss than free water loss

      (3) Adrenal insufficiency
      (4) Salt-losing renal failure
  d. CNS signs
      (1) Muscle twitching
      (2) Hyperactive tendon reflexes
      (3) Convulsions
      (4) Hypertension
  e. Acute hyponatremia—onset of symptoms occur when $[Na^+] < 130$ mEq/L; gradual hyponatremia—symptoms occur when $[Na^+] < 120$ mEq/L
  f. Evaluation
      (1) Serum and urine osmolarity
      (2) Urine sodium to see if renal loss (>20 mEq/L) or nonrenal loss (<10 mEq/L)
  g. Treatment
      (1) Treat the underlying cause of the hyponatremia.
      (2) Free water restriction is usually sufficient unless the cause is hypovolemic hypotonic hyponatremia. In this case, the patient should be given saline infusions.
      (3) Use hypertonic sodium infusions only if the patient becomes acutely hyponatremic and is profoundly symptomatic. Serum sodium should (usually) only be corrected to 125 mEq/L.
      (4) Raise serum sodium 2 mEq/L/hr using a rate of 3% NaCl:

$$\frac{\{2 \text{ mEq/L} \times 0.6(\text{body weight in kg})\}}{513 \text{ mEq/L}} \times 1000$$
$$= \text{ml/hr of 3\% NaCl}$$

      (5) Stop hypertonic saline when symptoms resolve since the risks of rapid correction of hyponatremia are permanent brain damage, seizures, and pontine myelinolysis.
      (6) Note that low serum sodium concentration can be an artifact of measurement. Hyperlipidemia and hyperproteinemia result in exclusion of sodium from a water-free space in the plasma sample.
2. Hypernatremia
  a. Etiology
      (1) Renal water loss secondary to inadequate ADH secretion (diabetes insipidus)

(2) Insensitivity of renal collecting duct to ADH (nephrogenic diabetes insipidus)

(3) Evaporation through the skin and from burn defects or profuse sweating from sepsis (sweat is hypotonic)

(4) Evaporation through the lungs (e.g., inadequate vaporization of air in a ventilated patient)

b. Symptoms: Restlessness, weakness, delirium, and maniacal behavior

c. Signs

(1) Dry sticky mucous membranes

(2) Decreased salivation

(3) Decreased lacrimation

(4) Red swollen tongue

(5) Elevated body temperature

d. Evaluation and treatment

(1) Slowly replace the lost water after calculation of water deficit:

$$\text{Water deficit} = 0.6 \text{ (body weight in kg)} \frac{[Na^+]}{140} - 1$$

(2) If an intracranial process is suspected, check urine and serum osmolarity. Diabetes insipidus results in dilute urine (<200 mOsm) despite a concentrated serum (>320 mOsm).

(3) If patient is alert and given access to water, desmopressin (1-deamino-8-arginine vasopressin; DDAVP) is an ADH analogue that can be given intranasally (2 to 4 µg bid) as a long-term management to prevent complications of polyuria (bladder distention, hydroureter, and hydronephrosis).

(4) If patient is not alert or is unable to have free access to water due to other injuries, replace the lost free water slowly and begin DDAVP 5 U SC q4h.

(5) If the cause is nephrogenic diabetes insipidus, give the patient thiazide diuretics and initiate salt restriction.

B. Potassium

The daily requirements are 0.5 to 1.0 mEq/kg/day, and the normal serum potassium concentration is 3.5 to 5.0 mEq/L.

1. Hypokalemia

   a. Etiology

[Handwritten margin note: Na mEq to correct = [Na+] − 140 → replace 0.5 mEq/hr. ÷ by 2 (for 0.5 mEq/hr.) 50. 0.5 for ♀]

(1) Renal loss

(2) Diuretics

(3) Osmotic diuresis (as in diabetic ketoacidosis)

(4) Hyperaldosteronism

(5) Renal tubular acidosis

(6) Gastrointestinal loss (vomiting, diarrhea, fistula)

(7) Artifact of alkalosis: Correction factor for potassium is 0.6 mEq/L K^+ = 0.1 pH unit

b. Symptoms: Weakness, ileus, tetany, vasoconstriction, and cardiac arrhythmias (especially with digoxin)

c. Treatment

(1) Oral potassium if possible

(2) Intravenous potassium at a maximum rate of 20 to 40 mEq/hr; replacement depends on total deficit:

Serum K^+ (mEq/L)	K^+ Deficit (mEq)
3-4	100-200 mEq
2-3	200-400 mEq

2. Hyperkalemia

a. Etiology

(1) Inadequate renal excretion of potassium: Renal failure, hypoaldosteronism, or diuretics which inhibit potassium secretion

(2) Shift of potassium from the intracellular compartment (at the time of cell death)

b. Cardiac manifestations: ECG—changes progress from peaked T waves to prolonged PR interval, followed by decrease in P wave size; QRS complex widens, and T wave merges with QRS complex to form a "sine wave"; finally followed by ventricular fibrillation

c. CNS manifestations: Paralysis and confusion

d. Therapy: Depends on the severity of the hyperkalemia

(1) If ECG changes are present:

(a) Calcium gluconate: 10 ml of a 10% solution intravenously to stabilize the myocardial membrane and block the effect of potassium on the heart

(b) Insulin and glucose: 10 to 15 U regular Humulin in 50 to 100 ml of $D_{50}W$ intravenously to drive the potassium intracellularly until it is removed from the body

   (c) Potassium trapping resins: e.g., Kayexalate (20 to 60 g in 100 to 150 g sorbitol), orally or as a retention enema

   (d) Dialysis: Necessary in refractory cases

 (2) If potassium is 5.0 to 6.5 mEq/L, without ECG changes:

   (a) Monitor ECG and stop all potassium administration.

   (b) Treat underlying cause.

C. Calcium

The daily intake is 800 to 1200 mg/day (2% of adult body weight is calcium), and the normal plasma calcium is 9.0 to 10.5 mg/dl. The normal ionized calcium level is 1.12 to 1.23 mmol/L.

1. Calcium metabolism

   a. Calcium is nearly equally divided between the ionized (50%) and protein-bound phase (45%), with the remainder (5%) bound to lactate, bicarbonate, phosphate, sulfate, or citrate; 80% of protein-bound calcium is bound to albumin and the remainder to globulins. For every 1 g/dl decrease in albumin lower than 4.0 g/dl, subtract 1 mg/dl from the serum calcium.

   b. The distribution of calcium is a function of body fluid pH and albumin concentration. One pH unit change results in a 1.7 unit change in ionized calcium (mg/dl).

   c. The proximal small bowel is the site of active calcium absorption of most of the daily calcium intake. Passive calcium absorption occurs in the distal small bowel.

   d. There is a regulated renal excretion of calcium of 100 to 400 mg/day.

2. Hypocalcemia

   a. Etiology

      (1) Renal failure

      (2) Acute pancreatitis

      (3) Severe hypomagnesemia

      (4) Hypoparathyroidism

      (5) Vitamin D deficiency

   b. Symptoms: Tetany

      (1) Peripheral and perioral paresthesias

      (2) Carpal spasm

  (3) Seizures
  (4) Bronchospasm; laryngospasm
  (5) Chvostek's sign
  (6) Trousseau's sign
 c. Treatment
  (1) Acute management: Calcium gluconate IV (10 to 20 ml 10% solution) over 10 to 15 minutes, then titrate with IV drip (6 to 8 10-ml amps of 10% calcium gluconate in 1 L of D_5W)
  (2) Chronic management
   (a) Calcium carbonate: Initially 1 to 2 g PO tid, then 0.5 to 1 g PO tid
   (b) Vitamin D: Dihydroxy-vitamin D_3 (0.25 to 1 μg PO qd) or vitamin D_2 (50,000 to 100,000 U PO qd).
3. Hypercalcemia
 a. Etiology
  (1) Hyperparathyroidism
  (2) Malignancy (breast, lung, kidney, colon, thyroid, multiple myeloma)
  (3) Sarcoidosis
  (4) Vitamin D intoxication, vitamin A intoxication
  (5) Milk-alkali syndrome
  (6) Thyrotoxicosis
  (7) Adrenal insufficiency
  (8) Immobilization
  (9) Idiopathic hypercalcemia of infancy
  (10) Paget's disease
  (11) Thiazide diuretics
 b. Manifestations
  (1) Muscle weakness
  (2) Nausea and vomiting resulting in hypovolemia
  (3) Weight loss
  (4) Fatigue, drowsiness
  (5) Confusion
 c. Acute therapy (basic management principles): Focuses on restoring intravascular volume and maximizing renal clearance of calcium with nonthiazide diuretics
  (1) If serum calcium < 12 mg/dl, hydrate with normal saline solution and give low-dose diuretic.
  (2) If serum calcium > 15 mg/dl, rapidly volume load with 5 to 6 L of NS and administer high-dose

diuretic. Place a central venous catheter and maintain a CVP at 10 cm H_2O while carefully monitoring for hypokalemia, hypomagnesemia, and pulmonary edema.

(3) If serum calcium = 12 to 15 mg/dl, clinical judgment should determine the appropriate management based on the above algorithm.

d. Chronic therapy

(1) Mithramycin: Administer 25 µg/kg IV qd for 3 to 4 days and then repeat at one or more week intervals. The effects are seen within 12 hours, and risks include thrombocytopenia, hepatocellular necrosis, and decreased clotting factors.

(2) Corticosteroids: Administer hydrocortisone 250 to 500 mg IV q8h or prednisone 40 to 100 mg PO. The effects are seen in several days.

(3) Calcitonin: Administer 4 IU/kg and increase to 8 IU/kg q6h. Use if rehydration, salt loading, and furosemide fail.

(4) Phosphate: Phosphate is reserved as the final therapeutic option. Oral Neutra-phos 250 mg tid to qid or 100 ml Fleet retention enema can be used to elevate the serum phosphate level to reduce calcium mobilization from bone and decrease gut absorption of calcium. Oral supplementation is much safer than intravenous administration. IV supplementation (1500 mg over 6 to 8 hours) should be used only emergently and only to restore a normal phosphate level. The risks of IV phosphate are fatal hypocalcemia, renal cortical necrosis, metastatic calcification, and fatal shock. Never give intravenous phosphate if the patient is hyperphosphatemic.

D. Magnesium

The daily requirements are 300 to 400 mg/day, and the normal serum magnesium is 1.3 to 2.1 mEq/L.

1. Hypomagnesemia

a. Etiology

(1) Hypoparathyroidism after parathyroidectomy

(2) Renal magnesium wasting due to systemic and intrinsic renal disease

(3) Extracellular fluid expansion due to hyperaldosteronism and SIADH

(4) Osmotic diuresis due to glycosuria: Depletes magnesium body stores

b. Manifestations
   (1) Weakness
   (2) Muscle fasciculations
   (3) Tremors
   (4) Personality changes
   (5) Vertigo
   (6) Seizures

c. Treatment
   (1) Acute management: For seizures or tetany give 1 to 2 g of magnesium sulfate as 10% solution over 15 minutes, then 1 g IM q4-6h depending on clinical setting. If patellar reflexes are absent, stop replacement.
   (2) Chronic management: Administer magnesium oxide 1200 mg PO qd.

2. Hypermagnesemia
   a. Etiology: Poisoning after oral or rectal administration in the setting of renal failure
   b. Manifestations: Usually associated with magnesium > 4.0 (magnesium > 12 may be fatal)
      (1) Decreased reflexes
      (2) Flaccid paralysis
      (3) Hypotension
      (4) Hypothermia
      (5) Coma
      (6) Respiratory failure
   c. Treatment: 10 ml of 10% calcium gluconate repeated as necessary (calcium antagonizes magnesium's effect on nerves and muscle)

E. Phosphate

The daily requirements are 800 to 1200 mg/day, and the normal serum phosphate is 2.5 to 4.3 mg/dl.

1. Phosphate homeostasis
   a. Serum calcium and phosphate vary inversely.
   b. Most of the body stores are in the teeth and bones.
   c. Intestinal absorption of phosphate is 80% to 90% efficient.

2. Hypophosphatemia
   a. Etiology
      (1) Hyperparathyroidism

(2) Follows TPN administration if phosphate is not included initially

(3) Phosphate loss in the urine from renal tubular insufficiency

b. Symptoms

(1) Anorexia

(2) Dizziness

(3) Bone pain

(4) Muscle weakness

(5) Hyporeflexia

(6) Paresthesias

(7) Cardiac failure, respiratory failure

(8) Seizures

(9) Coma

c. Associated findings

(1) Rhabdomyolysis

(2) Decreased phagocytosis

(3) Platelet dysfunction

(4) Hemolysis

d. Treatment

(1) If the patient has mild hypophosphatemia (1 to 2.5 mg/dl), treat the cause and consider giving Neutra-phos 500 PO bid-tid.

(2) If the patient has severe hypophosphatemia (<1 mg/dl), give intravenous sodium or potassium phosphate 2.5 to 5 mg/kg in 100 D_5W over 6 hours at 17 ml/hr via a central venous catheter. Repeat this procedure until the phosphate level >2.0 mg/dl. The risks of IV phosphate include hypocalcemia, metastatic calcification, and hypotension.

3. Hyperphosphatemia

a. Symptoms: No definite symptoms, although prolonged elevations lead to abnormal calcium phosphate deposits

b. Treatment: Aluminum hydroxide antacids

V. ACID-BASE MANAGEMENT

Normal blood pH is maintained at 7.37 to 7.43 to allow optimal function of cellular enzymes, clotting factors, and contractile proteins. This regulation is possible because of intracellular buffers, extracellular buffers, and respiratory compensation. Normal values for arterial and venous blood are shown in Table 3-5.

TABLE 3-5.
Normal Acid-Base Values

	pH	H$^+$ (mEq/L)	Pco$_2$ (mm Hg)	HCO$_3^-$ (mEq/L)
Arterial	7.37-7.43	37-43	36-43	22-26
Venous	7.32-7.38	42-48	42-50	23-27

A. **Intracellular Buffers**
   1. Proteins, Hb, bone, and organic phosphates serve as intracellular buffers.
   2. Approximately 50% of the H$^+$ generated by nonvolatile acids diffuses within minutes to hours intracellularly where it is buffered by proteins, bone, and organic phosphates.
   3. H$_2$CO$_3$ is almost entirely buffered intracellularly by deoxygenated Hb within red cells.

B. **Extracellular Buffers**
   Bicarbonate-carbonic acid system
   1. In extracellular fluids, acids (inorganic acids such as hydrochloric, sulfuric, and phosphoric acids, and organic acids such as lactic, pyruvic, and keto acids) combine with sodium bicarbonate to form the sodium salt of the acid and carbonic acid.
   2. Carbonic acid then dissociates into water and CO$_2$, and CO$_2$ is excreted in the lungs. Because it is in equilibrium with CO$_2$, H$_2$CO$_3$ is called a volatile acid. The following equations represent this process:

$$HCl + NaHCO_3 \rightarrow H_2CO_3 + NaCl$$
$$H_2CO_3 \rightarrow H_2O + CO_2$$

   3. The acid anion is excreted by the kidney with hydrogen or ammonium ions. Extracellular fluid pH is determined by ratio of base bicarbonate to the amount of carbonic acid in the blood. At a pH of 7.4, this ratio is 20:1. Regardless of the absolute values, a ratio of 20:1 keeps the pH at 7.4. This process is defined by the Henderson-Hasselbalch equation:

$$pH = pKa + \log\left(\frac{[HCO_3^-]}{[H_2CO_3]}\right)$$

4. H_2SO_4 and H_3PO_4 are produced through protein catabolism and incomplete oxidation of fat and carbohydrates. Because they are not in equilibrium with CO_2, they are called nonvolatile acids. H_2CO_3 that is generated by oxidative metabolism cannot be buffered by the bicarbonate-carbonic acid system because the addition of H^+ and HCO_3^- regenerates H_2CO_3.

VI. ABNORMALITIES IN ACID-BASE METABOLISM

A. Respiratory Acidosis

Increase in serum P_{CO_2} secondary to hypoventilation

1. Mechanism: Increased $P_{CO_2} \rightarrow$ increased $H_2CO_3 \rightarrow$ decreased ratio $\rightarrow$ decreased pH.
2. Acute compensation: Intracellular buffers $\rightarrow$ increase in $[HCO_3^-]$ (1 mEq/L for each 10 mm Hg rise in CO_2). Any elevation of $[HCO_3^-]$ above 30 mEq/L suggests a metabolic alkalosis as well.
3. Chronic compensation: Acid salts are excreted by the kidneys over the next 2 to 3 days in exchange for bicarbonate. This leads to an increased ratio, which in turn leads to an increased pH. This process increases $[HCO_3^-]$ by 3 to 4 mEq/L for each 10 mm Hg rise in P_{CO_2}.
4. Differential diagnosis includes the following:
   a. Acute CNS suppression (drugs, stroke, sleep apnea, O_2 therapy in COPD)
   b. Chronic CNS suppression (tumor, obesity)
   c. Impaired respiratory muscle function
   d. Airway obstruction
   e. Impaired pulmonary gas exchange (pneumonia, ARDS, pneumothorax, COPD)
   f. Inadequate ventilator settings or ventilator dysfunction
5. Treatment: The decision to urgently intubate a patient should be based upon physical exam and should not require evaluation of the blood gas. Time spent waiting on the laboratory values in a patient who is dyspneic, obtunded, and with obvious signs of increased work of breathing (i.e., accessory muscle use, diaphragmatic breathing, and intercostal muscle retractions) only jeopardizes the patient.

B. Respiratory Alkalosis

Decrease in serum P_{CO_2} secondary to hyperventilation

1. Mechanism: Decreased $P_{CO_2} \rightarrow$ decreased $H_2CO_3 \rightarrow$ increased ratio $\rightarrow$ increased pH.

2. Acute compensation: Buffers (intracellular and extracellular) compensate allowing $[HCO_3^-]$ to decrease 1 to 2 mEq/L for each 10 mm Hg fall in P_{CO_2}. This compensation will allow $[HCO_3^-]$ to fall to as low as 18 mEq/L.

3. Chronic compensation: Acid salts are resorbed by the kidneys in exchange for bicarbonate, which is excreted. This leads to a decreased ratio, which in turn leads to a decreased pH. This allows $[HCO_3^-]$ to decrease 4 to 5 mEq/L for each 10 mm Hg fall in P_{CO_2}.

4. Differential diagnosis includes the following:
   a. Ventilator settings in excess
   b. Hypoxemia
   c. Sepsis
   d. Medications (salicylates, progesterone, catecholamines, theophylline)
   e. CNS process (CVA, infection, tumor, trauma)
   f. Cirrhosis
   g. Psychogenic hyperventilation

5. Symptoms: These include lightheadedness, cramps, circumoral numbness, acral paresthesias, and altered mental status.

6. Treatment: Assess ventilator settings and rule out hypoxemia. Consider the other diagnoses listed above, and address the underlying cause.

C. **Metabolic Acidosis**
   Decrease in serum HCO_3^- due to retention or gain of acid or a loss of bicarbonate

   1. Mechanism: Decreased $HCO_3^- \rightarrow$ decreased ratio $\rightarrow$ decreased pH.

   2. Acute compensation: Increased alveolar ventilation $\rightarrow$ decreased $P_{CO_2} \rightarrow$ decreased $H_2CO_3 \rightarrow$ restores ratio $\rightarrow$ increased pH. This compensation results in a 1 to 1.3 mm Hg fall in P_{CO_2} for each 1 mEq/L decline in $[HCO_3^-]$.

   3. Symptoms and signs: These include lethargy, confusion, cool extremities, arrhythmias, hyperkalemia, and pulmonary hypertension.

   4. Evaluation: Determine anion gap (anion gap = $[Na+] - ([Cl^-] + [HCO_3^-])$). Normal anion gap is 8 to 12 mmol/L.

   5. Differential diagnosis with normal anion gap includes the following:
      a. Increased acid load (citrate in blood transfusions or cell death)
      b. Decreased renal clearance of acid

    c. Distal renal tubular acidosis

    d. Adrenal insufficiency

    e. Hypoaldosteronism

    f. TPN

    g. Loss of bicarbonate

    h. GI fistula

    i. Diarrhea

    j. Proximal renal tubular acidosis

    k. Ureterosigmoidostomy

    l. Early renal failure

    m. Carbonic anhydrase inhibitors (acetazolamide)

6. Differential diagnosis with abnormal anion gap includes the following:

    a. Renal failure

    b. Lactic acidosis (normal lactate is 0.5 to 1.5 mEq/L)

    c. Ketoacidosis (diabetic ketoacidosis and starvation)

    d. Ingestion (ethylene glycol, salicylates, methanol, paraldehyde)

7. Treatment includes the following:

    a. Stabilize the intensive care patient while efforts to correct the underlying process proceed. Optimize the volume status, correct hypoxemia, and evaluate for sepsis, cardiac failure, and renal failure. Rule out diabetic ketoacidosis.

    b. Administer sodium bicarbonate if pH < 7.2 after calculation of base deficit:

$$\begin{aligned} \text{Base deficit} = &\ (\text{body weight in kg})(0.4) \\ &\times \{(\text{desired}[HCO_3^-] \text{ in mEq/L}) \\ &- (\text{measured } [HCO_3^-] \text{ in mEq/L})\} \end{aligned}$$

    c. Give half of the calculated deficit and then follow serial blood gases as you titrate the $NaHCO_3$ to raise pH > 7.2. Optimizing the volume status and oxygenation of the patient as well as treating the underlying cause will usually prevent the need for exclusive use of $NaHCO_3$ to completely correct the pH.

    d. If $NaHCO_3$ is given too aggressively, the CO_2 produced (upon buffering H^+) can diffuse intracellularly and result in myocardial intracellular acidosis and cardiac dysfunction. This CO_2 production and shift can also cause cerebral suppression.

e. Other side effects of $NaHCO_3$ administration include hypernatremia, hypokalemia, hyperosmolarity, and fluid overload. Monitor serum potassium after $NaHCO_3$ administration.

D. Metabolic Alkalosis

Increase in serum HCO_3^- secondary to a loss of fixed acid or a gain of bicarbonate

1. Mechanism: Increased HCO_3^- → increased ratio → increased pH.

2. Compensation (mainly renal): Acid salts (such as chloride) are resorbed by the kidneys in exchange for bicarbonate which is excreted. This leads to a decreased ratio, which in turn leads to a decreased pH.

3. Respiratory compensation (occasionally): Respiratory compensation → decreased alveolar ventilation → increased P_{CO_2} → increased H_2CO_3 → restores ratio → decreased pH. Appropriate compensation by hypoventilation leads to a 5 to 7 mm Hg rise for each 10 mEq/L elevation in HCO_3^-.

4. Evaluation: Determine the volume status of the patient by physical examination, urine output, and CVP monitoring. Hypovolemic patients typically have low urine chloride and will respond to saline therapy.

5. Differential diagnosis includes the following:
   a. Hypovolemic and low urine chloride (<10 mEq/L)
   b. Loss of gastric fluid (emesis or NG aspirate)
   c. Diuretic therapy which mediates a contraction alkalosis
   d. Hypomagnesemia
   e. Relief of prolonged hypercapnia COPD
   f. Bicarbonate therapy of organic acidosis
   g. Administration of bicarbonate-producing organic salts (citrate, lactate, acetate)
   h. Milk-alkali syndrome
   i. Severe hypokalemia
   j. Excess mineralocorticoid (exogenous steroids, Cushing's syndrome, ACTH-secreting tumors, hyperaldosteronism, renal artery stenosis)

6. Treatment includes the following:
   a. For all alkalotic states, hypokalemia must be avoided. Potassium is in competition with hydrogen ions for resorption of sodium at the level of the renal tubule. In alkalosis, preferential excretion of potassium in exchange for sodium allows conservation of hydrogen ions. If renal tubule potassium is insufficient due to low serum

potassium, then hydrogen ions cannot be resorbed and alkalosis will persist. In hypokalemic metabolic alkalosis (commonly seen after prolonged emesis) the renal tubule prioritizes sodium resorption to restore volume status. Consequently, potassium and hydrogen are excreted, which leads to "paradoxic aciduria" and further alkalosis. Volume and potassium replacement should be performed concurrently.

b. If hypovolemia and low urine chloride are present, correct volume state with saline infusion and appropriate potassium supplementation to raise potassium to 4.5 to 5.0 mEq/L.

c. Histamine antagonists can diminish hydrogen ion secretion in gastric contents.

d. If euvolemia and high urine chloride are present, eliminate the excess mineralocorticoid and correct potassium to 4.5 to 5.0 mEq/L or magnesium to 2.0 mEq/L.

e. If severe alkalosis is present, acetazolamide 250 to 500 mg IV can cause bicarbonate excretion.

f. As a final option in the setting of severe renal failure or life-threatening metabolic alkalosis (pH > 7.6, [HCO_3^-] > 40 mEq/L), give 0.1 N HCl via a central venous catheter after calculation of chloride deficit:

$$\text{Chloride deficit (mEq)} = (20\% \times \text{body mass}) \times$$
$$(\text{normal plasma chloride} - \text{actual plasma chloride})$$

g. Infuse 100 mEq of HCl/L at a rate no faster than 125 ml or 2 mEq/kg/hr. Slower infusions are preferable and serial ABGs are vital in monitoring these patients. Complications include hemolysis and tissue necrosis.

SUGGESTED READING

Bates B: *A guide to physical examination,* ed 3, Philadelphia, 1983, JB Lippincott.

Economou S et al: *Review of surgery,* Philadelphia, 1988, WB Saunders.

Lyerly HK, Gaynor JW, editors: *Handbook of surgical intensive care: practices of the surgical residents of the Duke University Medical Center,* ed 3, St. Louis, 1992, Mosby.

Petersdorf RG, editor: *Harrison's principles of internal medicine,* ed 10, New York, 1983, McGraw-Hill.

CARDIOPULMONARY *4* RESUSCITATION

Cary H. Meyers

I. **OBJECTIVE**

The objectives are prompt initiation and proper execution of resuscitation techniques. The highest hospital discharge rates are associated with basic life support (BLS) activation within 4 minutes and advanced cardiac life support (ACLS) activation within 8 minutes.

A. **Basic Life Support**

1. Community-based training in the prevention, recognition, and initial management of patients suffering from primary respiratory or cardiac arrest

2. Delivery of temporary airway and circulatory support to maintain tissue perfusion until personnel trained in ACLS arrive

B. **Advanced Cardiac Life Support**

1. ACLS includes specific training of health care providers (including paramedics, physicians, and nursing personnel) to continue BLS and stabilize the patient hemodynamically using appropriate pharmacologic and electrical therapy.

2. ACLS provider certification includes training and testing of health care personnel in the recognition and management of cardiac arrhythmias, in addition to use of airway adjuncts, defibrillator/cardioverter units, and transcutaneous and transvenous pacemakers.

II. **INDICATIONS**

A. **Respiratory Arrest**

1. Drowning

2. Electrocution

3. Foreign body airway obstruction

4. Drug overdose
5. CVA
6. MI
7. Smoke inhalation
8. Airway trauma

B. Cardiac Arrest
 1. CAD (most common); often associated with arrhythmias
    a. Ventricular tachycardia
    b. Ventricular fibrillation
    c. Asystole
    d. EMD
    e. Supraventricular tachycardia
 2. Hypovolemia
 3. Acute respiratory failure
 4. Hyperkalemia
 5. Severe acidosis
 6. Extreme derangements in body temperature

III. BASIC LIFE SUPPORT

The initiation of BLS begins with the assessment of the patient, determination of unresponsiveness, and activation of EMS; then the physician follows the ABCs of BLS.

A. Airway
 1. Make sure patient is in supine position.
 2. Open airway.
    a. Head tilt–chin lift
    b. Jaw-thrust maneuver
 3. Determine breathlessness—look and listen.
 4. If the patient resumes breathing, roll to decubitus position while maintaining airway patency.

B. Breathing
 1. Methods
    a. Mouth-to-mouth: Simplest technique which does not require special devices or assistance
    b. Mouth-to-mask: The use of a barrier device to protect the health care provider from patient secretions
    c. Bag-valve mask: Optimal method of supporting ventilation in the hospital setting as 100% oxygen may be delivered to the patient
    d. Cricoid pressure: Useful adjunct when an assistant is available to prevent gastric distension, regurgitation, and aspiration during CPR

    2. Goals of ventilation
      a. The goal tidal volume is 800 to 1200 ml
      b. Allow 1.5 to 2 seconds for exhalation.
      c. Deliver two initial breaths to determine whether there is upper airway obstruction, followed by 10 to 12 breaths per minute.

C. Circulation
    1. No pulse
    2. Guidelines for chest compressions
      a. Patient must be in a horizontal, supine, or Trendelenburg position.
      b. Use a backboard when available for more efficient chest compressions.
      c. Position your hands over the xyphoid process so that the heel of one hand rests on the sternum and the other hand is positioned over the first hand—fingers should be off the chest.
      d. With elbows locked and shoulders positioned directly over the hands, compress the chest 1.5 to 2 inches at a rate of 80 to 100 compressions per minute, using the hips as a fulcrum.
      e. Adequacy of chest compressions is judged by the presence of a carotid or femoral pulse.
      f. Chest compressions must be coupled with appropriate rescue breathing for successful resuscitation.
    3. One rescuer CPR (Fig. 4-1)
    4. Two rescuer CPR (Fig. 4-2)

IV. ADVANCED CARDIAC LIFE SUPPORT
A. Equipment
    1. Airway adjuncts
      a. Oxygen: Used as soon as possible
      b. Bag-valve mask: Useful alternative to mouth-to-mouth breathing as oxygen may be easily added into the circuit and disease transmission is less likely between rescuer and airway patient
      c. Oropharyngeal/nasopharyngeal airways: Should be used in patients who are not intubated to maintain airway patency
      d. Endotracheal intubation: Should be performed as soon as practical by appropriately trained personnel to isolate the airway from aspiration and to provide easy access for suctioning and drug delivery when needed

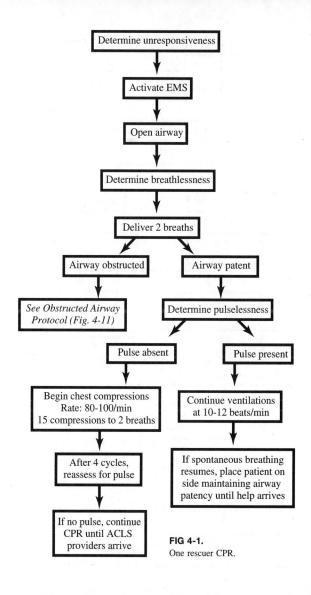

FIG 4-1.
One rescuer CPR.

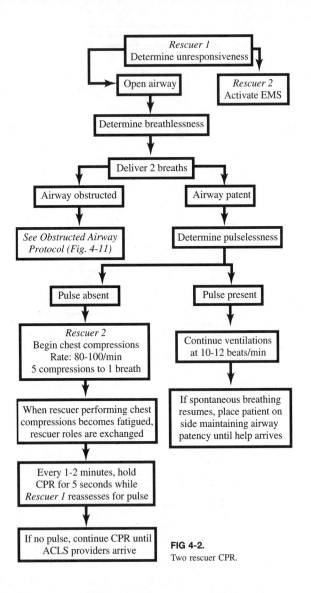

FIG 4-2.
Two rescuer CPR.

    e. Cricothyrotomy: Acceptable emergency airway in the setting of severe facial trauma

    f. Transtracheal high-frequency jet ventilation: Temporary alternative to cricothyrotomy using a specially designed jet ventilator–catheter circuit

2. Artificial circulation adjuncts

    a. Abdominal counterpulsation has been reported to improve hemodynamics during CPR and survival for in-hospital arrests; however, no survival benefit has become apparent for arrests in the field. This technique is not currently recommended due to insufficient clinical data.

    b. High frequency CPR (120 compressions/min) has been shown to improve hemodynamics, coronary perfusion, and survival in dogs; however, this method is not recommended by the AHA due to insufficient clinical trials.

    c. Pneumatically-driven automatic compression devices have been available for several years. These devices provide optimal rates and depths of chest compression but often become malpositioned during the course of an arrest, causing sternal/rib fractures or inadequate compressions.

    d. MAST trousers are often placed in the field by EMS personnel; however, there is no data to suggest improved outcome in the setting of cardiac arrest. Their routine use is not recommended.

    e. Open-cardiac massage provides better hemodynamics than closed-chest massage, but survival benefit has not been clearly shown in the literature. Open-cardiac massage has not been shown to be effective in patients when applied after 25 minutes of total arrest time. Specific indications for thoracotomy include penetrating chest trauma and pericardial tamponade.

    f. Percutaneous cardiopulmonary bypass is a promising new modality to support patients in cardiac arrest by accessing the femoral vessels. This is the only technique which unloads the heart and allows a period of time to evaluate and potentially treat the patient.

3. Monitor/defibrillator

    a. It is essential to perform ACLS algorithms and they should be applied as soon as possible.

    b. Appropriate application of the monitor to the patient and arrhythmia recognition are central to ACLS. Providers must recognize the following arrhythmias:

       (1) Sinus tachycardia
       (2) Sinus bradycardia
       (3) Ventricular tachycardia
       (4) Ventricular fibrillation
       (5) Premature ventricular complexes
       (6) Supraventricular tachycardia
       (7) Atrial fibrillation/flutter
       (8) Premature atrial complexes
       (9) Atrioventricular blocks
       (10) Junctional rhythm
       (11) Asystole
       (12) EMD

    c. Early defibrillation has been shown to improve survival in cardiac arrest due to ventricular fibrillation and should be instituted in the field. Quick-look paddles are sufficient to make the diagnosis of ventricular fibrillation, therefore blind defibrillation is not necessary or indicated.

    d. Defibrillation paddles should be positioned with one over the sternum and the other lateral to the left nipple at the midaxillary line. Acceptable alternatives include the use of a back paddle placed posteriorly behind the heart and an anterior paddle placed over the precordium. A conductive gel must be applied to the paddles prior to defibrillation to decrease the resistance at the paddle-skin interface.

4. Transcutaneous pacemaker

    a. Currently, transcutaneous pacing is the preferred approach when indicated acutely since conductive pacing electrodes are easily applied without interrupting CPR. Central venous access is not necessary while using this device, which is an important consideration in patients with a bleeding diatheses.

    b. Many new monitor defibrillators will incorporate a transcutaneous pacemaker which will allow hands-free defibrillation of the patient.

    c. Indications for emergent pacing are summarized in the box on the following page.

    d. Application of the transcutaneous pacemaker to the

Indications for Emergent Pacing

Hemodynamically unstable bradyarrhythmias (systolic BP < 80 mm Hg)
Bradycardia with malignant escape rhythms
Mobitz type II or complete heart block in the setting of acute MI
Overdrive pacing of refractory unstable tachyarrhythmias

patient with asystole or EMD is rarely effective in increasing cardiac performance.

B. Drug Therapy

1. Route of administration
   a. Peripheral access is the first choice during CPR and is usually a more than adequate route for administering necessary drugs.
   b. Central access, when available, provides faster drug delivery to the heart and peripheral circulation.
   c. In the temporary absence of IV access, use the endotracheal tube to deliver **A**tropine, **L**idocaine, **I**soproterenol, **E**pinephrine, and **N**aloxone (mnemonic = ALIEN).
   d. Intraosseous access is also a valid, temporary route to administer fluids and medications, especially in children.
2. Pharmacologic agents used in ACLS (Table 4-1).

C. Application of ACLS

Implementation of algorithms

1. Code organization
2. Universal approach to the patient (Fig. 4-3)
3. Ventricular fibrillation/pulseless ventricular tachycardia (Fig. 4-4)
4. Pulseless electrical activity/electromechanical dissociation (Fig. 4-5)
5. Asystole algorithm (Fig. 4-6)
6. Tachycardia algorithm (Fig. 4-7)
7. Bradycardia algorithm (Fig. 4-8)
8. Cardioversion algorithm (Fig. 4-9)
9. Algorithm for hypotension, shock, and pulmonary edema (Fig. 4-10)

V. AIRWAY OBSTRUCTION

A. Introduction

1. Taught within the context of BLS as most incidents occur in the field

TABLE 4-1.
Frequently Used Pharmacologic Agents

Drug	Action	IV Bolus	Drug/250 ml	Infusion
Adenosine	Depresses SA and AV nodes	6 mg, then 12 mg	—	—
Amrinone	Phosphodiesterase inhibitor	0.75 mg/kg over 2-3 min	—	2-20 µg/kg/min
Atropine	Vagolytic	0.5-1 mg every 2-3 min to 3 mg	—	—
Bretylium	Sympatholytic	5 mg/kg, then 10 mg/kg every 5 min to 30-35 mg/kg max	2 g	1-2 mg/min
Calcium chloride	Direct inotropic agent	2-4 mg/kg every 10 min	—	—
Diltiazem	Ca++ channel antagonist	0.25 mg/kg, then 0.35 mg/kg	250 mg	5-15 mg/hr
Dobutamine	β-Agonist	—	500 mg	2-20 µg/kg/min
Dopamine	Mixed α-, β-, DA-agonist	—	400 mg	2-20 µg/kg/min
Epinephrine	Mixed α-, β-agonist	1 mg every 3-5 min, then up to 0.1 mg/kg every 3-5 min	1 mg	0.01-0.15 µg/kg/min

Isoproterenol	β-Agonist	—	1 mg	2-10 µg/min
Lidocaine	Type Ib antiarrhythmic	1-1.5 mg/kg, then 0.5-1.5 mg/kg to 3 mg/kg max load	2 g	2-4 mg/min
Nitroglycerin	Direct vasodilator	—	100 mg	10-500 µg/min
Nitroprusside	Direct vasodilator	—	50-100 mg	1-10 µg/kg/min
Norepinephrine	Mixed α-, β-agonist	—	4 mg	0.02-0.20 µg/kg/min
Phenylephrine	α-Agonist	—	10 mg	1-5 µg/kg/min
Procainamide	Type Ia antiarrhythmic	20 mg/min to a max dose of 17 mg/kg	2 g	1-4 mg/min
Sodium bicarbonate	Corrects acidosis	1 mEq/kg, then 0.5 mEq/kg every 10 min	—	—
Verapamil	Ca++ channel antagonist	2.5-5 mg over 2 min, then 5-10 mg every 15-30 minutes to a max dose of 20 mg	—	—

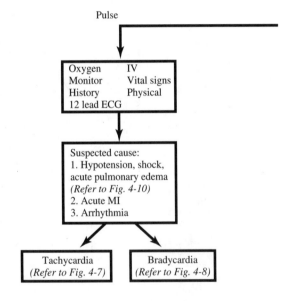

FIG 4-3.
Universal approach for adult ACLS.

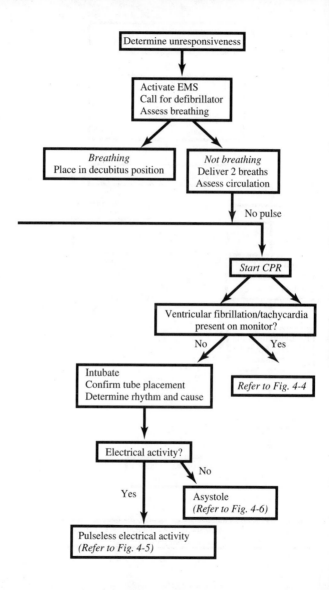

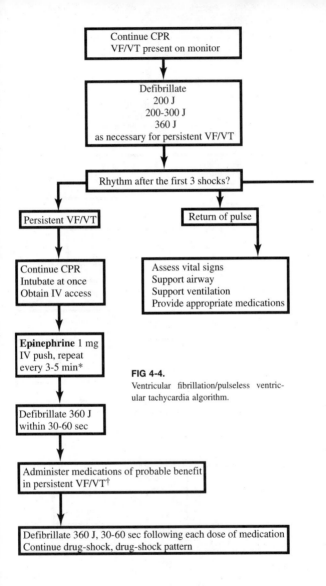

FIG 4-4.
Ventricular fibrillation/pulseless ventricular tachycardia algorithm.

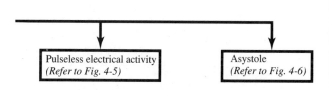

* **Sodium bicarbonate:** 1 mEq/kg IV is indicated early for hyperkalemia and contraindicated in hypoxic lactic acidosis. It may be useful
(1) if preexisting metabolic acidosis
(2) if tricyclic antidepressant overdose
(3) to alkalinize the urine in drug overdose
(4) if intubated and there is a long arrest interval
(5) if pulse returns after a long arrest interval.
†**Lidocaine:** 1.5 mg/kg IV bolus, repeat in 3-5 min to total dose of 3 mg/kg; then **bretylium:** 5 mg/kg IV bolus, repeat in 5 min with 10 mg/kg; **magnesium sulfate:** 1-2 g IV in torsades de pointes, suspected drop in Mg, or refractory VF

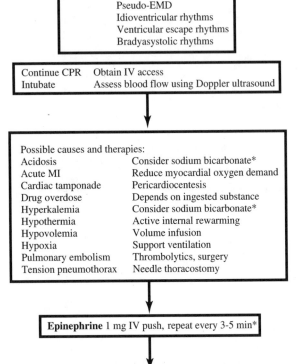

Includes:	EMD
	Pseudo-EMD
	Idioventricular rhythms
	Ventricular escape rhythms
	Bradyasystolic rhythms

Continue CPR	Obtain IV access
Intubate	Assess blood flow using Doppler ultrasound

Possible causes and therapies:

Acidosis	Consider sodium bicarbonate*
Acute MI	Reduce myocardial oxygen demand
Cardiac tamponade	Pericardiocentesis
Drug overdose	Depends on ingested substance
Hyperkalemia	Consider sodium bicarbonate*
Hypothermia	Active internal rewarming
Hypovolemia	Volume infusion
Hypoxia	Support ventilation
Pulmonary embolism	Thrombolytics, surgery
Tension pneumothorax	Needle thoracostomy

Epinephrine 1 mg IV push, repeat every 3-5 min*

Atropine 1 mg IV push, for bradycardia, repeat every 3-5 min to 0.04 mg/kg

Sodium bicarbonate: 1 mEq/kg IV is indicated early for hyperkalemia and contraindicated in hypoxic lactic acidosis. It may be useful (1) if preexisting metabolic acidosis, (2) if tricyclic antidepressant overdose, (3) to alkalinize the urine in drug overdose, (4) if intubated and there is a long arrest interval. *Contraindicated:* If pulse returns after long arrest interval.

FIG 4-5.
Pulseless electrical activity algorithm.

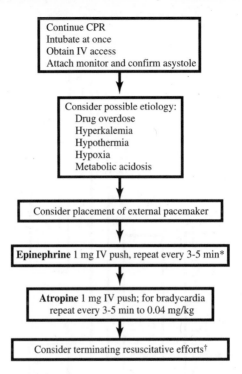

```
┌─────────────────────────────────────┐
│  Continue CPR                        │
│  Intubate at once                    │
│  Obtain IV access                    │
│  Attach monitor and confirm asystole │
└─────────────────────────────────────┘
                  │
                  ▼
    ┌───────────────────────────────┐
    │  Consider possible etiology:   │
    │    Drug overdose               │
    │    Hyperkalemia                │
    │    Hypothermia                 │
    │    Hypoxia                     │
    │    Metabolic acidosis          │
    └───────────────────────────────┘
                  │
                  ▼
┌─────────────────────────────────────┐
│ Consider placement of external       │
│ pacemaker                            │
└─────────────────────────────────────┘
                  │
                  ▼
┌─────────────────────────────────────┐
│ Epinephrine 1 mg IV push, repeat     │
│ every 3-5 min*                       │
└─────────────────────────────────────┘
                  │
                  ▼
┌─────────────────────────────────────┐
│ Atropine 1 mg IV push; for           │
│ bradycardia repeat every 3-5 min     │
│ to 0.04 mg/kg                        │
└─────────────────────────────────────┘
                  │
                  ▼
┌─────────────────────────────────────┐
│ Consider terminating resuscitative   │
│ efforts†                             │
└─────────────────────────────────────┘
```

*Sodium bicarbonate: 1 mEq/kg IV is indicated early for hyperkalemia and contraindicated in hypoxic lactic acidosis. It may be useful (1) if preexisting metabolic acidosis, (2) if tricyclic antidepressant overdose, (3) to alkalinize the urine in drug overdose, (4) if intubated and there is a long arrest interval.
Contraindicated: If pulse returns after long arrest interval.
Epinephrine: 1 mg IV every 3-5 min. If this fails, consider the following:

   Intermediate dosing: 2-5 mg IV every 3-5 min
   Escalating dose: 1 mg, 3 mg, 5 mg IV every 3-5 min
   High dose: 0.1 mg/kg IV every 3-5 min

†Consider arrest interval and persistence of asystole despite successful intubation.

FIG 4-6.
Asystole algorithm.

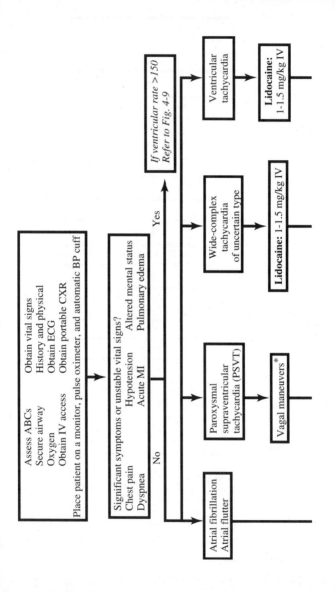

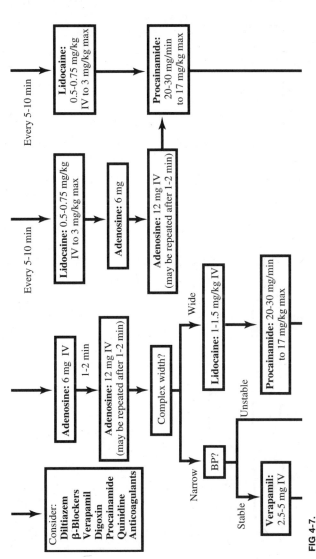

(Continued.)

FIG 4-7.
Tachycardia algorithm.

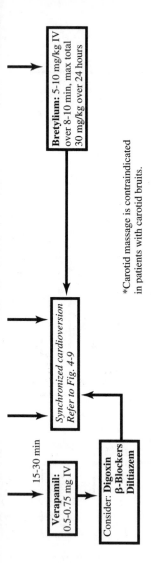

Bretylium: 5-10 mg/kg IV over 8-10 min, max total 30 mg/kg over 24 hours

Synchronized cardioversion Refer to Fig. 4-9

Verapamil: 0.5-0.75 mg IV

15-30 min

Consider: **Digoxin β-Blockers Diltiazem**

*Carotid massage is contraindicated in patients with carotid bruits.

FIG 4-7, cont'd

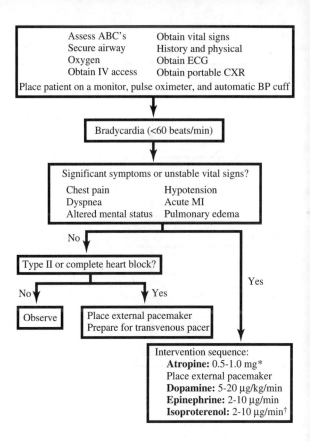

Assess ABC's   Obtain vital signs
Secure airway   History and physical
Oxygen   Obtain ECG
Obtain IV access   Obtain portable CXR
Place patient on a monitor, pulse oximeter, and automatic BP cuff

Bradycardia (<60 beats/min)

Significant symptoms or unstable vital signs?

Chest pain   Hypotension
Dyspnea   Acute MI
Altered mental status Pulmonary edema

No

Type II or complete heart block?

No

Observe

Yes

Place external pacemaker
Prepare for transvenous pacer

Yes

Intervention sequence:
Atropine: 0.5-1.0 mg*
Place external pacemaker
Dopamine: 5-20 µg/kg/min
Epinephrine: 2-10 µg/min
Isoproterenol: 2-10 µg/min†

*Atropine: Not effective in the denervated transplanted heart.
Consider placement of an external pacemaker or cactecholamine
infusion. Otherwise, repeat dose every 3-5 min up to a maximum
of 0.04 mg/kg.
†Isoproterenol: Use with extreme caution, especially if
myocardial ischemia/infarction is the suspected etiology of the
bradycardia, since isoproterenol will increase myocardial oxygen
consumption.

FIG 4-8.
Bradycardia algorithm.

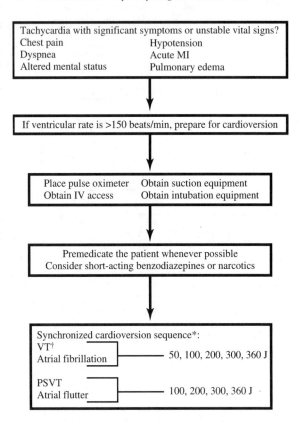

Tachycardia with significant symptoms or unstable vital signs?
Chest pain   Hypotension
Dyspnea   Acute MI
Altered mental status   Pulmonary edema

↓

If ventricular rate is >150 beats/min, prepare for cardioversion

↓

Place pulse oximeter   Obtain suction equipment
Obtain IV access   Obtain intubation equipment

↓

Premedicate the patient whenever possible
Consider short-acting benzodiazepines or narcotics

↓

Synchronized cardioversion sequence*:
VT†
Atrial fibrillation ———— 50, 100, 200, 300, 360 J

PSVT
Atrial flutter ———— 100, 200, 300, 360 J

*If clinical conditions deteriorate and there are delays in
synchronization, go to unsynchronized shocks.
†Polymorphic VT should be treated like VF: 200, 200-300,
then 360 J

FIG 4-9.
Cardioversion algorithm.

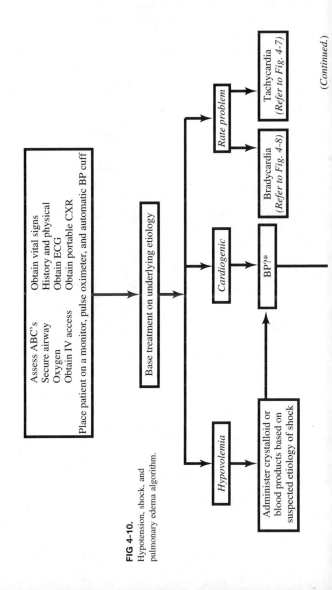

FIG 4-10.
Hypotension, shock, and pulmonary edema algorithm.

Assess ABC's   Obtain vital signs
Secure airway   History and physical
Oxygen   Obtain ECG
Obtain IV access   Obtain portable CXR
Place patient on a monitor, pulse oximeter, and automatic BP cuff

Base treatment on underlying etiology

Hypovolemia

Administer crystalloid or blood products based on suspected etiology of shock

Cardiogenic

BP?*

Rate problem

Bradycardia
(Refer to Fig. 4-8)

Tachycardia
(Refer to Fig. 4-7)

(Continued.)

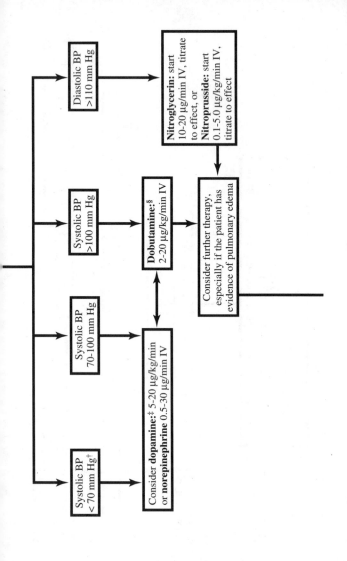

Systolic BP <70 mm Hg[†]

Consider **dopamine**:[‡] 5-20 µg/kg/min or **norepinephrine** 0.5-30 µg/min IV

Systolic BP 70-100 mm Hg

Systolic BP >100 mm Hg

Dobutamine:[§] 2-20 µg/kg/min IV

Diastolic BP >110 mm Hg

Nitroglycerin: start 10-20 µg/min IV, titrate to effect, or **Nitroprusside:** start 0.1-5.0 µg/kg/min IV, titrate to effect

Consider further therapy, especially if the patient has evidence of pulmonary edema

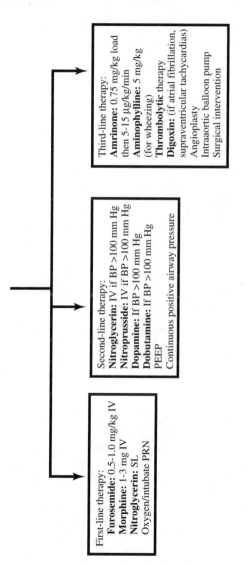

First-line therapy:
Furosemide: 0.5-1.0 mg/kg IV
Morphine: 1-3 mg IV
Nitroglycerin: SL
Oxygen/intubate PRN

Second-line therapy:
Nitroglycerin: IV if BP >100 mm Hg
Nitroprusside: IV if BP >100 mm Hg
Dopamine: If BP >100 mm Hg
Dobutamine: If BP >100 mm Hg
PEEP
Continuous positive airway pressure

Third-line therapy:
Amrinone: 0.75 mg/kg load then 5-15 μg/kg/min
Aminophylline: 5 mg/kg (for wheezing)
Thrombolytic therapy
Digoxin: (if atrial fibrillation, supraventricular tachycardias)
Angioplasty
Intraaortic balloon pump
Surgical intervention

*Initiate invasion hemodynamic monitoring if possible.
†Consider a 250-500 ml fluid bolus prior to initiating inotropic support.
‡Dopamine should be used preferentially to norepinephrine to stabilize BP.
§Avoid dobutamine when systolic BP < 100 mm Hg.

FIG 4-10, cont'd

2. May be associated with cardiac arrest and often erroneously blamed on a heart attack ("café coronary")

B. Etiology
1. Intrinsic
   a. Tongue
   b. Epiglottis
   c. Blood/emesis
2. Extrinsic
   a. Food (usually meat)
   b. Small toys, round objects in children

C. Risk Factors
1. Inability to adequately chew food
   a. Poor dentition
   b. Neurologic deficit
   c. Young children, infants
2. Dentures
3. Elevated blood ethanol levels

D. Diagnosis
1. The patient is unable to ventilate and is clutching the neck (universal distress sign).
2. Airway obstruction must be differentiated from heart attack, seizure, stroke, and drug overdose.
3. Symptoms include coughing, wheezing, and inability to phonate. If gas exchange worsens with increasing distress, stridor, and cyanosis, treat as a total airway obstruction.
4. Do not interfere with patient's efforts to expectorate the foreign body. If the patient is unsuccessful in clearing the foreign body, activate EMS.

E. Treatment
1. Heimlich maneuver
   a. Administer brisk abdominal thrusts resulting in an artificial cough by transmitting pressure from the abdomen to the diaphragm and thorax.
   b. Ideally this maneuver is performed from behind the patient with the fist of one hand placed with the thumb against the abdominal wall. The other hand is placed on top of the fist and a brisk upward abdominal thrust is delivered.
   c. If the patient is supine, the rescuer should straddle the victim and use the heel of one hand with the other hand on top to perform abdominal thrusts.
   d. Hands must be positioned in the midline above the

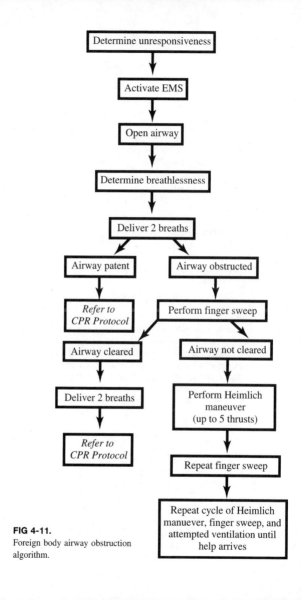

FIG 4-11.
Foreign body airway obstruction algorithm.

umbilicus and below the xyphoid process to prevent potential complications.

2. Chest thrusts
   a. Reserved for gravid and markedly obese patients
   b. Similar to performing chest compressions during CPR
3. Finger sweep
   a. Reserve this method for the unconscious victim.
   b. Open the airway by grasping the tongue and mandible and lifting the mandible.
   c. Use the index finger of the other hand to sweep the oropharynx of any foreign body or emesis.
4. Recommended sequence for unconscious patient (Fig. 4-11)

VI. SPECIAL CONSIDERATIONS
A. Complications of CPR
1. Rib fracture
2. Sternal fracture
3. Pneumothorax
4. Hemothorax
5. Fat emboli
6. Liver and spleen lacerations
7. Gastric distention/regurgitation
B. Risk of Disease Transmission During CPR
1. Saliva has not been shown to be a vector for HIV or hepatitis B virus transfection; however, tuberculosis, herpes simplex, and bacterial pathogens may be transmitted through mouth-to-mouth resuscitation.
2. Recommendations include the following:
   a. Latex gloves and a face shield or bag-valve mask device should be used when possible.
   b. If the patient is suspected of having tuberculosis, rescuers should undergo appropriate screening tests for tuberculosis with prophylactic therapy for converters.
   c. Early intubation is encouraged when appropriate personnel and equipment are available.

SUGGESTED READING

Cummins RO, editor: *Textbook of advanced cardiac life support,* 1994, American Heart Association.

Emergency Cardiac Care Committee and Subcommittees AHA: Guidelines for cardiopulmonary resuscitation and emergency cardiac care, III: adult advanced cardiac life support, *JAMA* 268:2242-2250, 1992.

Feneley MP et al: Influence of compression rate on initial success of resuscitation and 24 hour survival after prolonged manual cardiopulmonary resuscitation in dogs, *Circulation* 77:24-250, 1988.

Geehr EC, Lewis FR, Auerbach PS: Failure of open-heart massage to improve survival after prehospital nontraumatic cardiac arrest, *N Engl J Med* 314:1189-1190, 1986.

Hartz R et al: Clinical experience with portable cardiopulmonary bypass in cardiac arrest patients, *Ann Thorac Surg* 50:437-441, 1990.

Krischer JP et al: Complications of cardiac resuscitation, *Chest* 92:287-291, 1987.

Paradis NA, Martin GB, Goetting MG: Simultaneous aortic, jugular bulb, and right atrial pressures during cardiopulmonary resuscitation in humans: insights into mechanisms, *Circulation* 80:361-368, 1989.

Rudikoff MT et al: Mechanisms of blood flow during cardiopulmonary resuscitation, *Circulation* 61:345-352, 1980.

Stults KR et al: Prehospital defibrillation performed by emergency medical technicians in rural communities, *N Engl J Med* 310:219-223, 1984.

Zoll PM et al: External noninvasive temporary cardiac pacing: clinical trials, *Circulation* 71:937-944, 1985.

PROCEDURES 5

Thomas A. D'Amico

I. **CENTRAL VENOUS CATHETERIZATION**
A. **Indications**
Central venous catheterization is used to administer fluids, vasoactive drugs, drugs that irritate veins, and total parenteral nutrition; to obtain vascular access when peripheral access is poor; to perform hemodialysis; to perform plasmapheresis; and to gain access to the central venous compartment and right heart for physiologic monitoring.

B. **General Approach**
1. Central venous cannulation is performed as a sterile procedure, and requires adequate patient preparation and the following equipment: 18-g needle and guidewire (several centimeters longer than the catheter to be placed); catheter (single-, double-, or triple-lumen) or 8F introducer-sheath combination; povidone-iodine solution; cap, mask, sterile gloves, and sterile towels; lidocaine (1% solution without epinephrine).
2. Prior to placement, obtain a chest film for the purpose of comparison to subsequent films.
3. For internal jugular vein and subclavian vein cannulation, the patient should be supine in the Trendelenberg position (15°) to distend the veins and to reduce the incidence of air embolism. Turn the patient's head away from the desired side of cannulation. Wear the cap, mask, and sterile gloves, prepare the skin with povidone-iodine solution, and drape the field with sterile towels. Determine the length for catheter placement (catheter tip in the superior vena cava) by measuring from the point of insertion to the angle of Louis (Fig. 5-1).

C. **Technique**
The Seldinger (guidewire) technique is preferable to the catheter-over-needle technique and may be used for central venous as well as arterial access.

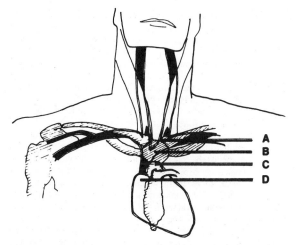

FIG 5-1.
Superficial anatomic landmarks used to determine the depth of central venous catheters. **A,** Sternoclavicular joint–subclavian vein. **B,** Manubrium–brachiocephalic vein. **C,** Angle of Louis–superior vena cava. **D,** 5 cm inferior to Angle of Louis–right atrium. (From Kaye W: *Intravenous techniques.* In *Textbook of advanced cardiac life support,* Dallas, 1981, American Heart Association.)

1. Infiltrate the desired area with lidocaine. Puncture the skin with the 18-g needle mounted on a 10-ml syringe, maintaining constant negative pressure, and advance slowly until blood appears. Upon entering the vein, disengage the syringe and cover the needle with a sterile gloved finger in order to minimize bleeding and to prevent air embolism.

2. Insert the wire through the needle and advance slowly into the vein. The wire should pass with minimal resistance over its entire length. Remove the needle over the guidewire. Pass a dilator over the guidewire into the vein, retaining control of the guidewire at all times in order to prevent embolization of the wire. Remove the dilator over the guidewire.

3. To pass a single-, double-, or triple-lumen catheter, thread the catheter over the guidewire and into the vein to the measured depth, taking particular care not to contaminate any part of the catheter. Remove the wire through the catheter and cap all ports. To insert an introducer and sheath, enlarge the puncture site to 1 cm with a sterile blade. Pass the introducer and sheath together over the wire. Slow and gentle pressure will usually safely advance the introducer into the vein. Allowing the introducer to warm and soften in the circulation for a moment may permit easier passage. When certain of correct placement, remove the introducer and wire through the sheath, and immediately cap the sheath with its previously flushed connector. Aspirate and flush all ports of the catheter or sheath to ascertain intraluminal placement. Secure the catheter to the skin with a suture. Dress the venipuncture site with povidone-iodine ointment, sterile gauze, and clear polyurethane.

4. Verify the location of the catheter with a chest film immediately after placement. Catheters should descend toward the heart, and the tip should be found in the superior vena cava or at the cavo-atrial junction. Also inspect the film for the presence of pneumothorax.

D. Internal Jugular Vein

1. Anatomy: As the internal jugular vein emerges at the base of the skull, it enters the carotid sheath posterior to the internal carotid artery and continues posterior and lateral to the common carotid artery until it crosses anterior to the common carotid artery near its termination. The internal jugular vein is medial to the sternocleidomastoid muscle superiorly, crossing deep to it and emerging at the triangle between the sternal and clavicular heads of the sternocleidomastoid. It continues behind the clavicular head where it joins the subclavian vein (Fig. 5-2).

2. Central approach: Identify the triangle formed by the sternal and clavicular heads of the sternocleidomastoid muscle (Fig. 5-3). Palpate the adjacent carotid artery pulse and retract the carotid medially with gentle digital pressure. Insert the needle at the apex of the triangle of the sternocleidomastoid, directing the needle inferiorly and laterally along the medial aspect of the clavicular head toward the ipsilateral nipple. If the vein is not entered on

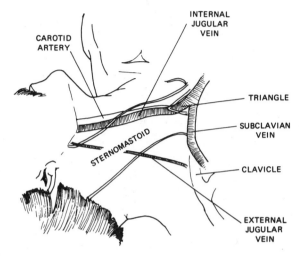

FIG 5-2.
Anatomy of the internal jugular vein. (From Kaye W: *Intravenous techniques.* In *Textbook of advanced cardiac life support,* Dallas, 1981, American Heart Association.)

the first pass (3 to 4 cm), maintain negative pressure in the syringe while slowly withdrawing the needle (in difficult cases a 22-g "seeker" needle may be useful in locating the jugular vein prior to inserting the 18-g needle). If venous blood is encountered, remove the syringe and follow the Seldinger technique as described above. If venous blood is not encountered, reassess the landmarks and make a second pass. If arterial blood is encountered, immediately remove the needle and maintain pressure over the artery for 10 minutes before resuming.

3. Posterior approach: Introduce the needle deep to the lateral border of the sternocleidomastoid muscle, 5 cm superior to the clavicle, and just superior to the junction of the sternocleidomastoid and the external jugular vein (Fig. 5-4). Direct the needle inferiorly and anteriorly toward the suprasternal notch. If the vein is not entered on the first

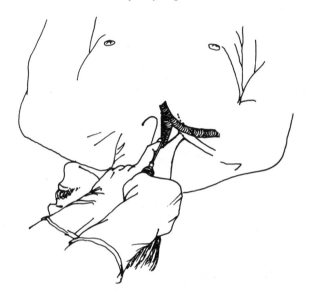

FIG 5-3.
Anatomic landmarks for cannulation of the internal jugular vein using the central approach. (From Kaye W: *Intravenous techniques.* In *Textbook of advanced cardiac life support,* Dallas, 1981, American Heart Association.)

pass (5 cm), maintain negative pressure in the syringe while slowly withdrawing the needle. If venous blood is encountered, remove the syringe and follow the Seldinger technique as described previously. If venous blood is not encountered, reassess the landmarks and make a second pass. If arterial blood is encountered, immediately remove the needle and maintain pressure over the artery for 10 minutes before resuming.

E. **Subclavian Vein**

1. Anatomy: The subclavian vein crosses over the first rib anterior to the anterior scalene muscle which separates the subclavian vein and artery. The subclavian vein continues posterior to the medial third of the clavicle (to which it is

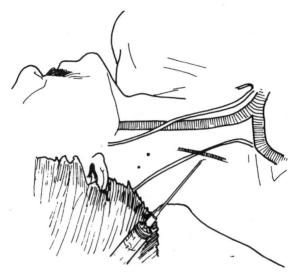

FIG 5-4.
Anatomic landmarks for cannulation of the internal jugular vein using the posterior approach. (From Kaye W: *Intravenous techniques.* In *Textbook of advanced cardiac life support,* Dallas, 1981, American Heart Association.)

attached) to join the internal jugular vein deep to the sterno-costoclavicular joint (Fig. 5-5).

2. Infraclavicular approach: The ideal point for needle insertion is 1 cm inferior to the junction of the middle and medial thirds of the clavicle. Direct the needle superiorly and medially, just deep to the clavicle and over the first rib, toward the suprasternal notch (Fig. 5-6). If the vein is not entered on the first pass (5 cm), maintain negative pressure in the syringe while slowly withdrawing the needle. If venous blood is encountered, rotate the needle 90° so the bevel faces inferiorly. Remove the syringe and follow the Seldinger technique as described previously. If venous blood is not encountered, reassess the landmarks and make a second pass. If arterial blood is encountered, remove the

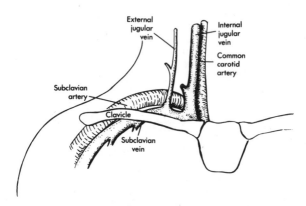

FIG 5-5.
Anatomy of the subclavian vein. (From Sladen A: *Invasive monitoring and its complications in the intensive care unit,* St. Louis, 1990, CV Mosby.)

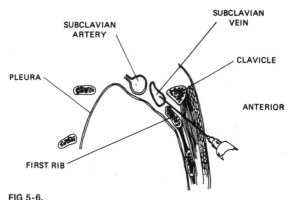

FIG 5-6.
Sagittal section through the medial third of the clavicle. (From Kaye W: *Intravenous techniques.* In *Textbook of advanced cardiac life support,* Dallas, 1981, American Heart Association.)

needle immediately. Due to the anatomy of the subclavian artery, arterial compression for hemostasis is not possible. Thus the patient must be observed closely for signs of hemodynamic compromise, which indicate hemorrhage. Hemostasis usually occurs and the patient is not endangered.

F. Complications

Complications arise in 1% to 20% of procedures overall, including pneumothorax (5% to 10%), arterial puncture (2% to 9%), hematoma formation, hemothorax, air embolism, hemomediastinum, brachial plexus injury, trachial laceration, subclavian vein thrombosis, sepsis, and death.

G. Special Considerations

1. The success rate for internal jugular vein cannulation is 60% to 80%, and for subclavian vein cannulation it is 85% to 95%. The complication rate for internal jugular vein cannulation is 5% to 20%, and for subclavian vein cannulation it is 6% to 10%.

2. If air is encountered during an unsuccessful attempt at central venous catheterization, obtain a chest film prior to attempting to cannulate the contralateral site to avoid undetected bilateral pneumothorax.

3. A 4 mm Hg gradient across a 20-g catheter permits air flow at 90 ml/sec, emphasizing the importance of correct patient positioning and other precautions against air embolism. To treat suspected air embolism, place the patient in the left lateral decubitus position, administer 100% oxygen, and attempt to aspirate the air through the catheter.

4. Central venous catheters should be changed over a wire (if the site is not infected) or replaced every 3 to 5 days to minimize infectious and thromboembolic complications. In cases of suspected catheter-borne infections, remove the catheter and submit its tip under sterile condition for culture.

5. The internal jugular vein is the preferred site in patients with bleeding disorders. Coagulopathy or thrombocytopenia may increase the incidence of hemorrhagic complications and are therefore relative contraindications to cannulation of the subclavian vein.

6. The subclavian vein is the preferred site for long-term

central venous access, since it provides greater patient comfort and facilitates catheter care.

7. Retrograde passage of the catheter into the internal jugular vein may occur after attempted cannulation of the subclavian vein. Manual compression of the internal jugular vein or rotation of the patient's head toward the side of cannulation while passing the guidewire may prevent this complication. When retrograde passage occurs, remove the catheter and attempt cannulation again.

II.   PULMONARY ARTERY CATHETERIZATION
A.   Indications
PA catheterization is used to provide continuous hemodynamic monitoring in an unstable or potentially unstable patient utilizing CVP, pulmonary arterial systolic and diastolic pressures, PCWP, and cardiac output; to guide the fluid management in complicated patients; to sample mixed venous (pulmonary arterial) blood for oxygen content; and to gain access to the right ventricle for cardiac pacing.

B.   General Approach
1. PA catheterization is performed as a sterile procedure and requires the following equipment: Supplies for catheter sheath placement including sterile gowns and sterile drapes; pulmonary artery catheter (7F); transducer, oscilloscope, and monitor (all calibrated); and cardiac defibrillator, lidocaine, and atropine (at bedside).
2. In preparation for the procedure, the patient is monitored continuously with a continuous ECG and should have a functioning intravenous catheter in place for treatment of cardiac dysrhythmias. Sterile preparation is performed as previously described, which includes utilizing a cap, mask, sterile gown, sterile gloves, sterile drapes, and preparing the skin.

C.   Technique
1. Cannulate the internal jugular vein or the subclavian vein using the Seldinger technique as described previously, and insert the catheter sheath. After securing the sheath, ensure that the PA catheter has been properly flushed and that the balloon is functional. Thread the catheter through its sterile protective sleeve.
2. With the balloon deflated, insert the catheter through the sheath to a depth of 20 cm; at this point the tip will be

beyond the end of the sheath and in the right atrium. Inflate the balloon and advance the catheter slowly while inspecting the ECG for dysrhythmias and the pressure tracing for the succession of characteristic waveforms (Fig. 5-7). Once the proper position has been reached (pulmonary capillary wedge), the balloon is deflated. At this point, the tracing should return to that of the PA. After the catheter has been successfully positioned, draw the protective sleeve over it and secure the connector.

3. Verify the position. The disappearance of the characteristic PA waveform when the balloon is inflated and its prompt return when the balloon is deflated is mandatory. In addition, the oxygen saturation of blood samples drawn with the balloon inflated should be greater than that of systemic arterial blood. Obtain a chest film to ascertain that the tip of the catheter is in a main branch of the PA. Also inspect the film for the presence of pneumothorax.

D. Complications

Complications associated with the PA catheter include cardiac dysrhythmias (premature ventricular contractions, ventricular tachycardia, ventricular fibrillation, and right bundle branch block), pulmonary hemorrhage, pulmonary infarct, catheter entanglement, cardiac perforation, valvular damage, endocarditis, and sepsis.

E. Special Considerations

The presence of left bundle branch block in the patient prior to placement is a relative contraindication to the use of a PA

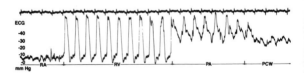

FIG 5-7.

Succession of pressure waveforms observed during the advancement of pulmonary artery catheter through the right atrium (RA), right ventricle (RV), pulmonary artery (PA), and to the pulmonary capillary wedge (PCW) position. (From Kaye W: *Intravenous techniques.* In *Textbook of advanced cardiac life support,* Dallas, 1981, American Heart Association.)

catheter since its passage may result in complete heart block. Fluoroscopic guidance may facilitate the passage of the catheter into the PA in difficult cases.

III. ARTERIAL CATHETERIZATION
A. Indications
Arterial catheterization is used to monitor arterial pressure continuously in any condition in which the factors influencing cardiac function may change rapidly (hypertensive crisis, shock, hemodynamic instability, administration of vasoactive or inotropic agents, and positive-pressure ventilation), and to provide access for frequent arterial blood samples.

B. General Approach
1. Arterial catheterization is performed as a sterile procedure and requires the following equipment: Appropriately sized catheter-over-needle; flexible guidewire; povidone-iodine solution; cap, mask, sterile gloves, and sterile towels; lidocaine (1% solution without epinephrine); pressure tubing, transducer and monitor.
2. Although the catheter-over-needle technique is acceptable, particularly for the radial artery, the Seldinger technique is preferred for femoral and axillary arterial cannulation. An introducer needle may be used, or the guidewire may be passed through the catheter prior to advancing the catheter entirely into the artery.

C. Radial Artery
1. The equipment includes a 20-g (2-inch) catheter-over-needle, an arm board and roll of gauze, and other supplies as listed above.
2. Assess collateral circulation by performing the Allen test. Occlude the radial and ulnar arteries digitally until blanching of the hand is noted. Release the ulnar artery. Ulnar collateral circulation is considered inadequate if more than 5 seconds elapse before blushing of the hand occurs, in which case another site is selected.
3. For proper placement, support the patient's hand in dorsiflexion with a roll of gauze under the wrist. Secure the palm and lower arm to the board. Use sterile precautions as previously described. Palpate the radial artery just proximal to the head of the radius. Insert the 20-g needle-catheter at a 30° angle to the skin with the bevel down. Advance the catheter and needle until blood appears

at the hub of the needle. Maintain the position of the needle and advance the catheter into the artery. If arterial blood is not encountered, reassess the landmarks and make a second pass. If arterial blood is encountered, but the catheter cannot be passed, immediately remove the needle and maintain pressure over the artery for 10 minutes before resuming. If the artery cannot be cannulated in three attempts, discontinue the procedure and choose another site. Once the catheter has been successfully passed, remove the needle and attach the hub of the catheter to the pressure tubing. Secure the catheter to the skin with a suture or tape. Apply povidone-iodine ointment to the puncture site and cover with a sterile dressing.

D. **Femoral Artery**

1. The equipment includes an 18-g (4-inch) catheter-over-needle, a razor and surgical soap, and other supplies as listed above.

2. The femoral artery is found at the midpoint of a line between the anterior superior iliac spine and the symphysis pubis. Medial to the femoral artery is the femoral vein; lateral to the femoral artery is the femoral nerve. Scrub and clip the groin area and prepare the skin with povidone-iodine solution. Use sterile precautions as previously described. Infiltrate the skin with lidocaine.

3. For proper placement, enter the skin at a 45° angle with the catheter-over-needle or the needle alone (Seldinger technique). If the Seldinger technique is chosen, the wire must pass without any resistance, indicating that it is intraluminal and that it has not dissected. If the artery is not entered on the first pass (3 to 4 cm), maintain negative pressure in the syringe while slowly withdrawing the needle. If arterial blood is encountered, remove the syringe and follow the Seldinger technique as previously described. If arterial blood is not encountered, reassess the landmarks and make a second pass. If arterial blood is encountered, but the guidewire cannot be passed, immediately remove the needle and maintain pressure over the artery for 10 minutes before resuming. If the artery cannot be cannulated in three attempts, discontinue the procedure and choose another site. Once the catheter has been successfully passed, remove the needle or wire and attach the hub of the catheter to the pressure tubing. Secure the

catheter to the skin with a suture. Dress the site with povidone-iodine ointment, sterile gauze, and clear polyurethane.

E.   Dorsalis Pedis Artery

1. The equipment includes a 20-g (2-inch) catheter-over-needle and other supplies as listed above.

2. The dorsalis pedis artery, the extension of the anterior tibial artery, is found on the dorsum of the foot, parallel and lateral to the extensor hallucis longus. In 12% of the population, the dorsalis pedis artery is absent. Demonstrate the presence of collateral flow by assessing the flow in the posterior tibial artery by palpation, or by using a Doppler flow meter. Maintain sterile conditions as previously described. Infiltrate the skin with lidocaine.

3. For proper placement, palpate the dorsalis pedis artery, and insert the 20-g needle-catheter at a 30° angle to the skin with the bevel down. Advance the catheter and needle until blood appears at the hub of the needle. Maintain the position of the needle and advance the catheter into the artery. If arterial blood is not encountered, reassess the landmarks and make a second pass. If arterial blood is encountered, but the catheter cannot be passed, immediately remove the needle and maintain pressure over the artery for 10 minutes before resuming. If the artery cannot be cannulated in three attempts, discontinue the procedure and choose another site. Once the catheter has been successfully passed, remove the needle and attach the hub of the catheter to the pressure tubing. Secure the catheter to the skin with a suture or tape. Apply povidone-iodine ointment to the puncture site and cover it with a sterile dressing.

F.   Axillary Artery

1. The equipment includes an 18-g (6-inch) catheter-over-needle, a razor and surgical soap, and other supplies as listed above.

2. The axillary artery is the continuation of the subclavian artery entering the axilla at the lateral border of the first rib; at the teres major muscle, it becomes the brachial artery. The axillary sheath contains the axillary artery, axillary vein, and the brachial plexus (Fig. 5-8). Interruption of flow in the axillary artery will not lead to ischemia in the arm because of extensive collateral flow from the

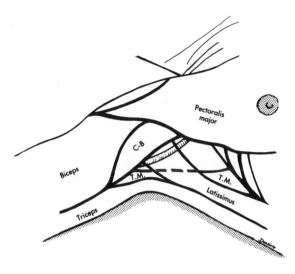

FIG 5-8.
Anatomic landmarks for cannulation of the axillary artery. *C-B,* coracobrachialis muscle; *T.M.,* teres major muscle. (From Sladen A: *Invasive monitoring and its complications in the intensive care unit,* St. Louis, 1990, CV Mosby.)

thyrocervical trunk and the subscapular artery. Hyperabduct, externally rotate, and immobilize the arm. Shave the axilla and prepare the skin with povidone-iodine solution. Maintain sterile conditions as previously described. Infiltrate the skin with lidocaine.

3. For proper placement, enter the skin as high as possible in the axilla with the catheter-over-needle or needle alone (Seldinger technique). If the Seldinger technique is chosen, the wire must pass without any resistance, indicating that it is in the lumen and that it has not dissected. If the artery is not entered on the first pass (5 cm), maintain negative pressure in the syringe while slowly withdrawing the needle. If arterial blood is encountered, remove the syringe and follow the Seldinger

technique as described above. If arterial blood is not encountered, reassess the landmarks and make a second pass. If arterial blood is encountered, but the guidewire cannot be passed, immediately remove the needle and maintain pressure over the artery for 10 minutes before resuming. If the artery cannot be cannulated in three attempts, discontinue the procedure and choose another site. Once the catheter is successfully passed, remove the needle or wire and attach the hub of the catheter to the pressure tubing. Secure the catheter to the skin with a suture. Dress the site with povidone-iodine ointment, sterile gauze, and clear polyurethane.

G. **Complications**

Complications of arterial cannulation include thrombosis (temporary, 10% to 15%), thromboembolism, distal ischemia, hemorrhage, hematoma, infection, arteriovenous fistula, and neurological complications (brachial plexus).

H. **Special Considerations**

Change arterial catheters over a wire if the site is not infected, or replace every 3 to 5 days to minimize infectious and ischemic complications. Remove a catheter immediately when signs of distal ischemia appear. Brachial artery cannulation is not recommended, because of its inadequate collateral circulation and unacceptably high incidence of complications. Risk factors for ischemic complications include female sex, low cardiac output state, use of vasoconstricting agents, multiple failed attempts to cannulate, peripheral vascular disease, and prolonged duration of cannulation.

IV. **ENDOTRACHEAL INTUBATION**

A. **Indications**

Endotracheal intubation is used when an unconscious patient cannot be ventilated with conventional methods, to protect the airway in an unresponsive patient, for respiratory insufficiency, for cardiopulmonary arrest, or to hyperventilate a patient with elevated intracranial pressure.

B. **General Approach**

1. Endotracheal intubation may be performed electively (e.g., in a patient with progressive respiratory insufficiency), or emergently (e.g., in a patient in cardiopulmo-

nary arrest). In either case, endotracheal tube placement should be performed promptly yet carefully and requires the following equipment: Laryngoscope; endotracheal tubes of various sizes; malleable stylet; rigid pharyngeal suction apparatus and flexible tracheal suction catheter; bag-valve-mask ventilation unit; and an oxygen source.

2. The ideal position for direct visualization of the glottic opening requires the alignment of three axes: (1) the mouth, (2) the pharynx, and (3) the trachea. Extend the head and flex the neck to obtain this alignment known as the "sniffing position."

C. **Technique**

Orotracheal approach

1. Prior to attempting endotracheal intubation, hyperventilate the patient with 100% oxygen with the face mask. Suction the oropharynx. Standing at the head of the patient, hold the laryngoscope in the left hand and open the patient's mouth with the right hand. Insert the blade of the laryngoscope in the right side of the mouth, displace the tongue to the left, and advance the blade in the midline to the base of the tongue. If a curved blade is used, advance the tip into the valecula exposing the glottic opening. If a straight blade is used, insert the tip under the epiglottis directly.

2. At this point, the epiglottis, the arytenoid cartilage, the vocal cords, and the glottic opening should be visualized clearly. The upper airway and trachea may be anesthetized with lidocaine 4% aerosolized solution (5 ml). Place the endotracheal tube under direct vision through the vocal cords, advancing the cuff 2 cm past the vocal cords into the trachea. If intubation has not been achieved after 30 seconds, ventilate the patient again with 100% oxygen with the face mask. Once intubation is successful, inflate the cuff and ventilate the patient with 100% oxygen manually, auscultating the axillae bilaterally. If breath sounds are clear and equal, secure the tube to the patient's face and initiate mechanical ventilation.

3. If gurgling sounds are present, indicating esophageal intubation, immediately remove the tube and ventilate the patient with the face mask prior to another attempt. If breath sounds are observed to be greater on the right, indicating right mainstem bronchus intubation, deflate the

cuff, withdraw the tube slightly, and reinflate the cuff. If auscultation reveals equal breath sounds bilaterally, secure the tube. After initiating mechanical ventilation, obtain a chest film to verify correct positioning of the tip of the endotracheal tube. In addition, obtain an arterial blood sample to verify adequate oxygenation and ventilation.

D.   Complications

Complications of orotracheal intubation, which occur more frequently in the emergent setting, include oropharyngeal and dental trauma, tracheal laceration or rupture, vocal cord injury, avulsion of the arytenoid cartilage, esophageal perforation, vomiting and aspiration, intubation of the right mainstem bronchus, and intubation of the pyriform sinus.

E.   Special Considerations

A "difficult" airway may be encountered and is characterized by laryngeal edema, upper airway trauma, trachea not in the midline, a tumor obstructing the airway, and limited range of motion at the cervical or temporomandibular joints. Assume that all patients have a full stomach and take precautions against aspiration during intubation; maintain the patient's protective reflexes by withholding heavy sedation, and instruct an assistant to apply cricoid pressure during the procedure. For patients with a suspected or known spinal injury, orotracheal intubation is contraindicated. Blind nasotracheal intubation may be attempted for airway control; otherwise, cricothyroidotomy is recommended. A malleable stylet may facilitate intubation in some patients.

V.   EMERGENT CRICOTHYROIDOTOMY

A.   Indications

An emergent cricothyroidotomy is used for immediate airway management after trauma to the oropharynx that precludes direct visualization of the glottic opening, immediate airway management after unsuccessful endotracheal intubation, and upper airway obstruction.

B.   General Approach

1. Although the technical details are critical, the success of emergent cricothyroidotomy depends on sound judgement concerning the timing of the procedure. Anticipation of the possible necessity of this approach to airway management contributes to its success. For the most expedient placement, the following equipment is required: Knife blade

and handle; povidone-iodine or other antiseptic solution; pediatric endotracheal tube or 14-g catheter-over-needle; bag-valve ventilation unit; and oxygen source.

2. The patient must be supine with the head extended. The standard precautions for sterility should be attempted, although the emergent nature of this procedure usually does not permit complete surgical preparation. If possible, the area should be prepared with povidone-iodine solution.

C. **Technique**

1. Palpate the cricothyroid membrane between the thyroid and cricoid cartilages. Incise the skin vertically and insert the knife through the cricothyroid membrane. Insert the knife handle through the cricothyroidotomy and rotate 90°. Insert the pediatric endotracheal tube through the opening, inflate the cuff, and begin ventilation with the bag-valve unit and 100% oxygen.

2. As an alternative, puncture the cricothyroid membrane with a catheter-over-needle and remove the needle. Mount the hub of the catheter with the barrel of a 12-ml syringe, which serves as a connector for ventilation.

D. **Complications**

Complications of emergent cricothyroidotomy include hemorrhage, perforation of the esophagus, and inability to cannulate the trachea.

E. **Special Considerations**

Assume that all trauma patients requiring cricothyroidotomy have a cervical spine injury and take all necessary precautions to protect the spinal cord. Cricothyroidotomy is the procedure of choice when emergency surgical airway access is necessary and is associated with a lower complication than emergent tracheostomy. After cricothyroidotomy in an emergent setting, airway control may be converted electively to a standard tracheostomy.

VI. THORACENTESIS

A. **Indications**

Thoracentesis is used to obtain a sample of pleural fluid for diagnosis or to drain a restricting pleural effusion and relieve respiratory compromise.

B. **General Approach**

1. Thoracentesis is performed as a sterile procedure, and requires the following equipment: 18-g catheter-over-

needle, stopcock, 20-ml syringe; extension tubing and collecting vessel; providone-iodine solution and sterile drapes; and lidocaine (1% solution without epinephrine).

2. If possible, the patient is placed in the sitting position, with the arms supported on a bedside table. As an alternative, place the patient in the supine position, with the head of the bed elevated to 90°. Locate the fluid level by percussion. Perform thoracentesis two interspaces below the percussed fluid level but not lower than the eighth intercostal space. Prepare the skin with povidone-iodine solution and drape the field.

C. **Technique**

1. Infiltrate the skin with lidocaine using a 25-g needle. Anesthetize the deeper tissues with a 20-g needle including the periosteum of the rib below the chosen intercostal space. While aspirating the syringe to avoid intravascular injection of lidocaine, enter the pleural cavity over the superior aspect of the rib, avoiding the intercostal neurovascular bundle. Administer lidocaine through the pleura; subsequent aspiration should confirm the presence of pleural fluid.

2. Remove the needle and reenter the pleural space with the catheter-over-needle attached to a syringe. Remove the needle, covering the hub of the catheter to prevent pneumothorax. Mount the stopcock and the 20-ml syringe to the catheter. For diagnostic purposes, aspirate fluid directly. For drainage of a large effusion, connect the extension tubing to the stopcock, so the pleural fluid can be withdrawn into the syringe and ejected through the tubing into a collecting container. Upon completion of the procedure, place a small sterile dressing.

3. Obtain a chest film to document the removal of the pleural fluid. In addition, inspect the film for the presence of pneumothorax.

D. **Diagnosis**

The pleural fluid is collected under sterile conditions and analyzed for differential cell count, gram stain and bacterial culture, fungal and mycobacterial culture, cytology, protein and glucose, amylase, LDH, and pH.

E. **Complications**

Complications include pneumothorax, hemothorax, and puncture of the lung, liver, or spleen.

VII. TUBE THORACOSTOMY

A. Indications

Tube thoracostomy is used for the following: Pneumothorax (greater than 20% in magnitude); hemothorax, hydrothorax, or chylothorax; prophylaxis for high risk patients prior to positive pressure ventilation; or prophylaxis after penetrating thoracic injury.

B. General Approach

1. Tube thoracostomy is performed as a sterile procedure and requires the following equipment: Thoracostomy tube (24 to 28F for pneumothorax; 28 to 36F for hemothorax); povidone-iodine solution; cap, mask, sterile gown, gloves, towels, and drapes; lidocaine (1% solution without epinephrine); sterile instruments (knife, scissors, Kelly clamp); and collection-suction apparatus.

2. Place the patient in the supine position. The preferred site for tube thoracostomy is the fifth intercostal space in the anterior axillary line. Prepare the skin with povidone-iodine solution. Wear cap, mask, sterile gown, and sterile gloves. Create a sterile field with towels and drapes.

C. Technique

1. Measure the chest tube from the desired insertion site to the apex, and mark the chest tube with a suture. Infiltrate the skin with lidocaine using a 25-g needle. Anesthetize the deeper tissues using a 20-g needle including the periosteum of the ribs above and below the chosen intercostal space. While aspirating the syringe to avoid intravascular injection of lidocaine, enter the pleural cavity over the superior aspect of the rib, avoiding the intercostal neurovascular bundle. Administer lidocaine through the pleura, and subsequent aspiration should confirm the presence of pleural air or fluid.

2. Remove the needle and incise the skin one interspace below the desired site of insertion. Create a subcutaneous tunnel with blunt dissection using the Kelly clamp. Enter the pleural space with the tip of the clamp, just over the superior margin of the rib; open the clamp, spreading the pleura. With a gloved finger, confirm penetration into the chest by palpating the lung, sweeping away pleural adhesions if present. Grasp the tip of the thoracostomy tube with the Kelly clamp, and insert both into the pleural space. Direct the tube posteriorly and superiorly for

drainage of hemothorax or hydrothorax or anteriorly for pneumothorax. Ensure that the last hole in the tube is within the thoracic cavity. Secure the tube to the chest wall with a suture. Cover the wound with a sterile dressing consisting of petrolatum-soaked gauze and sponges.

3. Inspect the collecting system for an adequate water seal and measure the amount of drainage. Inspect and secure all connections. Obtain a chest film to assess the position of the catheter and the evacuation of air or fluid from the thoracic cavity.

D.   Complications

Complications include hemorrhage, laceration of the lung, infection, cardiac injury, subcutaneous placement, re-expansion pulmonary edema, and intraperitoneal placement.

E.   Special Considerations

Trocar tube thoracostomy is associated with a high complication rate and therefore is not recommended.

VIII. PERICARDIOCENTESIS

A.   Indications

Pericardiocentesis is used to relieve cardiac tamponade emergently in patients with respiratory distress or progressive hypotension, or to obtain fluid for diagnostic study.

B.   General Approach

1. Pericardiocentesis is performed as a sterile procedure with complete monitoring available, and requires the following supplies: 16-g (4-inch) needle, short-beveled; 50-ml syringe; sterile alligator connector (for ECG V-lead); povidone-iodine solution; cap, mask, sterile gown, gloves, towels, and drapes; and lidocaine (1% solution without epinephrine).

2. If the indication for pericardiocentesis is cardiac tamponade, the infusion of volume intravenously will improve cardiac performance until the pericardium can be drained.

3. Place the patient in the supine position. Continuous ECG monitoring is mandatory. Prepare the skin with povidone-iodine solution. Wear cap, mask, sterile gown, and sterile gloves. Create a sterile field with towels and drapes.

C.   Technique

Paraxiphoid approach

1. Connect the ECG V-lead to the needle with the sterile alligator clip. ST segment elevation during the procedure

indicates ventricular contact with the needle, and PR segment elevation suggests atrial contact.

2. Infiltrate the skin and subcutaneous tissue to the left of the xiphoid process with lidocaine. Insert the needle 1 cm to the left of the xiphoid at a 30° angle to the frontal plane while continuously aspirating the syringe. Advance the needle while observing the ECG. If grossly bloody fluid is obtained, assess it for coagulation. Clotting suggests intracardiac penetration, whereas pericardial fluid should not coagulate. If successfully entered, the pericardium should be completely drained. This may require the placement of a catheter, either through the needle, or using a guidewire.

D. Complications

Complications include cardiac dysrhythmias, cardiac puncture, myocardial laceration, coronary artery laceration, air embolism to a cardiac chamber or coronary artery, pneumothorax, and hemorrhage.

E. Special Considerations

The pericardial sac normally contains only 50 ml of fluid; in the acute setting, it can accommodate an additional 100 ml before cardiac tamponade results. Pericardiocentesis to remove bloody fluid after trauma is a temporary maneuver and should be followed by thoracotomy.

IX. PARACENTESIS

A. Indications

Paracentesis is used in patients diagnosed with unexplained ascites, when there is suspicion of spontaneous bacterial peritonitis, and for relief of severe ascites causing respiratory compromise.

B. General Approach

1. Paracentesis is performed as a sterile procedure and requires the following equipment: 20-g catheter-over-needle, stopcock, 50-ml syringe; extension tubing and collecting vessel; povidone-iodine solution; sterile gloves and sterile drapes; and lidocaine (1% solution without epinephrine).

2. Place the patient in the supine position. Confirm the presence of fluid by percussion. The preferred site for paracentesis is lateral to the rectus abdominis muscle in the lower abdomen. Prepare the skin with povidone-iodine solution and drape the field.

C. **Technique**
1. Infiltrate the skin with lidocaine using a 25-g needle. Anesthetize the deeper tissues with the 20-g needle, making the needle track discontinuous using the z-track technique. While aspirating the syringe, advance the needle through the fascia and into the peritoneum until ascitic fluid returns; remove the needle.
2. Insert the catheter-over-needle in the same manner; when ascitic fluid is encountered again, advance the catheter and remove the needle. Attach a three-way stopcock and the 50-ml syringe.
3. For diagnostic purposes, aspirate fluid directly. For drainage of massive ascites, connect extension tubing to the stopcock, so fluid may be withdrawn into the syringe and ejected through the tubing into a collecting container. Upon completion of the procedure, a sterile dressing is placed.

D. **Diagnosis**
The ascitic fluid is collected under sterile conditions and may be analyzed for differential cell count, gram stain and bacterial culture, fungal and mycobacterial culture, cytology, protein and glucose, amylase, LDH, and pH.

E. **Complications**
Complications include hemorrhage, infection, bowel perforation, bladder perforation, persistent ascitic leak, and hypotension (secondary to withdrawal of excessive volume).

X. **PERITONEAL DIALYSIS: INSERTION OF THE TENCKHOFF CATHETER**

A. **Indications**
Peritoneal dialysis is used for the temporary management of acute renal insufficiency or the long-term management of end-stage renal disease with continuous ambulatory peritoneal dialysis.

B. **Tenckhoff Catheter**
The Tenckhoff catheter is a flexible silicone rubber tube with an inner diameter of 2.6 mm and an outer diameter of 5 mm. It is comprised of three segments: The intraperitoneal segment (11 to 15 cm); the intramural segment (5 to 7 cm); and the external segment. The intraperitoneal segment has multiple 0.5 mm perforations; the intramural segment includes 1 or 2 Dacron cuffs.

C.   **General Approach**

1. The bedside insertion of the peritoneal dialysis (Tenck-hoff) catheter is performed as a sterile procedure and requires the following equipment: Tenckhoff catheter and obturator; detachable trocar and obturator; priming trocar or priming catheter; Faller guide; povidone-iodine solution; cap, mask, sterile gown, gloves, towels, and drapes; lidocaine (1% solution without epinephrine); sterile instruments (knife, scissors, clamps, forceps); and peritoneal dialysis fluid and administration tubing.

2. Contraindications to the insertion of a peritoneal dialysis catheter at the bedside include extreme obesity and previous abdominal surgery.

3. Place the patient in the supine position. The preferred site for placement is in the midline, inferior to the umbilicus. Prepare the skin with povidone-iodine solution. Wear a cap, mask, sterile gown, and sterile gloves, and create a sterile field with towels and drapes.

D.   **Technique**

1. Infiltrate the skin and subcutaneous tissue with lidocaine. Make a 3-cm midline incision 2 cm inferior to the umbilicus. Using blunt dissection, identify the linea alba and provide upward traction with a suture or a clamp. Enter the peritoneum with a catheter-over-needle or trocar. Connect the priming catheter or trocar to the administration tubing and instill approximately 2 L of dialysis solution.

2. Lubricate the Tenckhoff catheter, its obturator, and the Dacron cuffs with sterile saline; insert the obturator into the Tenckhoff catheter. Remove the priming catheter or trocar and insert the detachable trocar and obturator. After correct positioning within the peritoneum, remove the obturator from the trocar.

3. Insert the Tenckhoff catheter and its obturator through the trocar into the peritoneum, directing the catheter deeply into the pelvis. Remove the trocar over the catheter, and then detach it. Remove the obturator from the catheter, and position the inner Dacron cuff to rest at the fascial level. Test the catheter for patency. Secure the catheter to the fascia.

4. Create an exit site lateral and inferior to the entrance with a stab wound so that the subcutaneous cuff is 2 cm below

the skin; this site should be just large enough for the catheter. Create a subcutaneous tunnel with the Faller guide, and carefully pull the end of the catheter through the tunnel; insert the titanium connector. Suture the insertion wound and apply sterile dressings.

E.   **Complications**
Bleeding from the abdominal wall, recognized as bloody effluent, occurs in 30% of the cases. Other complications include dialysis solution leaks (15% to 35%), inadequate drainage, extraperitoneal extravasation, intestinal perforation, and peritonitis.

F.   **Special Considerations**
Other types of peritoneal dialysis catheters, such as any of the rigid dialysis catheters, may be placed at the bedside; however, the Tenckhoff catheter appears to be the safest and the most widely used. The most common etiology of early catheter failure is omental entanglement resulting from placement anteriorly in the peritoneum rather than deeper in the pelvis.

XI.   **SENGSTAKEN-BLAKEMORE TUBE**
A.   **Indication**
The Sengstaken-Blakemore tube is used to compress endoscopically proven variceal hemorrhage by tamponade of the gastroesophageal junction.

B.   **General Approach**
1. Adequate fluid resuscitation should take precedence over attempts to treat upper gastrointestinal bleeding and should be accomplished with two large-bore intravenous catheters in the forearm.
2. After adequate fluid resuscitation is achieved, the placement of a Sengstaken-Blakemore tube may be performed in conjunction with other therapeutic modalities in the management of variceal hemorrhage, such as the administration of vasopressin (0.2 to 0.4 U/min IV).
3. The placement of a Sengstaken-Blakemore tube is performed with continuous ECG monitoring, and supplemental oxygen available and will require the following equipment: Sengstaken-Blakemore tube; suction apparatus; 50-ml syringe; pressure manometer; a nasogastric tube; Ewalt tube; lubrication; and supplies for endotracheal intubation.

C. Technique

1. Place the patient in the left lateral decubitus position. Empty the stomach by passing a large orogastric or Ewalt tube. Test the balloons of the Sengstaken-Blakemore tube carefully prior to insertion; lubricate the tube well.

2. Pass the tube nasally to the 50-cm mark. Fill the gastric balloon with 150 to 200 ml air or a dilute radiocontrast solution. Clamp the tube. Using gentle traction, withdraw the tube until resistance is encountered at the gastroesophageal junction. Secure the tube to the patient's face under minimal traction.

3. Irrigate the distal tube with saline. In the absence of continued bleeding, leave the esophageal tube deflated. If bleeding has not ceased, inflate the esophageal balloon to 40 torr.

4. Pass a nasogastric tube through the contralateral nostril until resistance is sensed at the level of the esophageal balloon. Continuously aspirate the blind esophageal segment to prevent regurgitation and aspiration of esophageal secretions.

5. Obtain a chest film to confirm correct positioning.

D. Management

1. The esophageal tube may remain deflated in the absence of bleeding, but should be inflated to 40 torr if bleeding ensues in the first 24 hours after placement.

2. The balloon(s) of the Sengstaken-Blakemore tube remain inflated for 24 hours, and are then deflated if no further bleeding has occurred.

3. The tube may be removed after a second 24-hour period without bleeding.

E. Complications

Complications include esophageal rupture secondary to malposition of the gastric balloon; aspiration of blood, gastric secretion, or saliva; and refractory variceal hemorrhage.

F. Special Considerations

Consider intubation in all cases of altered consciousness, shock, or complex medical problems.

SUGGESTED READING

Berk JL, Sampliner JE, editors: *Handbook of critical care,* Boston, 1990, Little, Brown.

Civetta JM, editor: *Intensive care therapeutics,* New York, Appleton-Century-Crofts, 1980.

Civetta JM, Taylor RW, Kirby RR, editors: *Critical care,* Philadelphia, 1988, JB Lippincott.

Daldec DL, Krome RL: Thoracostomy, *Emerg Med Clin North Am* 4:441, 1986.

Dauphinee K: Orotracheal intubation, *Emerg Med Clin North Am* 6:699, 1988.

Kaye W: *Intravenous techniques.* In *Textbook of advanced cardiac life support,* Dallas, 1981, American Heart Association.

Nolph KD, editor: *Peritoneal dialysis,* Dordecht, the Netherlands, 1989, Kluwer Academic.

Putterman C: Central venous catheterization, *Acute Care* 12:219, 1986.

Sladen A: *Invasive monitoring and its complications in the intensive care unit,* St. Louis, 1990, CV Mosby.

Taylor RW, Civetta JM, Kirby RR, editors: *Techniques and procedures in critical care,* Philadelphia, 1990, JB Lippincott.

Walls RM: Cricothyroidotomy, *Emerg Med Clin North Am* 6:725, 1988.

PART TWO

PATHOPHYSIOLOGY

THE CARDIAC SYSTEM $\quad$ 6

Jeffrey S. Heinle

I. GENERAL PRINCIPLES

A. Cardiac Physiology

1. The heart is an efficient muscular pump with the highest basal oxygen extraction of any organ in the body.

2. Myocardial Do_2 is increased by increases in coronary blood flow (coronary vasodilatation) since oxygen extraction is already maximal. This is important in ischemic heart disease since fixed coronary lesions prevent increases in coronary blood flow, and lead to a supply/demand mismatch.

3. The majority of coronary blood flow occurs during *diastole,* therefore diastolic pressure and the length of diastole become important factors.

4. The typical cardiac cycle is depicted in Figure 6-1.

5. The heart is innervated by both the parasympathetic (vagus) and sympathetic (postganglionic, paravertebral) nervous systems. Parasympathetic tone predominates at rest.

B. Cardiac Output

The cardiac output (CO) is the amount of blood ejected by the ventricle per minute and is the product of stroke volume (SV) and heart rate (HR):

$$CO \text{ (L/min)} = SV \text{ (L/beat)} \times HR \text{ (beats/min)}$$

The following four determinants can be manipulated to improve cardiac output:

1. Preload

   a. The Frank-Starling Law of the Heart states that increasing preload (or filling) of the ventricle increases stretch of the myofibrils. This leads to an increase in

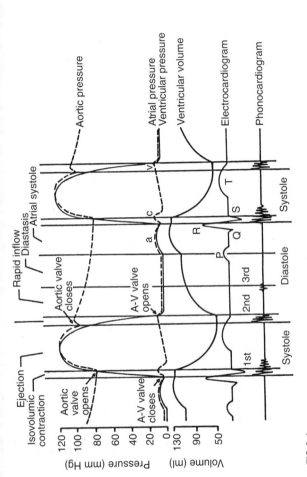

FIG 6-1.
The cardiac cycle. (From Guyton AC: *Textbook of medical physiology,* ed 8, Philadelphia, 1991, WB Saunders.)

tension and an increased force of contraction, which leads to increased stroke volume and cardiac output. However, the increase in tension also leads to an increase in MVO_2.

b. The LVEDV, or preload, is approximated by the LVEDP, which itself is approximated by the PCWP (except in the presence of mitral valve disease or pulmonary hypertension).

c. Ventricular filling occurs during diastole, and the majority of filling occurring during the first third of diastole, which is the time of rapid filling immediately following opening of the AV valve. (See Fig. 6-1.) Diastolic ventricular filling is impaired when the heart rate exceeds 120 beats/min.

d. Ventricular filling from atrial systole is responsible for approximately 30% of the ventricular volume and up to 20% of cardiac output.

e. In summary, preload can be increased by volume infusion, keeping the heart rate <120 beats/min and maintaining sinus rhythm.

2. Afterload
   a. Afterload is defined as the tension the ventricle must overcome before it can begin ejection.
   b. The major determinant of afterload for the left ventricle is aortic pressure.
   c. Decreasing afterload will increase the SV and cardiac output, and decrease MVO_2 because a decrease in tension is generated.

3. HR
   a. The principal control is through the autonomic nervous system (acetylcholine from the parasympathetic system, and catecholamines from the sympathetic system).
   b. Local factors (temperature, pH, atrial stretch, aortic arch, and carotid sinus baroreceptors) also play an important role.
   c. Increasing HR increases cardiac output as long as the rapid phase of diastolic filling is not impaired. Increases in HR will also increase MVO_2.

4. Contractility
   a. Contractility is defined as the force of contraction for a given myocardial fiber length.
   b. Contractility is affected by endogenous catechol-

amines, calcium concentration, and inotropic agents (through their effects on intracellular calcium concentration).

   c. An increase in the contractile state leads to an increased SV and cardiac output but also results in an increase in MVo_2.

C. **Cardiac Receptors**

An understanding of the cardiac adrenergic receptors (Table 6-1) is important to understand the use of inotropic and vasopressor agents. These receptors work through adenyl cyclase and cyclic AMP to control calcium channels in the cell membrane, therefore affecting the intracellular calcium concentration.

   1. Beta-receptors (β)
      a. β_1: Found predominantly in atrial and ventricular myocardium and have both chronotropic and inotropic effects
      b. β_2: Found in smooth muscle and glandular tissue; cause smooth muscle relaxation leading to arteriolar vasodilatation as well as bronchial smooth muscle relaxation
   2. Alpha-receptors (α)
      a. α_1: Postsynaptic receptors found predominantly on vascular smooth muscle (arterioles) with fewer receptors found in the myocardium; inotropic and vasopressor effects
      b. α_2: Presynaptic receptors which inhibit neurotransmitter (catecholamine) release
   3. Dopaminergic receptors
      a. Found in the renal and mesenteric vascular beds

TABLE 6-1.

Adrenergic Receptors

Receptor	Location	Action
α_1	Myocardium	(+) Inotropy
	Vascular smooth muscle	Vasoconstriction
α_2	Vascular smooth muscle	Vasoconstriction
β_1	Myocardium	(+) Chronotropy & inotropy
β_2	Skeletal muscle arterioles	Relaxation
	Visceral arterioles	Relaxation
	Bronchial muscle	Relaxation

From Parmley WW, Chatterjee K, editors: *Cardiology: physiology, pharmacology, diagnosis,* vol 1, 1991.

b. Cause vasodilatation leading to increased renal blood flow and glomerular filtration rate

D. Pharmacologic Agents

1. Adrenergic receptor effects of common pharmacologic agents (Table 6-2)
2. Hemodynamic effects of common pharmacologic agents (Table 6-3)
3. Phosphodiesterase inhibitors (amrinone, milrinone)
   a. Mechanism of action
      (1) In the myocardium, inhibition of phosphodiesterase leads to increased intracellular cAMP, increased contractility, and increased rate of myocardial relaxation.
      (2) In the periphery, phosphodiesterase inhibitors produce vasodilatation.
   b. Important hemodynamic effects include increased SV and cardiac output, decreased SVR, decreased pulmonary vascular resistance, and decreased PA pressures.
   c. Because there is no significant increase in MVO_2 with the use of these agents, they are excellent drugs for the treatment of heart failure.

TABLE 6-2.

Effect of Sympathomimetic Agents on Adrenergic Receptors

	Site of Action				
	Heart		Peripheral Vasculature		
	Contractility	Heart Rate	Vasoconstriction	Vasodilatation	
	β_1	β_1	α	β_2	DA*
Dopamine					
<5 µg/kg/min	—	—	—	—	++
5-10 µg/kg/min	++	+	—	—	—
>10 µg/kg/min	+++	+	+++	—	—
Dobutamine	+++	+	+	+	—
Epinephrine	+++	+++	++	++	—
Norepinephrine	++	++	+++	—	—
Isoproterenol	+++	+++	—	+++	—
Phenylephrine	—	—	+++	—	—

From Parmley WW, Chatterjee K, editors: *Cardiology: physiology, pharmacology, diagnosis,* vol 1, 1993.
*DA = Dopaminergic receptors on renal and splanchnic vasculature.

d. Indications for their use in the ICU setting are heart failure with elevated LVEDP, low cardiac output, and poor peripheral perfusion despite other therapy (inotropes, IABP).

e. The major side effect is hypotension due to decreased peripheral vascular resistance. Other side effects include arrhythmias and thrombocytopenia (amrinone).

4. Dosages of common pharmacologic agents (Table 6-4)

TABLE 6-3.

Hemodynamic Effects of Common Pharmacologic Agents

	Cardiac Output	HR	MAP	SVR	PCWP
Dopamine					
<5 μg/kg/min	↔	↔	↔	↔	↔
5-10 μg/kg/min	↑↑	↑	↑↑	↑↔	↑↔
>10 μg/kg/min	↑	↑↑	↑↑	↑↑↑	↑
Dobutamine	↑↑↑	↑↔	↓↔	↓	↓↔
Epinephrine	↑↑	↑↑↑	↑↔	↓	↑↔
Norepinephrine	↑↓↔	↑↔	↑↑↑	↑↑↑	↑↔
Isoproterenol	↑↑↑	↑↑↑	↓↓	↓↓↓	↓↓
Phenylephrine	↓↔	↓↔	↑↑	↑↑↑	↑↔
Amrinone	↑↑↑	↑↔	↓↔	↓	↓
Milrinone	↑↑↑	↑↔	↓↔	↓	↓
Nitroglycerin	↑↓↔	↑↔	↓↓	↓↓	↓↓↓
Sodium nitroprusside	↑	↔	↓↓↓	↓↓↓	↓

From Parmley WW, Chatterjee K, editors: *Cardiology: physiology, pharmacology, diagnosis,* vol 1, 1993.

TABLE 6-4.

Inotropic Agents

	Dosages (μg/kg/min)		
	Low	Medium	High
Dopamine	<5	5-10	>10
Dobutamine (Dobutrex)	<5	5-10	>10
Epinephrine (Adrenalin)	0.01-0.05	0.05-0.20	>0.20
Norepinephrine (Levophed)	0.02-0.10	0.10-0.20	>0.20
Isoproterenol (Isuprel)	0.01-0.05	0.05-0.10	>0.10
Phenylephrine (Neosynephrine)	0.6-1	1-2.0	>2
Amrinone (Inocor)	5	10-15.0	>15
Milrinone (Primacor)	0.30-0.50	0.50-0.75	>0.75

5. Afterload-reducing agents (Table 6-5)
E. **Hemodynamic Parameters (Table 6-6)**

II. ISCHEMIC HEART DISEASE
A. **Introduction**
   1. CAD remains the leading cause of death in the US. Acute manifestations (unstable angina, acute MI, sudden death) of

TABLE 6-5.

Afterload-Reducing Agents

Medication	Dosage
Mixed arteriolar and venous vasodilators	
Sodium nitroprusside (Nipride)	IV: 1-7 µg/kg/min
α-Blocker: prazosin (Minipres)	PO: 1-2 mg tid
ACE inhibitor: captopril (Capoten)	PO: 6.25-12.5 mg tid (up to 25-50 mg tid)
Arteriolar vasodilators	
Hydralazine (Apresoline)	PO: 10-40 mg qid
	IM: 10-50 mg q4h
	IV: 10-20 mg (repeat as necessary)
Venous vasodilators	
Nitroglycerin	IV: 0.1-2 µg/kg/min

TABLE 6-6.

Hemodynamic Parameters and Derived Indices

	Normal Values	Calculation*
Hemodynamic Parameters		
Cardiac output (CO)	4-6 L/min	—
Pulmonary capillary wedge pressure (PCWP)	2-12 mm Hg	—
Pulmonary artery pressure (PAP)	15-30/3-12 mm Hg	—
Right ventricular pressure	15-30/0-8 mm Hg	—
Central venous pressure (CVP)	0-8 mm Hg	—
Derived Indices		
Cardiac index (CI)	2.5-4 L/min/m^2	CO/BSA
Mean arterial pressure (MAP)	70-105 mm Hg	dbp + (sbp − dbp)/3
Systemic vascular resistance (SVR)	800-1200 dyne-sec/cm^5	[(MAP − CVP)/CO] × 80
Pulmonary vascular resistance (PVR)	45-130 dyne-sec/cm^5	[(MPAP − PCWP)/CO] × 80

*dbp = diastolic blood pressure, sbp = systolic blood pressure, MPAP = mean pulmonary artery pressure.

ischemic heart disease occur as the first evidence of the disease in approximately 30% of patients with CAD.

2. CAD secondary to atherosclerosis is the most common form of heart disease and accounts for the majority of operative mortality due to heart disease.

3. The basic pathophysiology is an imbalance between myocardial oxygen delivery and consumption due to fixed lesions in the coronary arteries, or less commonly, to coronary vasospasm.

4. Risk factors for atherosclerotic CAD include male gender, increasing age, elevated serum total cholesterol or LDL fraction, hypertension, tobacco use, diabetes mellitus, and a family history of CAD.

5. Medical therapy is aimed at improving oxygen supply and demand mismatch by increasing oxygen supply and decreasing oxygen demand (Table 6-7).

   a. Nitrates

     (1) Nitrates cause vascular smooth muscle relaxation.

     (2) Venous dilatation leads to venous pooling and a decrease in venous return resulting in a decrease in preload and a decrease in MVo_2.

TABLE 6-7.

Common Antianginal Agents and Dosages

Nitrates	
Nitroglycerin	Sublingual: 0.3-0.6 mg (repeat q5min × 3)
	Topical: 1-2″ q4-6h or 0.1-0.6 mg/hr q24h
	Intravenous: 0.1-3 µg/kg/min
Isosorbide dinitrate	10-20 mg PO tid or qid or
	20-40 mg PO q6-12 h (extended release)
Calcium channel blockers	
Diltiazem (Cardizem)	120-260 mg PO daily in 3 or 4 divided doses
Nifedipine (Procardia)	10-30 mg PO tid
Verapamil (Calan, Isoptin)	240-480 mg PO daily in 3 or 4 divided doses
Amlodipine (Norvasc)	5-10 mg PO qd
β-Blockers	
Nonselective	
Propranolol (Inderal)	10-20 mg PO tid or qid
Nadolol (Corgard)	40-80 mg PO qd
β_1 selective	
Metoprolol (Lopressor)	50-200 mg PO q12h
Atenolol (Tenormin)	25-200 mg PO qd

> > (3) Coronary vasodilatation leads to an increase in subendocardial blood flow.
> > (4) The overall result is a decrease in oxygen demand and an increase in oxygen supply.
>
> b. β-Blockers
> > (1) Decrease BP, HR, and contractility
> > (2) Decrease oxygen demand
>
> c. Calcium channel blockers
> > (1) Reduce afterload and decrease contractility (decrease MVo_2)
> > (2) Cause coronary artery dilatation, especially in coronary vasospasm (improve supply)

B. Preoperative Management

1. Evaluation

   a. Medical history

   > (1) Anginal symptoms include chest pressure or heaviness with radiation to the neck, jaw, or arm.
   > (2) Determine whether there is a history of prior MI, especially if recent.
   > (3) Assess stability of anginal symptoms and patient's functional status.
   > (4) Symptoms should be distinguished from other causes of chest pain including pneumonia, gastrointestinal pathology, pulmonary embolism, acute aortic dissection, pericarditis, or costochondritis.

   b. Physical examination

   > (1) Vital signs
   > (2) Cardiac examination with attention to presence of murmurs and gallops (especially an S_3 which may indicate a failing heart)
   > (3) Evidence of elevated CVP (jugular venous distention)
   > (4) Evidence of CHF (rales, pedal edema)
   > (5) Extracardiac evidence of atherosclerosis (bruits, diminished peripheral pulses)

   c. ECG

   > (1) Evidence of prior MI or acute ischemia (Q waves, ST-T wave changes including ST elevation or depression, and T wave inversion)
   > (2) Arrhythmias
   > (3) Conduction system abnormalities

    d. CXR
      (1) Assess heart size.
      (2) Assess pulmonary status including pulmonary vascularity, Kerley lines, or underlying pulmonary pathology.
    e. Functional or anatomical assessment of severity of CAD: May require radionuclide angiography, stress ECG, or coronary angiography in some patients

  2. Management
    a. Optimize medical therapy.
    b. Control arrhythmias (Section V).
    c. Continue cardiac medications up to the time of surgery.

  3. Cardiac risks of noncardiac surgery
    a. Risk of perioperative MI
      (1) In patients without known heart disease, risk is approximately 0.2%.
      (2) In patients with known CAD, risk is 4% to 5%.
      (3) The mortality rate of a postoperative MI is approximately 40% to 50%.
    b. Risk of cardiac death or recurrent MI in patients with a history of MI
      (1) MI > 6 months prior to surgery: 5%
      (2) MI 3 to 6 months prior to surgery: 11%
      (3) MI < 3 months prior to surgery: 30%
      (4) Therefore should delay elective surgery for 6 months following a MI
    c. Risk factors
      (1) Perioperative cardiac risk can be estimated based on criteria identified by Goldman (Table 6-8).
      (2) Cardiac risk increases with increasing Goldman class (Table 6-9).
      (3) Several of these factors may be amenable to preoperative intervention, and if possible surgery should be delayed until these factors are optimized.

C. Intraoperative Management
  1. Use intraoperative and postoperative invasive hemodynamic monitoring (arterial line and pulmonary artery catheter) for patients with unstable angina, recent MI, Goldman class III or IV risk index, CHF, or significant valvular heart disease.
  2. Pay meticulous attention to intraoperative hemodynamic stability and avoid sustained periods of hypotension or hypertension.

TABLE 6-8.

Cardiac Risk Index

Cardiac Risk Factor	Points
History	
Age > 70 yr	5
MI within previous 6 mo	10
Physical Exam	
S_3 gallop, JVD, or left heart failure	11
Important valvular aortic stenosis	3
ECG	
Nonsinus rhythm or premature atrial contractions	7
>5 premature ventricular contractions/min	7
General medical status (if any of following present)	3
K < 3 mEq/L; HCO_3^- < 20 mEq/L	
BUN > 50 mg/dL; Cr > 3 mg/dL	
Po_2 < 60 mm Hg; Pco_2 > 50 mm Hg	
Abnormal AST; cirrhosis; chronic liver disease	
Chronically bed-ridden	
Operation	
Intraperitoneal, intrathoracic, aortic	3
Emergency	4

From Goldman L: *Assessment and management of the cardiac patient before, during, and after cardiac surgery.* In Parmley WW, Chatterjee K, editors: *Cardiology,* vol 3, Philadelphia, 1991, JB Lippincott.

TABLE 6-9.

Cardiac Risk by Class

Class	Points	Major Cardiac Complications (%)	Cardiac Death (%)
I	0-5	0.7	0.2
II	6-12	5	2
III	13-25	12	2
IV	>25	22	56

From Goldman L: *Assessment and management of the cardiac patient before, during, and after cardiac surgery.* In Parmley WW, Chatterjee K, editors: *Cardiology,* vol 3, Philadelphia, 1991, JB Lippincott.

    3. Use perioperative intravenous nitrates in patients with significant CAD.

D. Postoperative Management

    1. Avoid postoperative pain and agitation with judicious use of narcotics and benzodiazepines.

    2. Avoid rapid changes in BP.

3. The risk of postoperative MI is highest immediately postoperatively and the third through the fifth postoperative days as activity increases and fluid shifts occur. Follow patients identified as being at risk closely throughout this period.

E. **Management of Cardiac Ischemia/Acute MI**

1. MI occurs when acute thrombosis of the coronary artery leads to myocardial ischemia and cell death. Cell death begins about 20 minutes after coronary artery occlusion, and complete cell death in the area at risk occurs in 4 to 6 hours.

2. Diagnosis of MI includes the following considerations:
   a. May be painless in up to 50% of cases
   b. Should be suspected in any patient with unexplained chest discomfort, hypotension, new onset arrhythmias, mental status changes, or evidence of cardiac failure/ pulmonary edema
   c. History and physical exam
      (1) History of CAD, substernal chest pressure, neck/ arm pain, nausea
      (2) Hypotension, rales, S_3 gallop, new murmur, mental status changes
   d. ECG: ST elevation or depression, T wave changes, appearance of Q waves
   e. Cardiac isoenzymes
      (1) Total CK may be elevated for a variety of reasons (recent surgery, intramuscular injection, trauma, CPR), but the MB isoenzyme fraction is specific for myocardial injury.
      (2) CK-MB is elevated as early as 4 to 6 hours following an MI, peaks at 24 hours, and returns to normal in approximately 72 hours.
      (3) LDH is elevated as early as 10 to 12 hours following an MI, peaking at 48 to 72 hours.

3. Management
   a. Rapid assessment and transfer to SICU for ECG and hemodynamic monitoring
   b. Bed rest
   c. Prompt pain relief
      (1) Sublingual nitroglycerin, intravenous nitroglycerin infusion
      (2) Morphine (1 to 2 mg IV q30min PRN)

(3) Judicious use of benzodiazepines to control anxiety and agitation

d. Oxygen administration—oxygen saturation monitoring (pulse oximetry, ABG)

e. Pharmacologic agents for persistent ischemia (See Table 6-7.)

   (1) Increase coronary blood flow.

      (a) Nitrates

      (b) Calcium channel blockers if vasospasm suspected

   (2) Decrease O_2 demand

      (a) Decrease preload: Nitrates

      (b) Control heart rate: β-Blockers

      (c) Decrease afterload: Nitrates, nitroprusside, β Blockers, calcium channel blockers

      (d) Decrease contractility: β-Blockers, calcium channel blockers

      (e) Use caution: When administering β-blockers and calcium-channel blockers in patients with low left ventricular ejection fraction and congestive heart failure

      (f) Use caution: When administering nonspecific β-blockers in patients with bronchospastic disease because of their effects on β_2-receptors

   (3) Use antiplatelet agents (aspirin) to prevent platelet aggregation.

   (4) Consider anticoagulation with heparin to prevent propagation of thrombosis and limit infarct size.

   (5) Consider IABP placement.

   (6) Consider thrombolytic therapy (Table 6-10).

      (a) Thrombolytics may be indicated within 4 to 6 hours of onset of symptoms in a patient with a

TABLE 6-10.

Thrombolytic Agents in Acute MI

Drug	Dosage (Intravenous)
Streptokinase	1.5×10^6 IU/60 min
Urokinase	1.5×10^6 IU bolus, then 1.5×10^6 IU/90 min*
Tissue plasminogen activator	15 mg bolus, 50 mg/30 min, then 35 mg/60 min (total = 100 mg/90 min)

*Not FDA approved for IV use in acute MI.

classic history of MI and ST elevation of > 1 mm in two contiguous leads to salvage myocardium.

  (b) Caution must be used with these agents in the postoperative period because of the risk of bleeding; in general, these agents are not used within 14 days after surgery.

f. Ongoing ischemia despite the above measures: Should consider coronary revascularization

g. Prophylactic lidocaine: No longer routinely administered; current recommendation is to use only if life-threatening ventricular arrhythmias, ventricular tachycardia, or frequent PVCs are present (Section V)

h. Laboratory data
  (1) ECG on admission and q8h × 24 hours
  (2) CK isoenzymes on admission and q8h × 24 hours
  (3) LDH isoenzymes on admission and q12h × 48 to 72 hours
  (4) CBC and serum electrolytes including calcium and magnesium levels
  (5) ABG
  (6) Chest radiograph to assess cardiac size and presence of pulmonary congestion or edema

i. Monitoring
  (1) Perform frequent physical examinations for evaluation of BP and HR as well as evidence of CHF and new murmurs.
  (2) Provide ECG monitoring.
    (a) 12-lead to evaluate for improvement of ST-T wave changes
    (b) Continuous monitoring for identification of arrhythmias or heart block
  (3) Invasive monitoring may be required if the patient is hemodynamically unstable, if there is a question of intravascular volume status, or if intravenous pharmacologic agents are required. This may include placement of an intraarterial catheter, PA catheter, or urinary bladder catheter.

F. Complications of Acute Myocardial Infarction
  1. Arrhythmias (Section V)
  2. CHF/pulmonary edema (Section III)

3. Cardiogenic shock (See Chapter 2.)
   a. Cardiogenic shock is due to inadequate tissue perfusion because of to pump failure.
   b. The mortality rate in acute MI > 50%.
   c. Findings include hypotension, elevated filling pressures, low cardiac output, and oliguria.
   d. Management includes invasive hemodynamic monitoring with intraarterial PA, and urinary catheters.
   e. The goals of management are improvement in ventricular performance and cardiac output, maintenance of systemic arterial pressure and tissue perfusion, preservation of myocardium, and limitation of infarct size.
   f. Specific treatment includes the following:
      (1) Optimize preload by the judicious use of volume administration based on the physical exam and ventricular filling pressures.
      (2) Administer inotropic and vasopressor agents (Tables 6-3 and 6-4). Begin with a first-line drug such as dopamine or dobutamine, and titrate to achieve the desired effect. If this is inadequate, add second-line therapy, such as epinephrine, norepinephrine, or a phosphodiesterase inhibitor.
      (3) Insert an IABP if there is evidence of persistent ischemia and hemodynamic instability. Beneficial effects of the IABP include an increase in coronary peripheral perfusion while decreasing afterload.
4. RV infarction
   a. RV infarct may complicate inferior MI and lead to RV failure.
   b. Significant RV infarct is notable for jugular venous distention in the absence of pulmonary congestion.
   c. Because of hypotension and elevated right sided cardiac pressures, an RV infarct may be confused with pericardial tamponade. Echocardiography can be helpful in this setting.
   d. Initial therapy involves the general treatment of acute MI as outlined above, as well as the administration of intravenous fluids to support the failing RV.
   e. If there is no improvement with initial therapy, consider the administration of dobutamine or phosphodiesterase inhibitors because of their beneficial effects on the pulmonary vasculature. (See Tables 6-3 and 6-4.)

5. Pericarditis (Dressler's syndrome)
   a. Common following acute MI
   b. Characteristic chest pain which is increased by a recumbent position and by respiration
   c. Characteristic pericardial rub on physical examination
   d. Important to differentiate from postinfarction angina
   e. Autoimmune phenomenon treated symptomatically with NSAIDs
6. Postinfarction VSD/papillary muscle rupture/ventricular free wall rupture
   a. VSD and papillary muscle rupture are both heralded by new onset of a systolic murmur and often present with hypotension and significant heart failure.
   b. The diagnosis is suspected in VSD by a step up in O_2 saturation from the RA to the RV (due to the left to right shunt) and in papillary muscle rupture by severe mitral regurgitation with large v waves on the PCWP tracing.
   c. The diagnosis is confirmed by echocardiography.
   d. Initial treatment is focused on pharmacologic afterload reduction as well as the use of IABP to reduce the amount of mitral regurgitation or left to right shunting.
   e. These are surgical emergencies and urgent repair is often indicated.
   f. Ventricular free wall rupture has a peak incidence on the second to eighth day after the infarction and is characterized by a sudden tearing pain associated with hypotension and evidence of cardiac tamponade.

III. CONGESTIVE HEART FAILURE AND PULMONARY EDEMA
A. Congestive Heart Failure
1. Pathophysiology
   a. CHF is the inability of the heart to maintain a cardiac output adequate to meet the metabolic needs of the organs. It represents the failure of the heart as a pump and may result in cardiogenic shock.
   b. In general, CHF is due to a loss of functional myocardium secondary to ischemic heart disease, cardiomyopathy, or chronic valvular heart disease. Both systolic and diastolic dysfunction may be involved.
2. Diagnosis
   a. Symptoms: May be acute or chronic

(1) Due to congestion: Peripheral edema, orthopnea, paroxysmal nocturnal dyspnea, dyspnea on exertion, nocturia

(2) Due to decreased cardiac output: Fatigue, weakness, poor exercise tolerance, confusion

b. Physical findings

(1) Tachycardia, hypotension

(2) Pulmonary congestion: Rales, expiratory wheezes, tachypnea

(3) Vasoconstriction: Peripheral cyanosis, cool extremities, diminished peripheral pulses

(4) Jugular venous distention, hepatomegaly, hepatojugular reflux, peripheral edema

(5) S_3 gallop

c. Laboratory data

(1) Hypoxemia

(2) Metabolic acidosis

(3) Hyponatremia

d. CXR

(1) Cardiomegaly

(2) Cephalization of pulmonary vasculature or frank pulmonary edema

e. Assessment of ventricular function: Echocardiography, radionuclide imaging, cardiac catheterization (including right heart catheterization)

f. Differential diagnosis

(1) Pulmonary signs and symptoms

(a) Pneumonia

(b) COPD, asthma flare

(c) ARDS, volume overload

(2) Cardiomegaly: Pericardial effusion

(3) Hypotension

(a) Volume depletion

(b) PE

(c) Sepsis

3. Etiology

a. Hypertension is the most common cause.

b. CAD is the second most common cause.

c. Less common causes include other types of cardiomyopathy and valvular heart disease.

4. Treatment in the ICU

a. Supportive

(1) Bed rest

(2) Supplemental oxygen

(3) Treatment of complicating derangements (such as infection, anemia, or diabetes mellitus) which may have led to decompensation of previously stable CHF

b. Improvements in myocardial contractility

(1) Digoxin remains as a cornerstone of therapy.

(a) Loading (12 to 15 µg/kg; 10 µg/kg in renal failure): Give one half of dose initially then one fourth of the dose q2-4h × 2 doses.

(b) Maintenance (0.125 to 0.375 mg/day): Monitor HR, ECG, and digoxin levels to avoid digoxin toxicity.

(2) Utilize inotropic agents if required.

c. Reduction of CHF symptoms

(1) Dietary sodium restriction (<2 g/day)

(2) Fluid restriction (<2 L/day)

(3) Diuretic therapy

(a) Furosemide: The initial dose is 20 mg IV, and the dose should be doubled and administered every 4 to 6 hours until a satisfactory diuresis is obtained. The maximum dose is 200 mg (larger doses may be associated with significant toxicity).

(b) Ethacrynic acid: This loop diuretic can be used as an alternative to furosemide. The initial dose is 25 mg IV, and subsequent doses can be increased in 25-mg increments until satisfactory diuresis obtained.

d. Afterload reduction

(1) Afterload-reducing agents can substantially improve cardiac output and forward flow in the setting of decreased cardiac output, pulmonary congestion, and high SVR. They are also useful in patients with hypertension and in patients whose CHF is secondary to regurgitant valvular disease.

(2) Some commonly used afterload-reducing agents are listed in Table 6-5.

(3) In the acute setting, nitroprusside is often used to initiate therapy. It is a potent vasodilator with a short half-life, which makes it an excellent agent in

this setting. After stabilization, the patient can be converted to long term oral therapy.

(4) ACE inhibitors (captopril, enalapril, benazepril) affect the renin-angiotensin system. Captopril is probably still the most commonly used, starting at a dose of 6.25 to 12.5 mg PO q8h and increasing as needed to control BP.

(5) Calcium channel blockers, especially nifedipine, have a starting dose of 10 mg PO q6h, titrating to control BP up to 120 mg/day.

B. Pulmonary Edema

1. Pathophysiology
   a. Pulmonary edema is the increase in extravascular lung water resulting from a transudation of fluid into the alveoli. The accumulation of fluid in the alveoli prevents effective gas exchange.
   b. Pulmonary edema can be a result of cardiac or extracardiac sources.
      (1) Cardiogenic pulmonary edema: Elevation in LVEDP due to heart failure leads to an increase in hydrostatic capillary pressure and transudation of fluid across the capillary wall.
      (2) Noncardiogenic pulmonary edema includes the following considerations:
         (a) Altered permeability of the alveolar capillary membrane, as seen in sepsis and ARDS, allows for transudation of protein and fluid across the membrane and into the alveoli.
         (b) Low plasma oncotic pressure, as seen in malnutrition and with low serum albumin, also allows for transudation of fluid across the capillary membrane.

2. Diagnosis
   a. Symptoms
      (1) Dyspnea, orthopnea
      (2) Cough
      (3) Fatigue
      (4) Altered mental status, agitation
   b. Signs
      (1) Tachypnea, tachycardia
      (2) Rales
      (3) Jugular venous distention, peripheral edema

    c. Laboratory data

      (1) ABG reveals hypoxemia (decreased Pao_2) with normal or low $Paco_2$.

      (2) CXR demonstrates cephalization of the pulmonary vasculature, enlarged hilar vessels, and interstitial edema.

3. Supportive therapy

    a. Utilize supplemental oxygen and endotracheal intubation if indicated by persistent hypoxia, labored respiration, or inability to control secretions.

    b. Assess the circulation; if perfusion is inadequate or patient is hypotensive, invasive monitoring with an intraarterial line and PA catheter should be considered.

    c. Establish venous access and place urinary catheter.

    d. Provide bed rest with head of the bed elevated.

    e. Obtain laboratory data (ABG, CBC, electrolytes, CXR).

    f. Provide a 12-lead ECG and provide continuous ECG monitoring.

    g. Utilize invasive hemodynamic monitoring if indicated.

4. Decreased pulmonary congestion

    a. Morphine 1 to 4 mg IV q15min (causes venous pooling and decreases preload, also allays anxiety)

    b. Diuretics

    c. Vasodilator therapy

      (1) Venodilators (IV nitroglycerin) cause venous pooling and are potent preload-reducing agents.

      (2) Afterload-reducing agents (IV nitroprusside) are effective in patients with low cardiac output and high SVR, and effectively reduce LVEDV and pulmonary hydrostatic pressure. They should be titrated until cardiac output improves or hypotension occurs.

5. Inotropic agents

    a. First-line drugs include dopamine and dobutamine. Dobutamine is an excellent agent because of its effects on the vasculature (decreased SVR and pulmonary vascular resistance), but it can cause hypotension and may not be appropriate in a patient that is already hypotensive.

    b. Second-line drugs include epinephrine and phosphodiesterase inhibitors. Phosphodiesterase inhibitors may

be especially useful if right heart failure is present.
6. Afterload-reducing agents
   a. Nitroprusside is the agent of choice because of its rapid action and short half-life.
   b. The IABP can be considered in cases of severe LV failure that are resistant to the above measures.
   c. Control HR and maintain sinus rhythm to improve cardiac output.
7. Identification and treatment of underlying or precipitating factors (e.g., tachyarrhythmias, malignant hypertension, valvular disease, fluid overload, acute MI, allergic reaction)

IV. VALVULAR HEART DISEASE
A. Aortic Stenosis
1. Classification of acquired aortic stenosis
   a. Calcific (>60%)
   b. Degenerative (24%)
   c. Rheumatic (12%)
2. Pathophysiology
   a. Pressure overload on the LV leads to LV hypertrophy.
   b. LV hypertrophy and eventual failure lead to a decrease in LV compliance and increased LVEDP.
   c. The LV cavity is small and is sensitive to small changes in preload.
   d. The atrial contribution is important to filling and therefore to cardiac output.
   e. These patients are prone to arrhythmias and are sensitive to ischemia secondary to the LV hypertrophy.
3. Diagnosis
   a. History
      (1) Most often, there is a long symptom-free latent period with the onset of symptoms typically in the fifth and sixth decades.
      (2) The classic triad includes the following:
         (a) Angina: Present in over 60% of patients with severe aortic stenosis, 50% of whom also have underlying CAD
         (b) Dyspnea on exertion: Because of inadequate cardiac output
         (c) Syncope: Because of a fixed cardiac output, peripheral vasodilatation may lead to diminished cerebral perfusion pressure

b. Physical exam
   (1) Physical findings: May be minimal, especially in end-stage, low output disease
   (2) Arterial pulse: Characterized by slow upstroke and small volume
   (3) LVH: May be manifested by a pronounced apical impulse or LV lift
   (4) Aortic ejection murmur
      (a) Crescendo/decrescendo
      (b) Heard best at the base, especially in the right second intercostal space
      (c) Referred to carotids
c. Laboratory findings
   (1) ECG (LV hypertrophy)
   (2) CXR
      (a) Cardiomegaly may be seen late in the disease, but often the cardiac silhouette is normal.
      (b) The aortic valve calcifies.
   (3) Echocardiography
      (a) Morphologic information about the valve
      (b) Can estimate the aortic gradient; significant stenosis indicated by systolic gradients > 50 mm Hg
   (4) Cardiac catheterization
      (a) Performed in patients > 40 years of age because of high incidence of coexisting CAD
      (b) Can estimate aortic valve area; considered severe if < 1 cm^2/m^2

4. Management
   a. Maintain adequate preload.
   b. Maintain sinus rhythm, consider arrhythmia prophylaxis, and avoid tachycardia.
   c. Avoid low SVR and peripheral vasodilatation, which accentuate the gradient across the valve.
   d. The cardiac output remains relatively "fixed," therefore vasopressors may be needed to restore systolic blood pressure in the hypotensive patient.
   e. Antibiotic prophylaxis for endocarditis is required. (Section IV, F)

B. Aortic Insufficiency
1. Etiologies
   a. Rheumatic (45%)

b. Annuloaortic ectasia (18%)

c. Endocarditis (18%)

2. Pathophysiology

 a. Volume overload is a result of regurgitant filling across the incompetent valve.

 b. Compensation occurs by LV dilatation and LV hypertrophy.

 c. Because of the dilatation, there is an increase in LV compliance. Large LV volume changes are associated with small changes in intracavitary pressure, therefore LAP and PCWP are less helpful in managing these patients.

 d. Ejection fraction is normal until LV function deteriorates.

 e. Chronic aortic insufficiency may be well tolerated for long periods of time.

 f. In contrast, acute aortic insufficiency is poorly tolerated because the regurgitant fraction fills a ventricle which is not as compliant. LVEDP rises rapidly and CHF and pulmonary edema occur early.

3. Diagnosis

 a. History

 (1) Chronic aortic insufficiency may be asymptomatic or mildly symptomatic for a long period of time, but it carries a poor prognosis once symptomatic.

 (2) The symptoms are the same as those of pulmonary venous hypertension (dyspnea on exertion, orthopnea).

 b. Physical exam

 (1) Wide pulse pressure (the "water hammer" pulse)

 (2) LV apical impulse displaced laterally

 (3) Early diastolic decrescendo murmur radiating to apex

 (4) Possible systolic ejection murmur

 (5) Possible Austin Flint murmur (an apical, mid-diastolic, fluttering murmur due to regurgitant jet on the anterior leaflet of the mitral valve)

 (6) Rales

 c. Laboratory findings

 (1) ECG: LV enlargement and hypertrophy

 (2) CXR: LV enlargement; may also demonstrate LA enlargement and pulmonary venous congestion

       (3) Echocardiography: LV enlargement and function, aortic valve vegetations in endocarditis; regurgitant jet demonstrated by color flow Doppler

       (4) Cardiac catheterization: Also demonstrates the regurgitation and LV enlargement and should be performed in any patient > 40 years of age to exclude CAD

  4. Management

    a. Treatment is focused on reducing the regurgitant fraction by afterload reduction and the treatment of CHF and pulmonary edema. (See Table 6-5 and Section III.)

    b. The use of the IABP is contraindicated because it may increase the severity of the regurgitation during balloon inflation.

    c. Antibiotic prophylaxis against endocarditis is required.

C. Mitral Stenosis

  1. Classification: Most common cause is rheumatic heart disease, which may produce mixed stenosis and incompetence

  2. Pathophysiology

    a. Mitral stenosis is the obstruction to flow of blood from the LA to the LV across the mitral valve.

    b. LV is "protected" (there is no pressure or volume overload).

    c. However, the obstruction to flow leads to elevated LA pressures and LA enlargement.

    d. Increasing LA pressure leads to pulmonary venous congestion and pulmonary edema.

    e. Increasing LA pressure also leads to pulmonary hypertension with RV overload and dilatation and eventual RV failure. This may eventually lead to tricuspid regurgitation.

    f. LA dilatation predisposes to atrial arrhythmias, especially atrial fibrillation, which can decrease cardiac output by 20% in these patients.

    g. Tachycardia may also increase the severity of the symptoms (decrease in diastolic filling time and therefore decrease in preload)

    h. Although there is normal LV thickness, volume, and systolic and diastolic function, cardiac output cannot be increased in times of stress or when afterload is acutely reduced.

  i. Systemic arterial emboli from LA thrombus may occur in up to 10% of patients with LA enlargement and atrial fibrillation

3. Diagnosis
   a. History
      (1) The primary symptom is dyspnea; patients are often asymptomatic until disease is severe.
      (2) With exertion, tachycardia, or atrial fibrillation, the patient may develop sudden pulmonary edema.
      (3) Other symptoms include orthopnea, paroxysmal nocturnal dyspnea, and fatigability.
   b. Physical examination
      (1) Loud S_1, opening snap, low pitched diastolic rumble with presystolic crescendo (if the patient is in sinus rhythm)
      (2) May be a palpable RV lift
      (3) May be signs of pulmonary congestion (on pulmonary examination)
   c. Laboratory findings
      (1) ECG
         (a) LA enlargement (p-mitrale)
         (b) RV hypertrophy
         (c) Atrial fibrillation (common)
      (2) CXR
         (a) LA enlargement
         (b) LV normal, but RV enlarged
         (c) Prominent pulmonary vasculature with cephalization of flow and pulmonary venous congestion
         (d) Possible mitral valve calcification
      (3) Echocardiogram
         (a) Mitral valve orifice size and gradient can be measured; an area < 0.8 cm^2/m^2 represents severe mitral stenosis.
         (b) RV function can be assessed.
         (c) Associated mitral regurgitation can be identified.
         (d) In patients with atrial fibrillation or LA enlargement, LA thrombus can be identified.
      (4) Cardiac catheterization
         (a) Utilize cardiac catheterization in patients > 40 years of age, since 25% will have CAD.

(b) Obtain hemodynamic data and confirm valve orifice size. An end-diastolic gradient > 10 mm Hg reveals significant mitral stenosis.

4. Management
   a. Maintain sinus rhythm and slow HR to improve LV filling.
      (1) Antiarrhythmic agents (Section V)
      (2) β-Blockers
   b. Diuresis and sodium restriction may improve symptoms.
   c. Avoid hypoxia and hypercarbia which cause pulmonary vasoconstriction.
   d. Anticoagulation should be considered for patients in chronic atrial fibrillation.
   e. Antibiotic prophylaxis for endocarditis is indicated.

D. Mitral Regurgitation
1. Classification
   a. Chronic mitral regurgitation
      (1) Rheumatic (isolated or associated with aortic valve disease)
      (2) Mitral prolapse or myxomatous degeneration
      (3) Ischemic papillary muscle dysfunction
   b. Acute mitral regurgitation
      (1) Infective endocarditis
      (2) Chordal rupture: "Idiopathic," ischemic
2. Pathophysiology
   a. Because of the incompetence of the mitral valve, a portion of the SV is directed into the LA. The amount of this regurgitant fraction is dependent on LV afterload and the pressure gradient between the LV and LA.
   b. Forward flow is reduced and therefore so is effective cardiac output.
   c. Over time, LV volume overload leads to LV dilatation and LV failure.
   d. LA pressure rises due to the regurgitant fraction, and with time pulmonary congestion and pulmonary edema will appear.
   e. Regurgitation also causes LA enlargement, which predisposes the patient to atrial arrhythmias.
   f. In acute MR, a small noncompliant LA is exposed suddenly to regurgitant volume, which leads to high LA

pressures, high pulmonary venous pressures, and pulmonary edema.

3. Diagnosis
   a. Acute mitral regurgitation: In the acute setting, there is a sudden appearance of severe pulmonary venous hypertension, pulmonary edema, hypotension, and decreased peripheral perfusion.
   b. Chronic mitral regurgitation is characterized by the following:
      (1) It is often asymptomatic until late in the disease.
      (2) Eventually fatigue, dyspnea, and pulmonary congestion will become manifest.
      (3) Late stages of mitral regurgitation are characterized by chronic CHF and cardiac cachexia.
   c. Physical examination
      (1) The pulse has a brisk upstroke.
      (2) On auscultation, there is a pansystolic, high pitched, systolic murmur heard best at the apex which radiates to the axilla.
      (3) Because of the large volume and rapid LV filling during diastole, an LV filling sound (S_3) and diastolic rumble may be heard.
      (4) Signs of severe mitral regurgitation include an overactive LV impulse at the apex signifying LV enlargement, and a precordial lift.
   d. Laboratory findings
      (1) ECG
         (a) LA enlargement
         (b) LV enlargement
         (c) Atrial fibrillation (common)
      (2) CXR
         (a) Cardiomegaly due to LA and LV enlargement
         (b) Lungs clear unless LV failure
      (3) Echocardiography
         (a) Determine severity of mitral regurgitation.
         (b) Determine etiology of mitral regurgitation.
         (c) Assess ventricular function.
      (4) Cardiac catheterization
         (a) The amount of regurgitation can be assessed on ventriculography.
         (b) The v wave of the LA and PCWP tracings will be prominent.

4. Management
   a. Reduce afterload to improve the forward output.
   b. Administer diuretics to improve the CHF symptoms.
   c. Provide inotropic support to aid the LV; dobutamine is an especially good agent because of its effect on reducing SVR.
   d. In the acute setting or in severe LV failure, an IABP may improve the hemodynamics significantly.
   e. Maintain sinus rhythm and control the HR to improve LV filling.
   f. Provide antibiotic prophylaxis for endocarditis.

E. **Prosthetic Valves**
   1. Tissue valves
      a. Examples: Carpentier-Edwards, Hancock, Ionescu-Shiley
      b. Advantages: Do not require long-term anticoagulation
      c. Disadvantages: Less durable, especially in the mitral position
   2. Mechanical valves
      a. Examples: St. Jude, Carbomedics, Medtronic-Hall, Bjork-Shiley, Starr-Edwards
      b. Advantages: Durability
      c. Disadvantages: Require long-term anticoagulation to prevent thromboembolic complications
      d. Other: Anticoagulation in the perioperative period
         (1) Warfarin should be discontinued 2 to 3 days preoperatively, and PT should be normalized prior to proceeding with surgery.
         (2) If there is a prosthetic mitral valve, anticoagulation with heparin IV infusion should be maintained until 6 hours prior to surgery.
         (3) Once hemostasis is achieved postoperatively (12 to 24 hours), IV heparin therapy should be started again and continued until warfarin anticoagulation is adequate.

F. **Antibiotic Prophlaxis for Endocarditis**
   1. Endocarditis prophylaxis is required in patients with the following conditions (high risk):
      a. Prosthetic cardiac valves
      b. Rheumatic or acquired valve disease
      c. Mitral valve prolapse with regurgitation

   d. Congenital cardiac defects
   e. Hypertrophic cardiomyopathy
   f. History of previous endocarditis
  2. Procedures that require prophylaxis in high-risk patients include the following:
   a. Dental procedures when gingival or mucosal bleeding is expected
   b. Tonsillectomy
   c. Surgery involving the following:
    (1) Respiratory mucosa
    (2) Intestinal mucosa
    (3) Gallbladder
    (4) Prostate
    (5) Urinary tract if infection present
    (6) Infected tissue
    (7) Vagina
   d. Rigid bronchoscopy
   e. Sclerotherapy of esophageal varices
   f. Esophageal dilatation
   g. Cystoscopy or urethral dilatation
   h. Vaginal delivery if infection present
  3. Information on antibiotic therapy for prophylaxis appears in Tables 6-11 and 6-12.
   a. See Table 6-11 for specific agents and dosages.
   b. See Table 6-12 for alternative agents and their dosages.

TABLE 6-11.

Endocarditis Prophylaxis

Site of Procedure	Prophylactic Regimens	
	Drug	Dosage
Dental/oral upper respiratory tract	Amoxicillin	3 g PO 1 hr prior to procedure then 1.5 g PO 6 hr later
Gastrointestinal	Ampicillin	2 g IV with—
Genitourinary	Gentamicin	1.5 mg/kg* IV 30 min prior then—
	Amoxicillin	1.5 g PO 6 hr later (or IV regimen 8 hr later)

From Dajani AS et al: Prevention of bacterial endocarditis: recommendations by the American Heart Association, *JAMA* 264:2919, 1990.
*Maximum dose not to exceed 80 mg

V. ARRHYTHMIAS
A. Introduction
1. Arrhythmias are common postoperatively (especially following cardiac and pulmonary surgery) and in critically ill patients with pulmonary or cardiac disease.
2. In the perioperative period, atrial distention, electrolyte imbalances, hypoxia, and high catecholamine states contribute to the development of arrhythmias.
3. The two basic mechanisms responsible for arrhythmias are the following:
   a. Enhanced automaticity: An abnormality in pacemaker activity
   b. Reentry: A circus movement of the electrical impulse due to an underlying abnormality in conduction and repolarization
4. Treatment is aimed at reversing precipitating causes and controlling the arrhythmia to improve cardiac output and

TABLE 6-12.

Alternative Endocarditis Prophylaxis

Alternative Regimens			
Site of Procedure	Reason	Drug	Dosage
Dental/oral upper respiratory tract	Amoxicillin/ penicillin allergy	Erythromycin	1.0 g 2 hr prior then 500 mg 6 hr later *or*
		Clindamycin	300 mg PO 1 hr prior then 150 mg PO 6 hr later
	NPO	Ampicillin	2 g IV/IM 30 min prior then 1.0 g IV/IM 6 hr later *or*
		Clindamycin	300 mg IV 30 min prior then 150 mg IV 6 hr later
	High risk/ penicillin allergy	Vancomycin	1.0 g IV 1 hr prior
Gastrointestinal	Ampicillin/ penicillin allergy	Vancomycin	1.0 g IV with—
Genitourinary		Gentamicin	1.5 mg/kg* IV 1 hr prior then repeat 8 hr later

From Dajani AS et al: Prevention of bacterial endocarditis: recommendations by the American Heart Association, *JAMA* 264:2919, 1990.
*Maximum dose not to exceed 80 mg

hemodynamic status. Antiarrhythmic agents and their dosages are listed in Table 6-13.

B. Diagnosis

1. Accuracy important since specific treatment based on the type of arrhythmia
2. A complete history and physical examination
   a. A history of previous palpitations or arrhythmias
   b. Current medications, including "recreational" drug use
   c. Historical or physical evidence of underlying cardiac or pulmonary disease
3. Laboratory evaluation
   a. CBC to evaluate anemia
   b. Serum electrolytes
   c. ABG to identify disturbances in pH, P_{CO_2}, and P_{O_2}
   d. Thyroid panel
   e. Serum drug levels when appropriate
4. CXR to exclude underlying pulmonary or pericardial pathology
5. ECG
   a. 12-lead to examine P wave and QRS morphology and to exclude myocardial ischemia and pericarditis
   b. Rhythm strip including leads a V_F and V_1, since they are the most helpful in identifying atrial activity
   c. Esophageal lead to help evaluate atrial activity
   d. Epicardial pacing wires to obtain atrial and ventricular ECGs in patients following cardiac surgery
      (1) Right atrial wires are attached to the right and left arm leads, and the other limb leads are placed in the normal position.
         (a) Lead I will give a bipolar atrial electrogram.
         (b) Leads II and III will provide unipolar atrial electrograms.
      (2) The regularity of the R-R interval, the AV-conduction ratio, and the presence of P waves and morphology can be determined.
6. May be both diagnostic and therapeutic benefits from maneuvers which increase vagal tone, increase the AV nodal refractory period, and slow ventricular rate; patient should be supine, have continuous ECG monitoring, and have IV access established prior to performing these maneuvers
   a. Carotid sinus massage

TABLE 6-13.
Common Antiarrhythmic Agents and Dosages

Class	Agent	Route	Dosage Loading	Dosage Maintenance	Comments
Ia	Quinidine	PO		324-628 mg q8-12h	Dosages are for gluconate preparation
	Procainamide	PO	750-1000 mg	500-1000 mg q6h	Maintenance dosages are for slow release preparation
		IV	500-1000 mg over 30-60 min	1-4 mg/min	Rapid loading may cause hypotension
Ib	Lidocaine	IV	1 mg/kg bolus	1-4 mg/min	
II	Propranolol	PO		10-60 mg q6-8h	Nonselective β-blocker
		IV	0.5-1.0 mg q15min up to 5 mg		
III	Atenolol	PO		25-200 mg qd	β₁-Selective
	Bretylium	IV	5-10 mg/kg over 10-20 min	1-2 mg/min	May cause hypotension
IV	Verapamil	PO		40-120 mg q6h	May cause hypotension; avoid use if impaired ventricle or with IV β-blocker administration
		IV	2.5-5 mg q2min up to 15 mg		
	Diltiazem	PO			See verapamil comments
		IV	0.25-0.35 mg/kg over 2 min	10 mg/hr	
Other	Digoxin	PO	0.5 mg then 0.25 mg q2-4h × 2 doses	0.125-0.5 mg qd	
		IV	same as PO	Same as PO	
	Adenosine	IV	6 mg bolus then 12 mg bolus if unsuccessful		Duration of action very short

(1) An ipsilateral carotid bruit is a relative contraindication to this maneuver.

(2) Perform this maneuver on the nondominant side first.

(3) Use gentle massage for 10 seconds.

(4) Never perform simultaneous bilateral massage.

b. The Valsalva maneuver can also be performed to increase vagal tone.

C. Sinus Bradycardia

1. May be a normal finding in well-trained athletes

2. Pathologic conditions include sick sinus syndrome, enhanced vagal tone, increased intracranial pressure, hypothyroidism, hypothermia, and drug use (especially β-blockers or calcium channel blockers)

3. Diagnosis—sinus rhythm below 60 beats/min; may be sinus arrhythmia

4. Treatment

   a. Asymptomatic patient: No specific therapy except to treat the underlying etiology

   b. Symptomatic patient

      (1) Administer atropine 0.5 to 1.0 mg IV; may repeat as needed.

      (2) Administer isoproterenol IV beginning at 1 μg/min; titrate to appropriate HR.

      (3) If epicardial pacing wires are present, provide temporary atrial pacing at 80 to 100 beats/min.

      (4) If pacing wires are not present, and the patient does not respond to pharmacologic interventions, a transcutaneous (Zoll) or transvenous pacemaker should be placed.

D. Premature Contractions

1. May be either insignificant or an indication of underlying pathology and potentially lethal arrhythmias

2. Common postoperatively and may indicate underlying myocardial or pericardial disease, electrolyte or acid-base disturbances, hypoxia, and central venous instrumentation

3. May originate from atrial, junctional, or ventricular regions of the heart

   a. Premature atrial contractions are characterized by an abnormal P wave followed by a normal QRS complex; AV conduction is variable.

   b. Premature junctional contractions result in a premature

QRS complex which is not preceded by a P wave. Retrograde P waves may be present, will have an abnormal morphology, and will be seen preceding, concurrent with, or following the QRS complex.

   c. Premature ventricular contractions originate distal to the bundle of His and are wide (>0.12 sec), abnormal QRS complexes which are not preceded by a P wave.

4. Treatment

   a. Asymptomatic patients without underlying heart disease require no specific therapy.

   b. Patients must be thoroughly evaluated and underlying precipitating metabolic abnormalities must be corrected.

   c. If premature atrial contractions are symptomatic and persistent despite correction of electrolyte abnormalities, they may be treated with Class Ia antiarrhythmic agents.

   d. If premature ventricular contractions are asymptomatic and occur <5 per minute, no specific therapy other than correcting predisposing conditions is required. If PVCs are frequent (≥6 per minute), multifocal, or occur in brief runs (≥3 PVCs), treatment is recommended.

      (1) Correct precipitating factor.

      (2) Provide acute treatment consisting of IV lidocaine or procainamide infusion.

      (3) Achieve chronic suppression with the use of Class Ia, Ic, and III agents.

E. Tachyarrhythmias (Table 6-14)

1. Atrial fibrillation

   a. Atrial fibrillation is frequently seen in the ICU and may be chronic (associated with valvular or ischemic heart disease) or acute. It frequently follows cardiac or pulmonary surgery, and prophylaxis may be indicated postoperatively following these procedures.

   b. It may be precipitated by postoperative stress (high catecholamine state), hypoxia, ischemia, pulmonary embolism, or thyrotoxicosis.

   c. Because of loss of atrial activity, the atrial contribution to diastolic ventricular filling, and rapid HRs, there is decreased filling of the LV and a decrease in cardiac output.

TABLE 6-14.
Tachyarrhythmias

Arrhythmia	Rate (beats/min)		Acute Treatment			Chronic Treatment	Comments
	Atrial	Ventricular	Unstable	Stable			
Sinus tachycardia	100–160	100–160	—	Correct underlying etiology; ±β-blocker		—	Often due to stress or trauma
Supraventricular tachycardia	120–250	120–250	dcCV	Adenosine, verapamil, Ia agent		Verapamil, β-blocker, Ia agent	Carotid massage and vagotonic maneuvers may terminate; avoid verapamil if etiology is accessory pathway
Atrial fibrillation	400–700	80–180	dcCV	Digoxin, verapamil, diltiazem, β-blocker		Add Ia agent	—
Atrial flutter	230–430	80–160	dcCV	Digoxin, verapamil, diltiazem, β-blocker		Add Ia agent	Frequently presents as regular rhythm at 150 beats/min (2:1 conduction)
Multifocal atrial tachycardia	100–180	100–180	—	Correct underlying disorder, verapamil		Correct underlying disorder, verapamil Ia agent	Multiple P wave morphologies; common with COPD
Ventricular tachycardia	—	100–220	dcCV	Lidocaine, Ia agent, bretylium			—

   d. ECG
      (1) Tachycardia: 100 to 180 beats/min
      (2) Irregular ventricular response
      (3) Absence of P waves
      (4) Disorganized atrial activity shown by atrial and
          esophageal ECG
   e. The hemodynamically unstable patient may be treated
      with synchronized DC cardioversion. Hemodynami-
      cally stable patients are treated medically to control
      ventricular rate and to chemically cardiovert to sinus
      rhythm.
      (1) Digoxin: 0.5 mg IV followed by 0.25 g IV q2-4h;
          up to 1.5 mg in 24 hours
      (2) Verapamil: 5 mg IV given every 5 minutes up to a
          total dose of 15 to 20 mg; may result in more rapid
          rate control than digoxin and may also result in
          cardioversion; administered with caution because
          of the chance of significant hypotension; adequate
          IV access and appropriate monitoring arranged
          prior to administration
      (3) Procainamide: Once rate control obtained, Type Ia
          agents administered to attempt cardioversion
      (4) Diltiazem: Administration as a continuous IV
          infusion recently introduced for the control and
          conversion of atrial tachyarrhythmias
      (5) Caution when administering β-blockers or calcium
          channel blocking agents to patients with a history
          of CHF; IV β-blockers and calcium channel
          blockers should not be administered concomitantly
          because of risk of precipitating complete heart
          block
      (6) Digoxin and a Type Ia agent included in chronic
          therapy
2. Atrial flutter
   a. The predisposing factors are similar to those of atrial
      fibrillation.
   b. The hemodynamic consequences are also similar to
      atrial fibrillation, with a decrease in LV filling and a
      decrease in cardiac output.
   c. ECG considerations include the following:
      (1) Flutter waves are best seen in the inferior leads but
          may not be apparent at rapid ventricular rates.

Carotid sinus massage or administration of adenosine may slow the rate so that the flutter waves can be identified.

(2) Atrial and esophageal leads will show the regular atrial activity at rates between 200 and 450 per minute.

(3) There is generally 2:1 AV conduction ratio present. In any patient with a regular, narrow, complex tachycardia at 150 beats/min, atrial flutter should be considered.

d. Treatment includes the following:

(1) Hemodynamically unstable: Synchronized DC cardioversion with 25 to 50 J initially

(2) Hemodynamically stable: Pharmacologic intervention similar to that for atrial fibrillation

(3) Patients with epicardial pacing wires: Rapid atrial pacing may result in cardioversion.

3. Paroxysmal supraventricular tachycardia

a. There are several different types caused either by reentry or increased automaticity. The rate is generally 120 to 250 beats/min and regular. The QRS complex is usually regular, but aberrant conduction may lead to QRS widening. Differentiation from ventricular tachycardia is imperative.

b. AV nodal reentry characteristics include the following:

(1) Most common type of supraventricular tachycardia

(2) Often abrupt onset and sudden termination

(3) Caused by a reentrant circuit in the AV node which leads to simultaneous retrograde depolarization of the atrium and antegrade depolarization of the ventricle (therefore, P waves often will not be visible)

c. AV nodal reentry secondary to an accessory pathway characteristics include the following:

(1) This is the next most common type of supraventricular tachycardia, due to an anomalous pathway directly connecting the atria and ventricle and bypassing the AV node.

(2) Orthodromic conduction is more common and leads to narrow complex tachycardia with P waves following the QRS complex.

(3) Antidromic conduction is less common. The QRS

complex will be wide and may be difficult to distinguish from ventricular tachycardia.

d. Hemodynamically unstable patients are treated with synchronized DC cardioversion with 10 to 50 J initially. Hemodynamically stable patients may be treated pharmacologically.

   (1) Vagal maneuvers prolong the refractory period of the AV node and may break the arrhythmia.

   (2) Adenosine (6 mg IV bolus; if unsuccessful, 12 mg IV bolus which may be repeated) also increases the refractory period and will often convert the arrhythmia.

   (3) Verapamil is effective for AV nodal reentry but should not be used if an accessory pathway is present, since it may actually enhance conduction through these pathways.

   (4) β-Blockers may be effective by increasing the AV node refractory period.

   (5) Type Ia agents may be effective.

4. Multifocal atrial tachycardia

   a. Due to several automatic atrial foci

   b. Commonly seen in COPD and severe pulmonary disease

   c. Several precipitating factors, including digitalis toxicity, theophylline administration, perioperative stress, hypoxia, electrolyte abnormalities, PE

   d. ECG which reveals a narrow QRS tachycardia (100 to 200 beats/min) and P waves of at least three different morphologies

   e. Treatment directed mainly at correcting underlying metabolic and electrolyte abnormalities, identifying and treating drug toxicities, and improving pulmonary function

5. Wide complex tachyarrhythmias (QRS complex > 0.12 seconds)—differential diagnosis includes ventricular tachycardia and atrial or supraventricular tachycardias with aberrancy or preexisting bundle branch block, and supraventricular tachycardia with antegrade accessory pathway conduction.

   a. Ventricular tachycardia

      (1) A life-threatening arrhythmia most often seen in the setting of ischemic heart disease

(2) Defined as three or more consecutive wide QRS complexes at a rate of >100 beats/min

(3) Sustained ventricular tachycardia defined as lasting more than 30 seconds

(4) Propensity to deteriorate into ventricular fibrillation

(5) Diagnosis made by ECG with wide complex tachycardia

(6) Findings favoring ventricular tachycardia over supraventricular tachycardia with aberrancy— QRS duration > 0.14 seconds, AV dissociation, fusion beats, left axis deviation, right bundle branch block with monophasic or biphasic QRS in lead V_1

(7) Treatment in the hemodynamically unstable patient—rapid intervention to prevent degeneration into ventricular fibrillation

    (a) Precordial thump while preparing for DC cardioversion

    (b) Synchronized DC cardioversion with 50 to 100 J initially, doubling the energy level if unsuccessful

    (c) If unsuccessful cardioversion, administer IV lidocaine (1 mg/kg) and repeat cardioversion

    (d) If unsuccessful, administer IV procainamide or bretylium and repeat cardioversion

(8) Treatment in the hemodynamically stable patient

    (a) IV lidocaine bolus (1 mg/kg) followed by IV infusion of 1 to 4 mg/min

    (b) If lidocaine ineffective, IV bretylium or procainamide

    (c) Must correct underlying precipitating factors, especially myocardial ischemia

  b. Ventricular fibrillation (See Chapter 4.)

VI. CARDIAC TAMPONADE
A. Etiology

1. A syndrome of impaired cardiac function due to increased intrapericardial pressures
2. Any process that results in a pericardial effusion (See box on p. 142.)
3. Most frequent causes include trauma, malignancy, uremia, and idiopathic pericarditis

Etiology of Cardiac Tamponade

Neoplasm—primary or metastatic (lung, breast, melanoma, lymphoma)
Infection—viral, bacterial, mycobacterial, fungal
Metabolic—uremia, myxedema
Trauma—blunt, penetrating, iatrogenic
Connective tissue diseases
Cardiovascular—postinfarction, postoperative, dissecting aortic aneurysm
Idiopathic

B. **Pathophysiology**
   1. The pericardium is a fibrous sac enclosing the heart and great vessels, normally containing less than 50 ml of fluid, with an average normal intrapericardial pressure of 0 mm Hg.
   2. Slow accumulation of fluid in the pericardial space may be well tolerated even at volumes in excess of 1 L. Rapid accumulation of fluid in the pericardial space leads to a rapid increase in pericardial pressure; small amounts of fluid (<200 ml) may lead to tamponade.
   3. Tamponade occurs when the fluid accumulation leads to increased intrapericardial pressure and impairment of diastolic filling of the ventricles.
   4. As intrapericardial pressure approaches RA pressure, RV diastolic filling decreases and RV output is decreased.
   5. With diminished right sided output, there is decreased pulmonary blood flow and diminished LV filling with subsequent decrease in left ventricular SV. This decrease in cardiac output may lead to hypotension and decreased peripheral perfusion.
   6. Compensatory mechanisms include increased ventricular ejection fraction, reflex tachycardia, increased SVR, and renal conservation of fluid to maintain intravascular volume.

C. **Diagnosis**
   1. Differential diagnosis (See box on p. 143.)
   2. Requires a high degree of suspicion and should be considered in any patient with unexplained hypotension, shock, cardiac arrest, or EMD
   3. Should be considered in patients with circulatory compromise in the setting of a disease process involving the pericardium

Differential Diagnosis of Cardiac Tamponade

Tension pneumothorax	Right heart failure
Hypovolemic shock	Congestive heart failure
Myocardial infarction	Constrictive pericarditis
Pulmonary embolism	

4. Symptoms—dyspnea, fatigue, agitation, air hunger
5. Signs
   a. Beck's triad: The classic findings of low systemic arterial pressure, elevated CVP, and muffled heart sounds; however, triad may not always be present
   b. Pulsus paradoxus: Exaggerated decrease in systolic blood pressure on inspiration
6. CXR—may show cardiac enlargement and a fat pad sign indicative of a pericardial effusion or may assist in ruling out other potential diagnosis
7. ECG—may demonstrate decreased voltages, nonspecific ST-T wave changes, evidence of pericarditis, or electrical alternans (uncommon)
8. Hemodynamic findings
   a. Arterial hypotension
   b. PA catheter—elevated CVP with equalization of CVP, RA, and PAD pressures
9. Echocardiography
   a. Most accurate method of detecting pericardial effusion
   b. May be helpful in identification of tamponade if abnormal respiratory variation in transvalvar flow velocities, bulging of intraventricular septum into the LV, or if diastolic collapse of the RV is seen
   c. If tamponade suspected on clinical grounds and patient is hemodynamically unstable, do not delay treatment awaiting echocardiographic evidence of pericardial effusion or tamponade

D. Treatment
1. Intravascular volume administration to increase to CVP and attempt to overcome pericardial pressure
2. Pericardiocentesis to decrease intrapericardial pressure; may be life-saving and should be considered in any patient

TABLE 6-15.

Indications for Pacing

Temporary	Permanent
Symptomatic bradycardia after acute MI	Sick sinus syndrome
Bifascicular or trifascicular block after acute anterior MI	Mobitz II AV block
Bridge to permanent pacing	Third-degree heart block
Following cardiac surgery	Low cardiac output syndrome
Low cardiac output syndrome	Bifasicular block after acute MI
	Symptomatic bilateral bundle branch block

who is hemodynamically unstable and in whom the diagnosis of tamponade is suspected. (See Chapter 5.)

VII. CARDIAC PACEMAKERS
A. Indications (Table 6-15)
B. Coding System
Three letter system
1. The first letter indicates the chamber paced, where:
   A = Atrium
   V = Ventricle
   D = Dual (both chambers)
2. The second letter indicates the chamber sensed: A, V, D, or O (if no chamber is sensed—asynchronous mode)
3. The third letter indicates mode of response once the signal is sensed, where:
   I = Inhibit the electrical output
   T = Trigger the electrical response
   D = Dual response where the atrium is triggered and the ventricle inhibited
4. Temporary pacemakers can function in the atrial demand mode, ventricular demand mode, or AV sequential mode, either synchronously or asynchronously.
C. Identifying Malfunction of a Pacemaker
1. If the answer to any of the following questions is no, the pacemaker is not functioning properly:
   a. Does the pacemaker impulse lead to electrical activation of the heart (capture)?
   b. Does the pacemaker sense the intrinsic electrical activity of the heart and prevent competing electrical activity?

      c. Does the pacemaker provide an appropriate heart rate for the clinical situation?

  2. If a temporary pacemaker appears to be malfunctioning, the temporary lead may need to be manipulated, the pacemaker cables may need to be changed, or the pacemaker generator may need to be adjusted.

  3. If a permanent pacemaker appears to be malfunctioning, seek cardiology consultation for complete interrogation of the pacemaker and possible reprogramming or replacement of the pacemaker or leads.

SUGGESTED READING

Abrams J, editor: Angina pectoris: mechanisms, diagnosis, and therapy, *Cardiol Clin* vol 9, 1991.

Ameli S, Shah SK: Cardiac tamponade: pathophysiology, diagnosis, and management, *Cardiol Clin* 9:665, 1991.

Braunwald E, editor: *Heart disease: a textbook of cardiovascular medicine,* ed 4, Philadelphia, 1992, WB Saunders.

Chatterjee K: Digitalis, catecholamines, and other positive inotropic agents. In Parmley WW, Chatterjee K, editors: *Cardiology: physiology, pharmacology, diagnosis,* vol 1, Philadelphia, 1993, JB Lippincott.

Dajani AS, et al: Prevention of bacterial endocarditis: recommendations by the American Heart Association, *JAMA* 264:2919, 1990.

Dowling RD, Griffith BP: *Cardiac Function.* In Simmons RL, Steed DL, editors: *Basic science review for surgeons,* Philadelphia, 1992, WB Saunders.

Goldman L: *Assessment and management of the cardiac patient before, during, and after noncardiac surgery.* In Parmley WW, Chatterjee K, editors: *Cardiology,* vol 3, Philadelphia, 1991, JB Lippincott.

Kirklin JW, Barratt-Boyes BG, editors: *Cardiac surgery,* ed 2, New York, 1993, Churchill Livingstone.

McEvoy GK, et al, editors: American hospital formulary service drug information 93, Bethesda, Md, 1993, American Society of Hospital Pharmacists, Inc.

Moreno-Cabral CE, Mitchell RS, Miller DC: *Manual of postoperative management in adult cardiac surgery,* Baltimore, 1988, Williams and Wilkins.

Perloff JK, editor: The cardiomyopathies, *Cardiol Clin* vol 6, 1988.

Sabiston DC, Spencer FC, editors: *Surgery of the chest,* ed 5, Philadelphia, 1990, WB Saunders.

Shah PK, editor: Acute cardiac care, *Cardiol Clin* vol 9, 1991.

Shapiro S, Brundage B: *Cardiac problems in critical care.* In Bongard FS, Sue DY, editors: *Current critical care diagnosis and treatment,* Norwalk, Conn, 1994, Appleton and Lange.

Wisler PL, Green FJ, Watanabe AM: *Cardiovascular adrenergic and muscarinic cholinergic receptors.* In Parmley WW, Chatterjee K, editors: *Cardiology: physiology, pharmacology, diagnosis,* vol 1, Philadelphia, 1991, JB Lippincott.

THE PULMONARY SYSTEM 7

Thomas A. D'Amico

I. PULMONARY PHYSIOLOGY

A. Anatomy

1. Conducting airways
   a. Trachea, mainstem bronchi, lobar bronchi, segmental bronchi, and terminal bronchioles
   b. Represent anatomic dead space and do not contribute to gas exchange
2. Respiratory zone
   a. Respiratory bronchioles, alveolar ducts, and alveolar sacs
   b. Comprises 300 million alveoli; a surface area for gas exchange of 50 to 100 m^2
   c. Alveolar cells
      (1) Type I pneumocytes: Responsible for gas exchange
      (2) Type II pneumocytes: Secrete surfactant (reduces the surface tension, increases compliance, decreases work of respiration)
      (3) Pulmonary fibroblasts

B. Lung Volumes (Fig. 7-1)

1. Tidal volume (V_T) is the volume of normal inspiration and normal expiration.
2. Inspiratory reserve volume (IRV) is difference between maximal inspiration and normal inspiration.
3. Expiratory reserve volume (ERV) is the difference between maximal expiration and normal expiration.
4. Residual volume (RV) is the volume remaining in the lung after maximal expiration.
5. Total lung capacity (TLC) is the volume in the lung after maximal inspiration.
6. Vital capacity (VC) is the volume expired between maximal inspiration and maximal expiration.

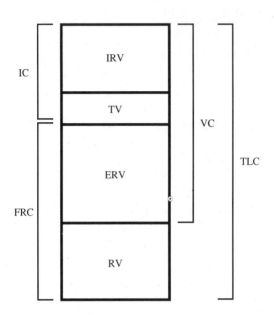

IRV: Inspiratory reserve volume
TV: Tidal volume
ERV: Expiratory reserve volume
RV: Residual volume
IC: Inspiratory capacity
FRC: Functional residual capacity
VC: Vital capacity
TLC: Total lung capacity

FIG 7-1.
Total lung capacity and physiologic lung volumes.

7. Inspiratory capacity (IC) is the volume inspired between normal expiration and maximal inspiration.

8. Functional residual capacity (FRC) is the volume of air in the lung at end-expiration (normal expiration).

C. **Respiratory Volumes**

1. Minute ventilation (V_E) is the volume of air inspired per minute.

2. Alveolar ventilation (V_A) is the fraction of V_E that reaches the alveoli and is available for gas exchange.

3. Dead space (V_d) is the fraction of V_E that is not available for gas exchange.

D. **Ventilation**

1. Pulmonary compliance

   a. Lung expansability is defined as the change in lung volume achieved by a given change in pressure.

   b. The lung is elastic and tends to collapse; the chest wall is expansile and tends to expand the lung.

   c. The FRC is the point of equilibrium between the two opposing forces.

2. Airway resistance

   a. Resistance to flow is defined as the pressure difference between the mouth and the alveoli divided by the flow rate.

   b. Resistance is proportional to the length of the airway and inversely proportional to the square of the radius of the airway.

E. **Perfusion**

1. Pulmonary vascular bed accommodates the entire cardiac output at a low perfusion pressure (15 mm Hg).

2. Alveolar hypoxia induces pulmonary vasoconstriction, increases pulmonary vascular resistance, and redistributes pulmonary blood flow.

3. Acidosis also induces pulmonary vasoconstriction, increases pulmonary vascular resistance, and redistributes pulmonary blood flow.

4. Fluid balance considerations include the following:

   a. Fluid balance across the capillary endothelium and alveolar epithelium is determined by capillary hydrostatic pressure, interstitial hydrostatic pressure, capillary osmotic pressure, and interstitial osmotic pressure.

   b. The ability of the capillary membrane to maintain its

osmotic pressure depends on preventing the passage of plasma proteins.

c. Normally there is a net flux of fluid out of the capillary into the interstitium, which is drained by pulmonary lymphatics; when capillary hydrostatic pressure increases and the capacity of pulmonary lymphatics is exceeded, pulmonary edema occurs.

F. Ventilation and Perfusion (V/Q) Matching

In the normal state, the distribution of ventilation parallels perfusion; V/Q mismatch is the most common cause of hypoxemia.

1. V/Q mismatch
   a. V/Q = 0: Alveoli are perfused but not ventilated; concentrations of O_2 and CO_2 in the alveoli are equal to the concentration in mixed venous blood ($Po_2 = 40$ mm Hg and $Pco_2 = 45$ mm Hg)
   b. V/Q < 1: Ventilation is less than perfusion, but gas exchange does occur; concentrations of O_2 and CO_2 in the alveoli are between those of mixed venous blood and normal arterial blood ($Po_2 = 40$ to 100 mm Hg and $Pco_2 = 40$ to 45 mm Hg)
   c. V/Q = 1: Ventilation matched by perfusion and normal gas exchange occurs; concentrations of O_2 and CO_2 in the alveoli are normal ($Po_2 = 100$ mm Hg and $Pco_2 = 40$ mm Hg)
   d. V/Q > 1: Ventilation exceeds perfusion and only a fraction of the ventilated lung takes part in gas exchange; concentrations of O_2 and CO_2 in the alveoli are between those of normal arterial blood and inspired gas ($Po_2 = 100$ to 150 mm Hg and $Pco_2 = 0$ to 40 mm Hg). The fraction of ventilation that does not take part in gas exchange contributes to the physiologic dead space.

2. Shunt
   a. A shunt is defined as mixed venous blood that does not participate in gas exchange. Shunts cause a decrease in arterial O_2 concentration, with minimal effect on CO_2. The effect on O_2 is not completely corrected by the administration of 100% O_2.
   b. Anatomic shunting refers to morphologic right-to-left shunts.

     c. Physiologic shunting refers to blood that passes through the pulmonary circulation without undergoing gas exchange.

     d. Shunt fraction is the ratio of blood flow through the shunt to the total flow. The normal shunt fraction is 1% to 2%.

G. Postoperative Pulmonary Dysfunction

  1. Atelectasis

     a. Supine positioning

     b. Mechanical ventilation

     c. Postoperative pain, splinting

  2. Respiratory depression

     a. Narcotics

     b. Benzodiazepines

  3. Bronchospasm secondary to airway instrumentation

  4. Pulmonary edema

  5. Impaired diaphragmatic function

  6. Residual neuromuscular relaxation

  7. Impaired cough

  8. Poor clearance of secretions

     a. Impaired ciliary function

     b. Mucus plugging

H. Work of Breathing

  1. Defined as the product of pressure and volume

  2. Requires V_{O_2}; may constitute up to 20% of the overall D_{O_2} in critically ill patients

  3. Components of work

     a. Elastic recoil of the lung and chest wall

     b. Frictional resistance of the airway

     c. Frictional resistance of the endotracheal tube and mechanical ventilator

II. PATHOPHYSIOLOGY OF ACUTE RESPIRATORY FAILURE

A. Hypercapnic Respiratory Failure

  1. Severe hypercapnia may cause respiratory acidosis, hypoxia, and cardiac dysfunction.

  2. O_2 must be administered in the setting of hypercapnia to correct hypoxia, and the goal of therapy is to correct hypoxemia without exacerbating the hypercapnia.

  3. Hypercapnic respiratory failure is difficult to treat without

endotracheal intubation and mechanical ventilation in patients with COPD, because the administration of O_2 may increase V/Q mismatching.

B. Respiratory Muscle Fatigue

1. Inability of the respiratory muscles to maintain adequate alveolar ventilation, because of limitations in energy supply or increased energy demand

2. Factors contributing to respiratory fatigue
   a. Inadequate energy storage
      (1) Malnutrition
      (2) Hypophosphatemia, hypomagnesemia, hypokalemia
      (3) Catabolic state (trauma, sepsis, malignancy)
   b. Inadequate energy delivery
      (1) Anemia
      (2) Hypoxia
      (3) Low cardiac output
   c. Excessive energy demand
      (1) Increased work of breathing
      (2) Decreased muscle efficiency

3. Characteristic sequence
   a. Rapid, shallow breathing
   b. Excessive use of accessory respiratory muscles during inspiration, producing paradoxical abdominal muscle relaxation
   c. Respiratory alternans (alternate recruitment of the diaphragm and other inspiratory muscles to defend fatigue)
   d. May be followed by bradypnea, heralding respiratory arrest

C. Acute Reactive/Obstructive Airway Disease

1. Increased airway resistance, respiratory muscle fatigue, and alveolar hypoventilation develop as a result of bronchoconstriction.
   a. Reversible airway obstruction
   b. Airway inflammation
   c. Airway hyperreactivity

2. Airway obstruction produces V/Q mismatching and increased alveolar-arterial oxygen differential ($AaDo_2$).

3. Early asthma is characterized by hyperventilation and hypocapnia; V/Q mismatching increases wasted ventilation and wasted respiratory effort.

4. Eventually, increased O_2 demand caused by increased respiratory work results in excessive CO_2 production; as respiratory muscles fatigue, $Paco_2$ increases.

5. When airway obstruction is severe, hypercapnia and respiratory acidosis may progress and hypoxia and respiratory arrest may follow.

6. Evaluation of acute reactive/obstructive airway disease includes the following:

   a. Assessment of frequency and severity of disease, including history of previous endotracheal intubation

   b. Determination of previous or current corticosteroid use; stress doses of steroids may be indicated

   c. Assessment of current medications

7. Management includes the following:

   a. Oxygen: Usually 25% to 40% to optimize oxygenation without exacerbating V/Q mismatching

   b. Inhaled bronchodilators (β_2-agonists): Albuterol, terbutaline, fenoterol, salbutamol

   c. Inhaled anticholinergics (ipratropium bromide): Decrease vagal tone and produce bronchial smooth muscle relaxation

   d. Intravenous corticosteroids: Reduce the inflammation associated with asthma

   e. Aminophylline: Increases the respiratory response to hypoxia and contributes to bronchodilatation; side effects—sinus tachycardia, ventricular arrhythmias, and seizures

   f. Endotracheal intubation and mechanical ventilation: In patients who do not respond appropriately to other therapy

D.   Chronic Obstructive Pulmonary Disease

1. Hypercapnia and hypoxemia during ARF complicating COPD are produced by alveolar hypoventilation and V/Q mismatching.

2. Low V/Q results from obstruction, secretions, airway edema, and smooth muscle contraction.

3. Although alveolar ventilation decreases, minute ventilation does not change, thus dead space ventilation increases.

4. Tidal volume and respiratory rate may increase in response to hypoxemia.

5. Airway resistance increases during ARF in patients with COPD, producing occult PEEP (auto PEEP), which may develop during spontaneous or mechanical ventilation
6. The physiologic consequences of occult PEEP include the following:
   a. Decreased venous return to the heart
   b. Decreased cardiac output
   c. Increased barotrauma

E. Adult Respiratory Distress Syndrome
1. ARDS is ARF characterized by noncardiogenic pulmonary edema and severe hypoxia secondary to intrapulmonary shunting.
2. The pathophysiology includes multifactorial activation of neutrophils, macrophages, and platelets, via complement activation or endotoxin release (Table 7-1).
3. The final common pathway of ARDS is the development of endothelial injury and increased permeability of the epithelium and endothelium.
4. Diffuse alveolar damage is observed with 3 pathologic stages, which include the following:
   a. Exudative stage (1 to 7 days): Alveolar and interstitial edema and hemorrhage, membrane hyalinization; damage greatest to the type I epithelial cell
   b. Proliferative stage (7 to 10 days): Fibrin deposition; type II pneumocyte, fibroblast, and inflammatory cell proliferation
   c. Fibrotic stage (14 days): Fibrosis within the interstitium, alveolar epithelium, and pulmonary vasculature
5. Manifestations: Pulmonary edema, reduced pulmonary

TABLE 7-1.

Risk Factors for the Development of ARDS

Risk Factor	Incidence of ARDS (%)
Sepsis	40-50
Aspiration	20-30
Multiple transfusions (10 U/6 hr)	20-30
Pulmonary contusion	15-20
Major fractures	5-10
Head trauma	5-10
Burns	2-5

compliance, increased airway resistance, increased physiologic dead space, and increased shunting

6. Clinical presentation: Dyspnea, tachypnea, hypoxia, pulmonary infiltrate

7. Incidence of nonpulmonary organ failure in patients with ARDS
   a. Renal: 40% to 50%
   b. Hepatic: 15% to 90%
   c. CNS: 10% to 30%
   d. GI: 10% to 30%
   e. Cardiac: 10% to 25%

8. Treatment of ARDS includes the following:
   a. Treatment of underlying cause
   b. Aggressive treatment of concomitant infections
   c. Usually requires supplemental oxygen in high concentrations because of increased pulmonary shunting
   d. May be necessary to use endotracheal intubation and PEEP; goal of therapy is to achieve O_2 saturation of 90% or greater while minimizing oxygen toxicity and barotrauma
   e. Optimization of Do_2 and Vo_2

9. The overall mortality rate of ARDS is 50% to 70%.
   a. When associated with sepsis, the mortality rate is 90%.
   b. When not associated with sepsis, the mortality rate is 10%.

F. Pneumonia (Section IV)

1. Produces hypoxia secondary to shunting (perfusion of consolidated pulmonary parenchyma, thus may be resistant to O_2 therapy

2. May cause particularly severe ARF in patients with underlying COPD, malnutrition, or when complicated by the development of ARDS

III. AIRWAY HEMORRHAGE
A. Presentation

1. Massive hemoptysis: 600 ml blood or more over 24 hours
   a. Massive hemoptysis is associated with a 15% to 50% mortality rate.
   b. The rate of bleeding with massive hemoptysis usually allows time for assessment, diagnosis, and effective medical management.

2. Exsanguinating hemoptysis: 150 ml/hr, with total blood loss exceeding 1000 ml
   a. Exsanguinating hemoptysis is associated with a mortality rate that is higher than 75%.
   b. Medical measures are unlikely to be successful with airway hemorrhage of this magnitude.

B. **Sources of Airway Hemorrhage in the ICU**
   1. Bronchial artery
      a. Bronchiectasis
      b. Tuberculosis
      c. Lung abscess
      d. Malignancy
      e. Necrotizing pneumonia
      f. Bronchitis
      g. Cystic fibrosis
   2. Pulmonary artery
      a. Tuberculosis
      b. Suppurative pulmonary disease
      c. Pulmonary arteriovenous fistula
      d. Malignancy
      e. PA rupture from catheter
   3. Innominate artery
      a. Tracheoinnominate fistula
      b. Tracheal resection
   4. Aorta
      a. Aortic dissection
      b. Aortic transection

C. **Initial Management**
   1. Prevent asphyxiation.
      a. Establish airway and administer humidified O_2.
      b. If site of bleeding is already known, turn the patient to the decubitus position with the bleeding side down to prevent hemorrhage into the contralateral lung.
   2. Resuscitate.
      a. Establish appropriate intravenous access and administer crystalloid solution.
      b. Type and cross match 6 U of blood.
      c. Assess and correct coagulation parameters including PT, PTT, fibrinogen, platelet count, and hematocrit.
   3. Characterize the source of bleeding.
      a. Measure rate and total volume of bleeding.
      b. Obtain a chest film.

    c. Consult a thoracic surgeon and arrange for bronchoscopy to be performed.

    d. Obtain appropriate airway cultures, and initiate broad spectrum antibiotics unless the source of the bleeding is known not to be suppurative.

D. Bronchoscopy

1. Indications for bronchoscopy include the following:
    a. To clear the airway of blood and clots and to restore adequate respiratory function
    b. To localize or lateralize bleeding
    c. To establish the etiology of the bleeding
    d. To initiate therapy
2. Rigid bronchoscopy may be performed in patients with acute massive hemorrhage; if it lateralizes the source of bleeding, endobronchial control may be achieved.
    a. Selective bronchial intubation
    b. Placement of dual lumen endotracheal tube
    c. Endobronchial tamponade with a Fogarty catheter
3. If rigid bronchoscopy does not lateralize bleeding and bleeding is not massive, flexible fiberoptic bronchoscopy is performed to visualize the lobar and segmental bronchial orifices (may be performed via rigid bronchoscope or via endotracheal tube).
4. Bronchoscopic examination identifies the bleeding source in approximately 90% of cases.
5. Adjunctive measures during bronchoscopy include the following:
    a. Selective segmental balloon tamponade during flexible bronchoscopy (4F Fogarty catheter)
    b. Endobronchial ice-cold saline lavage
    c. Endobronchial irrigation with topical epinephrine solution (0.2 ml of 1:1000 epinephrine diluted in 500 ml NS)

E. Arteriography and Embolization

1. Significant airway hemorrhage usually originates from the bronchial circulation; inflammatory pulmonary disease stimulates increased bronchial blood flow and stimulates growth of bronchial collaterals.
2. Diagnostic arteriography and therapeutic embolization of a dilated bronchial arteriole is often successful (75% to 85%) without significantly affecting nutritive blood flow.
3. Recurrence rate is 20%, thus successful embolization may

be followed by elective pulmonary resection in selected patients.

F. **Surgical Resection**

1. Surgical resection may follow successful embolization. It is most effective when bleeding has been localized to a single source and there are no contraindications to thoracotomy.
2. Placement of a dual lumen endotracheal tube is essential.
3. Surgical resection is the therapy of choice when the bleeding source is the pulmonary innominate artery

IV. NOSOCOMIAL PNEUMONIA

A. **Epidemiology**

1. Incidence is 5 to 50 cases per 1000 admissions
   a. 10 per 1000 general admissions
   b. 50 per 1000 ICU admissions
2. Risk factors
   a. Previous antibiotic therapy
   b. Surgery
   c. Hospitalization in ICU
   d. Mechanical ventilation
   e. Aspiration
   f. COPD
3. Mortality rate
   a. General mortality rate: 28%
   b. ICU mortality rate: 39%
   c. Mortality rate from pneumonia with gram-positive cocci: 15%
   d. Mortality rate from pneumonia with gram-negative cocci: 75%

B. **Diagnosis**

1. Positive cultures from the lower respiratory tract
   a. Sputum gram stain (organisms and >25 WBC/field) and culture
   b. Transtracheal aspiration
   c. Bronchoscopy (protected bronchial brush sample or bronchoalveolar lavage)
   d. Transthoracic aspiration
   e. Open-lung biopsy
2. Differential diagnosis
   a. ARDS
   b. Pulmonary edema
   c. Pulmonary embolism

      d. Pulmonary infarct

      e. Pulmonary hemorrhage

      f. Pulmonary contusion

      g. Atelectasis

      h. Sterile aspiration and chemical pneumonitis

      i. Malignancy

C. **Pathologic Agents**

    1. Gram-negative rods: 60% to 75%

      a. *Pseudomonas aeruginosa:* 15% to 30%

      b. *Acinetobacter* organisms: 10% to 15%

      c. *Proteus* organisms: 10% to 15%

      d. *Haemophilus* organisms: 10%

      e. *Escherichia coli:* 10%

      f. *Klebsiella* organisms: 10%

      g. *Serratia* organisms: 5%

    2. Gram-positive cocci: 25% to 35%

      a. *Staphylococcus aureus:* 25% to 30%

      b. *Streptococcus pneumoniae:* 10%

      c. Other streptococcal species: 10%

    3. Anaerobes: 2%

    4. *Candida albicans:* 10%

    5. Polymicrobial: 10% to 20%

D. **Treatment**

    1. Institutional micronial characteristics: May dictate early empiric coverage

      a. Common pathogens

      b. Patterns of microbial resistance

    2. Mildly to moderately ill patients: No sputum available, no recent surgery, not immunosuppressed, not mechanically ventilated

      a. Probable pathogens: *S. pneumoniae, Haemophilus influenzae, S. aureus*

      b. Empiric antibiotic coverage: Second-generation cephalosporin

    3. Moderately to severely ill: No sputum available, recent surgery, use of histamine antagonist, not mechanically ventilated

      a. Probable pathogens: Aerobic gram-negative rods

      b. Empiric antibiotic coverage: Third-generation cephalosporin; erythromycin if legionella is suspected

    4. Moderately to severely ill: Mechanically ventilated

      a. Probable pathogens: Aerobic gram-negative rods, including *P. aeruginosa;* suspect resistant microorganisms

  b. Empiric antibiotic coverage

    (1) Third-generation cephalosporin (with activity against *Pseudomonas* organisms) plus an aminoglycoside

    (2) Third-generation cephalosporin (with activity against *Pseudomonas* organisms) plus aztreonam

    (3) Imipenem

V.   PULMONARY MANIFESTATIONS OF TRAUMA

A.   Initial Evaluation

1. Physical examination

  a. Inspection: Penetrating trauma—entrance and exit wounds; blunt trauma—chest wall injuries, splinting, respiratory insufficiency

  b. Palpation: Tenderness, crepitus, fractures

  c. Auscultation: Breath sounds, rubs, "crunch" of pneumomediastinum

2. Chest radiograph: Pneumothorax, hemothorax, pneumomediastinum, widened mediastinum, pulmonary contusion, enterothorax, rib fractures, scapular fractures

B.   Pneumothorax

1. The treatment for a pneumothorax is a tube thoracostomy. (See Chapter 5.)

  a. May be therapeutic and diagnostic

  b. Primary goals are to prevent tension pneumothorax and fully reexpand lung

  c. May reveal unsuspected hemothorax

  d. Persistent, massive air leak suggestive of tracheobronchial injury

2. Management of pneumothorax takes precedence over treatment of other associated injuries after initial patient stabilization is achieved because of life-threatening potential.

C.   Tracheal and Bronchial Trauma

1. Etiology

  a. Penetrating trauma

  b. Blunt trauma (high-velocity deceleration injury)

2. Associated conditions

  a. Hemoptysis

  b. Hemothorax, pneumothorax, pneumomediastinum

  c. Multiple thoracic injuries (scapular fracture, multiple rib fractures, sternal fracture)

3. Diagnosis
   a. Massive air leak after tube thoracostomy
   b. Extraluminal position of endotracheal tube
   c. Bronchoscopic visualization
4. Treatment
   a. Patient stabilization; tube thoracostomy
   b. Selective bronchial intubation or dual lumen endotracheal intubation
   c. Minimization of airway pressure to limit barotrauma
   d. Surgical repair of the trachea or bronchus; may require pulmonary resection if injury is severe
5. Postoperative management
   a. Minimization of airway pressure to facilitate healing
   b. Aggressive pulmonary toilet
   c. Management of associated injuries

D. Pulmonary Contusion and Flail Chest
   1. Etiology
      a. Blunt trauma may produce severe thoracic injury, including flail chest.
      b. Flail chest is defined as fractures of three or more adjacent ribs at multiple sites, producing paradoxical chest wall movement.
   2. Diagnosis
      a. Inspection and palpation of paradoxical chest wall movement
      b. Radiographic evidence of multiple rib fractures and pulmonary contusion
   3. Pathophysiology
      a. Although paradoxical chest wall movement may be profound, pulmonary insufficiency associated with flail chest is related to the underlying pulmonary contusion.
      b. Pulmonary insufficiency associated with contusion is exacerbated by splinting and impaired respiratory excursion secondary to pain.
   4. Management
      a. Analgesia; may require placement of epidural catheter
      b. Aggressive pulmonary toilet and surveillance for the development of pneumonia
      c. Mechanical ventilation if above measures are unsuccessful in preventing pulmonary insufficiency
      d. Internal fixation/external splinting; rarely, if ever, required

VI. PULMONARY EMBOLISM

A. Evaluation of the Surgical Patient

   1. Low risk

      a. Age < 40 years

      b. Uncomplicated surgical procedure

   2. Moderate risk

      a. Age > 40 years

      b. Prolonged immobilization

      c. Obesity

      d. Malignancy

   3. High risk

      a. History of previous DVT or PE

      b. Surgery for pelvic malignancy

      c. Hip or major knee surgery

B. Risk Assessment (Table 7-2)

C. Prophylaxis

   1. Graduated compression stockings may be used in virtually all patients preoperatively, intraoperatively, and postoperatively.

   2. Intermittent pneumatic compression is recommended in all patients who are moderate or high risk; the mechanism of action is activation of the endogenous fibrinolytic system.

   3. Low-dose heparin (3000 to 5000 U SQ q6h) is used in selected high-risk patients who have no contraindication to anticoagulation.

D. Clinical Presentation

   1. Symptoms

      a. Dyspnea

      b. Pleuritic chest pain

      c. Hemoptysis

      d. Syncope

TABLE 7-2.

Risk of DVT or PE According to Patient Risk Groups

Clinical Manifestations	Patient Risk Groups		
	Low (%)	Moderate (%)	High (%)
Calf vein thrombosis	<10	10-40	40-50
Deep vein thrombosis	<1	2-10	10-25
Nonfatal pulmonary embolus	<0.1	1-2	5-10
Fatal pulmonary embolus	<0.01	0.1-1	1-5

    2. Signs
       a. Tachycardia
       b. Tachypnea
       c. Fever
       d. Hypotension
       e. Evidence of DVT

E. Diagnosis

    1. ABG analysis often demonstrates hypoxia and hypocarbia, although normal indices do not exclude PE.
    2. V/Q scans assess the matching of ventilation to perfusion.
       a. Normal V/Q scans effectively exclude significant PE.
       b. Low probability V/Q scans (<25% matched or mismatched defects) confer 10% probability of significant PE.
       c. Intermediate probability V/Q scans (25% to 50% matched defects) confer 30% probability of significant PE.
       d. High probability V/Q scans (>25% mismatched defects) confer 90% probability of significant PE.
    3. Pulmonary arteriography may be performed.
       a. If the V/Q scan has been interpreted as normal or low probability, surveillance and prophylaxis are continued.
       b. If the V/Q scan has been interpreted as intermediate probability, pulmonary arteriography is usually performed.
       c. If the V/Q scan has been interpreted as high probability, the patient is often treated definitively; pulmonary arteriography may be performed in patients with a relative contraindication to anticoagulation who require definite diagnosis prior to instituting therapy.

F. Treatment

    1. Systemic anticoagulation considerations include the following:
       a. Unless contraindicated, the patient is anticoagulated with IV heparin 5000 to 10,000 U bolus followed by a constant infusion at 10 to 15 u/kg, adjusted to keep PTT at 2.0 to 2.5 times control.
       b. Heparin is administered at therapeutic levels for 72 hours prior to conversion to oral anticoagulation.
       c. After conversion, warfarin is continued at least 3 to 6 months.

2. Fibrinolytic agents are usually reserved for hemodynamically significant PE.
3. The placement of a vena caval filter may be considered in high risk patients with documented DVT or PE.
   a. Considered mandatory in patients with contraindication to anticoagulation, such as recent neurologic surgery or concomitant gastrointestinal bleeding
   b. May be used adjunctively with anticoagulation in high-risk patients with refractory DVT or recurrent PE, despite heparin therapy

VII. BRONCHOSCOPY
A. Diagnostic
1. To investigate hemoptysis
2. To obtain cultures in suspected pulmonary infections
3. To determine the etiology of lobar collapse
4. To assess airway patency
5. To confirm or exclude tracheobronchial injury after trauma
6. To evaluate a patient with a pulmonary nodule; to obtain cytology; to stage lung cancer preoperatively
7. To evaluate a patient with suspected tracheoesophageal fistula
8. To evaluate a patient with suspected inhalation injury
B. Therapeutic
1. To aspirate retained secretions and mucous plugs
2. To remove foreign bodies
3. To perform endotracheal intubation in difficult cases

SUGGESTED READING

Hanowell LH, Junod FL, editors: *Pulmonary care of the surgical patient,* Mount Kisco, NY, 1994, Futura.

Russell JA: Pathophysiology of acute respiratory failure, *Chest Surg Clin North Am* 1:209, 1991.

Shamji FM, Vallieres, FM: Airway hemorrhage, *Chest Surg Clin North Am* 1:255, 1991.

THE RENAL SYSTEM

8

James R. Mault

I. INTRODUCTION

A. Normal Kidney Functions

1. Regulation of water and electrolyte balance
2. Excretion of metabolic wastes and foreign chemicals
3. Regulation of arterial BP
   a. The renin-angiotensin system
      (1) Renin
         (a) Produced by the juxtaglomerular apparatus
         (b) Catalyzes cleavage of angiotensinogen (secreted by liver) into angiotensin I
      (2) Angiotensin
         (a) Angiotensin I is converted into angiotensin II.
            (i) Enzymatic cleavage by ACE
            (ii) Occurs in vasculature of lungs or kidneys
         (b) Angiotensin II is a potent vasoconstrictor.
   b. Other vasoactive substances
      (1) Prostaglandins and kinins
      (2) Cause either vasoconstriction or vasodilation
4. Regulation of erythrocyte production
   a. Erythropoietin secretion by kidney
   b. Induces the production of erythrocytes in bone marrow
5. Regulation of vitamin D activity
   a. Conversion of vitamin D to the active form of vitamin D ($1,25$-dihydroxyvitamin D_3)
   b. Occurs in kidney

B. Basic Renal Processes

1. Glomerular filtration
   a. Glomerular filtration rate (GFR)
      (1) GFR is the amount of ultrafiltrate generated by the glomerulus per unit time.

(2) GFR is approximately 180 L/day in a 70-kg male.
(3) Typical concentrations of solutes after the various renal processes are listed in Table 8-1.
(4) Determinants of GFR include the following:
  (a) Permeability and surface area of the glomerular filter (relatively fixed)
  (b) Glomerular capillary hydraulic pressure
      (i) Most significant determinant of GFR
      (ii) Directly proportional to renal perfusion pressure
      (iii) Depends upon several factors
          aa. Systemic mean arterial pressure
          bb. Renal vascular resistance; increased by adrenergic stimulation and antidiuretic hormone, decreased by dopaminergic receptor stimulation and prostaglandins
          cc. Renal venous pressure
      (iv) Calculated by the formula:

$$RPP = \frac{MAP - RVP}{RVR}$$

where
RPP = renal perfusion pressure
MAP = systemic mean arterial pressure
RVP = renal venous pressure
RVR = renal vascular resistance

TABLE 8-1.

Daily Renal Solute Exchange

	Filtered	Reabsorbed	Secreted	Urine
Sodium (mEq)	25,200	25,050	—	150 (100 mEq/L)
Potassium (mEq)	720	720	100	100 (67 mEq/L)
Chloride (mEq)	18,000	17,870	—	130 (87 mEq/L)
Bicarbonate (mEq)	4,000	4,000	—	0
Urea (mM)	900	500	—	400 (267 mM)
Creatinine (mM)	15	—	—	15 (10 mM)
Glucose (mM)	900	900	—	0
Total solutes (mOsm)	49,735	49,040	140	910 (607 mOsm/L)
Water (ml)	180,000	178,500	—	1,500

    b. Composition of ultrafiltrate
      (1) Protein-free crystalloid solution
      (2) Electrolyte concentration nearly identical to that of the circulating plasma

2. Tubular reabsorption: Many of the filtered plasma solutes are either completely absent from the urine or present in substantially smaller quantities than were present in the initial ultrafiltrate. (See Table 8-1.) The reabsorption capabilities of the renal tubules are demonstrated further by the fact that 99% of the 180 L/day of ultrafiltrate is reabsorbed. Reabsorption of fluid and solutes in the tubule is accomplished by simple diffusion (concentration gradient), facilitated diffusion, active transport, or endocytosis.

3. Tubular secretion: Tubular secretion begins with simple diffusion of a substance out of the peritubular capillaries and into the interstitium. Transport into the tubule may be active or passive depending on the gradients of the particular solute. Tubular secretion plays a major role in hydrogen ion and potassium excretion.

II. CLINICAL ASSESSMENT OF RENAL FUNCTION
A. History and Physical
1. A history of uremia, hypertension, hematuria or proteinuria, and review of all medications should be obtained.
2. Signs suggestive of renal insufficiency include hypertension, alopecia, peripheral neuropathy, conjunctival calcification, band keratopathy, gynecomastia and/or testicular atrophy in males, peripheral edema, pericardial rub, and CHF.

B. Urinalysis
1. Urine output
    a. Under conditions of normal hydration, urine output should be within the range of 0.5 to 1.0 ml/kg/hr.
    b. High urine output *(polyuria)* may indicate diuretic use, diabetes mellitus, diabetes insipidus, acute renal failure, or certain types of chronic nephritis.
    c. Low urine output is described as either *oliguria* (urine output less than 400 ml/day in an adult) or *anuria* (absence of urine output). These may result from dehydration, cardiogenic shock, renal failure, or urinary outflow obstruction.

2. Urine pH
   a. Normal urine pH is 4.6 to 8.
   b. Acidic urine may be due to ketoacidosis, high protein diet, COPD, or various medications.
   c. Basic urine indicates urinary tract infection, renal tubular acidosis, diet, or bicarbonate therapy.
3. Urine specific gravity
   a. Specific gravity is normally between 1.003 and 1.030 and is a measure of the density of urine.
   b. Elevated specific gravity indicates dehydration, CHF, adrenal insufficiency, or SIADH.
   c. Decreased specific gravity reflects overhydration, diabetes insipidus, pyelonephritis, or glomerulonephritis.
   d. Specific gravity is an unreliable indicator of volume status or renal function in the presence of glycosuria, after use of intravenous radiographic contrast agents or in patients receiving diuretics.
   e. After a night of fluid restriction, a specific gravity >1.018 indicates appropriate tubular function and a requirement for increased intravascular volume.
4. Urine dipstick
   a. Glucose
      (1) Glucose is normally absent from urine.
      (2) Glucosuria reflects hyperglycemia resulting from diabetes mellitus, pancreatitis, shock, sepsis, steroids, hyperthyroidism, renal tubular dysfunction, or iatrogenic causes.
   b. Protein
      (1) Urine protein is normally 0 to 0.1 g/24 hrs.
      (2) Proteinuria, if detected by dipstick, should be quantified in a 24 hour urine collection prior to elective operation. Excretion in excess of 150 mg in 24 hours is indicative of significant renal parenchymal disease and warrants a more detailed evaluation prior to elective procedures.
   c. Ketones
      (1) Ketones are normally absent from urine.
      (2) Ketonuria is due to diabetic ketoacidosis, starvation, hyperthyroidism, fever, or pregnancy.
   d. Nitrite
      (1) Positive urine nitrite is indicative of urinary tract infection.

(2) Microscopic analysis and urine culture and sensitivity are indicated.

e. Bilirubin and urobilinogen

(1) Both bilirubin and urobilinogen are normally absent from urine.

(2) Positive urine bilirubin or urobilinogen indicates obstructive jaundice, hepatitis, cirrhosis, cholangitis, hemolysis, or suppression of intestinal flora by antibiotics.

f. RBCs and WBCs

(1) Neither red nor white blood cells are normally present in urine.

(2) Positive dipstick indicating hematuria or pyuria is an absolute requirement for microscopic analysis.

5. Microscopic analysis (sediment)

a. Hematuria: Microscopic hematuria may be a result of several factors, which include trauma, pyelonephritis, cystitis, prostatitis, nephrolithiasis, urinary tract cancer, coagulopathy, menses, polycystic kidneys, hemolytic anemia, transfusion reaction, or interstitial nephritis. (Section IV, C)

b. Pyuria

(1) The presence of greater than 10 WBCs per high power field is strong evidence of urinary tract infection. A clean-catch or straight-catheter urine sample should be obtained for urine culture and sensitivity. Elective operation is usually postponed if pyuria is documented.

(2) Other causes of pyuria occur with acute glomerular nephritis, urinary tract cancer, renal tuberculosis, or interstitial nephritis.

c. Epithelial cells: Identification of epithelial cells in urine occurs with acute tubular necrosis and necrotizing papillitis.

d. Casts

(1) Urinary casts are cylindrical masses of cellular elements derived directly from the kidney.

(2) The presence of erythrocyte casts suggests an acute glomerular nephritis, while the presence of leukocyte casts suggests nephritis or pyelonephritis.

(3) Identification of fatty casts with proteinuria is diagnostic of the nephrotic syndrome.

e. Crystals
   (1) In acidic urine, calcium oxylate and urate crystals may normally be present.
   (2) In alkaline urine, calcium carbonate and phosphate crystals may normally be present.
   (3) Cystine, sulfonamide, leucine, tyrosine, and cholesterol crystals in urine are abnormal.

6. Urine electrolytes and fractional excretion of sodium
   a. Normal urine electrolytes are listed in Table 8-1.
   b. A spot determination of urine electrolytes may be useful for assessment of intravascular volume status and aids in potassium supplementation. However, concentrations of electrolytes in urine may vary considerably with salt intake.
      (1) Urine sodium < 20 mEq/L suggests hypovolemia, shock, or hyponatremia.
      (2) Urine potassium < 10 mEq/L indicates hypokalemia or renal failure.
   c. Fractional excretion of sodium is a more reliable indicator of volume status and etiology of acute renal failure and is calculated by the formula:

$$FE_{Na} \ (\%) = \frac{U/P \ sodium}{U/P \ creatinine} \times 100,$$

   where:
   FE_{Na} = fractional excretion of sodium
   U/P sodium = ratio of urine and plasma sodium concentrations
   U/P creatinine = ratio of urine and plasma creatinine concentrations
      (1) In the presence of hypovolemia and hypoperfusion the renin-angiotensin system is activated, and the subsequent release of aldosterone will induce the kidney to reabsorb sodium. Therefore an FE_{Na} less than 1% is indicative of volume depletion.
      (2) An FE_{Na} elevation of greater than 3% is consistent with tubular injury or obstruction.
   d. Assessment of renal function or volume status by urine electrolytes is unreliable in the presence of a preexisting prerenal state (e.g., CHF, cirrhosis) with diuretic therapy or following the use of contrast dye.

C. **Plasma Creatinine and Creatinine Clearance (C_{Cr})**
 1. Creatinine is a metabolic end product of high energy phosphates in muscle. It is removed from the plasma mainly by glomerular filtration with only minor secretion by the proximal tubule. Therefore it is an accurate reflection of GFR.
 2. The plasma creatinine is determined by the rate of production (related to muscle mass) and the rate of excretion (related to GFR).
 3. As renal failure progresses, creatinine is a less reliable indicator of GFR as a result of increasing tubular secretion of creatinine. In these circumstances, other nonsecreted molecules, such as inulin, should be used to determine GFR.
 4. A gradual rise in plasma creatinine does not necessarily reflect continuing renal injury. A steady state level will take several days to develop and the creatinine will rise continually until a new plateau is reached.
 5. In patients with decreased muscle mass, the creatinine can remain within normal limits despite a significant impairment to renal function.
 6. C_{Cr} considerations include the following:
    a. GFR can be accurately assessed by measuring C_{Cr}. Predicted C_{Cr} is usually 90 to 150 ml/min but can be estimated from age (in years), body weight (in kg) and plasma creatinine (P_{Cr} in mg/100 ml) by the formula:

    $$C_{Cr} \text{ (ml/min)} = \frac{(140 - \text{age}) \times \text{wt}}{72 \times P_{Cr}} (\times 0.85 \text{ for females}).$$

    b. Actual creatinine clearance can be determined after a timed urine collection by the formula:

    $$C_{Cr} \text{ (ml/min)} = \frac{U_{Cr} \times U_{vol}}{P_{Cr} \times \text{time} \times \text{BSA}},$$

    where:
    U_{Cr} = urinary creatinine (mg/100 ml)
    U_{vol} = urine volume (ml)
    P_{Cr} = plasma creatinine (mg/100 ml)
    Time = minutes of urine collected
    BSA = body surface area (m^2)

    c. Many therapeutic agents require adjustment of dosage for patients with renal insufficiency. This adjustment is based on the ratio between the actual versus predicted creatinine clearance.

D. BUN

1. BUN (normal range is 10 to 20 mg/100 ml) is the end product of protein degradation via the urea cycle. It is freely filterable, but approximately 50% of filtered urea is reabsorbed. This reabsorption occurs passively and is dependent on water reabsorption to establish the diffusion gradient for urea. Therefore BUN reflects both the renal function and volume status of a patient.

2. As urea generation is directly dependent on protein intake and degradation, BUN may be unreliable as an indication of renal dysfunction in malnourished patients.

3. The relationship between BUN and renal function (GFR) is essentially loglinear. Therefore assuming constant fluid and nutritional balance, if an individual has a BUN of 10 mg/100 ml, a reduction in GFR of 50% is needed before the BUN becomes greater than 20 mg/100 ml.

E. U_{osm} and P_{osm}

1. Healthy kidneys excrete an osmolar load while retaining free water. If damage to the renal tubules occurs, this ability to excrete hyperosmolar urine becomes impaired, and urine and plasma osmolarity will approach equal values.

2. The maximal concentration of urine by the normal kidney is 1400 mOsm/L. Because approximately 910 mOsm of metabolic wastes are produced per day, if urine volume is inadequate (<30 ml/hr or <500 ml/day), these waste products will accumulate in the circulation due to impaired excretion.

3. Normal P_{osm} is 285 ± 15 mOsm/L.

4. Normal U_{osm} (40-700 mOsm/L) indicates the amount of solute in a given volume of urine.

5. The concentrating ability of the kidney, which indicates renal tubular function, correlates with the ratio between P_{osm} and U_{osm}. C_{osm} is represented by the formula:

$$C_{osm} \text{ (osm/min)} = \frac{U_{osm}}{P_{osm}} \times V \text{ (ml/min)},$$

where:

C_{osm} = osmolar clearance
V = urine volume (ml/min)

6. Free water clearance (C_{H_2O}) is calculated using the following formula:

$$C_{H_2O} = V - \frac{U_{osm} \times V}{P_{osm}}$$

a. C_{H_2O} is usually a negative number (less than -20) which becomes increasingly negative as renal concentration increases.
b. As renal tubular function decreases, concentrating ability falls and C_{H_2O} approximates zero (±10). C_{H_2O} may become positive ($>+20$) in diabetes insipidus or water intoxication.

7. P_{osm} may be falsely elevated due to osmotically active molecules present in excess amounts. These usually are glucose, urea, or alcohol. In the presence of hyperglycemia or elevated BUN, P_{osm} may be corrected by the formula:

$$\text{Osmolarity} = 2 \times [Na^+] + \frac{BUN(mg/dl)}{2.8} + \frac{Glucose(mg/dl)}{18}$$

III. CLINICAL MANAGEMENT OF HEMATURIA AND URINARY OBSTRUCTION
A. Hematuria
1. Microhematuria
   a. Accompanied by proteinuria or pyuria
      (1) Evaluate with urine culture (cath specimen preferable).
      (2) If culture is negative, consider tuberculosis, fastidious organisms, chlamydia, medical renal disease, or papillary necrosis.
   b. Unaccompanied by proteinuria
      (1) Rule out urolithiasis, urothelial malignancy, and renal cell carcinoma with intravenous pyelogram (or renal ultrasonography and retrograde pyelography in the presence of azotemia), urine cytology and cystoscopy. Table 8-2 lists various radiologic studies available to evaluate renal anatomy and function.
      (2) Also exclude trauma, coagulopathy, sickle cell trait, foreign body, or pseudohematuria.
      (3) "Benign" hematuria is a diagnosis of exclusion.

TABLE 8-2.

Radiological Evaluation of the Kidneys

Study	Anatomy	Function	Utility
Abdominal film	*	—	Nephrolithiasis, intraurinary air
Intravenous pyelogram	***	*	Nephrolithiasis, obstruction, pyelonephritis, tumors
Retrograde pyelogram	****	*	Obstruction, filling defects
Cystogram	****	**	Bladder and lower urinary tract anatomy and function
Ultrasound	***	—	Renal size, hydronephrosis, tumor, and nephrolithiasis
CT	****	*	Renal, retroperitoneal, and adrenal anatomy
Technetium scan	*	***	Renal blood flow and glomerular filtration
Arteriogram	****	****	Renal vasculature, upper and lower urinary tract

2. Gross hematuria
   a. Upper tract
      (1) Posttraumatic
         (a) There is a high index of suspicion with penetrating trauma, lower rib fracture, lumbar transverse process fracture or hemodynamic instability.
         (b) Assess bilateral function with intravenous pyelography or CT scan—urgent renal arteriography if no perfusion documented to renal unit.
         (c) Practice conservative management unless there is penetrating trauma with associated visceral injury, renal pedicle injury, expanding retroperitoneal hematoma with hemodynamic instability, or extensive urinary extravasation.
      (2) Nontraumatic—exclusion of malignancy, nephrolithiasis, arterial venous malformation, etc.
   b. Lower tract
      (1) Urethral
         (a) There is a high index of suspicion with pelvic fracture, blood at the external meatus, prostatic displacement on digital rectal examination, penetrating pelvic trauma, or "anuria."

    (b) Evaluate with retrograde urethrography. Perform a suprapubic cystostomy for partial or complete urethral disruption with delayed primary repair.
    (c) There is a high index of suspicion for associated injury (rectal, vascular) after pelvic trauma.
  (2) Bladder
    (a) Cystography with drainage film
    (b) Immediate repair for free intraperitoneal extravasation
    (c) Extraperitoneal extravasation managed with foley drainage alone in the absence of other lower tract pathology
c. Intractible vesical hemorrhage
  (1) Multiple blood transfusions are required to declare vesical hemorrhage as intractible. It is usually the result of advanced pelvic malignancy, radiation, or cyclophosphamide induced hemorrhagic cystitis.
  (2) The mainstay of therapy is correction of contributing or exacerbating factors (coagulopathy, thrombocytopenia, etc.) and thorough clot evacuation with fulguration of any discreet bleeding points. If bleeding persists, continuous bladder irrigation via large bore three-way foley catheter is indicated.
    (a) Irrigate initially with normal saline followed by 1% alum or 1% silver nitrate solution.
    (b) In recalcitrant cases, the addition of systemic alpha-amino caproic acid may be beneficial (1 g IV q1 × 4 followed by 1 g IV q4h).

B. Urinary Obstruction

1. Upper tract obstruction
  a. Pathophysiology
    (1) Complete unilateral ureteral obstruction with normal contralateral kidney results in elevation of pressure in pyelocaliceal system, diminution of renal blood flow, progressive impairment of renal function, and atrophy of obstructed kidney.
    (2) Recovery of function after relief of obstruction is dependent on duration of obstruction, morphology of renal pelvis, and presence or absence of infection.
    (3) Compensatory hypertrophy of contralateral kidney occurs and is most marked in neonates.

b. Etiology
   (1) Intrinsic
      (a) Stones
      (b) Tumor—95% transitional cell carcinoma
      (c) Sloughed papilla—primarily seen in diabetes, sickle cell disease, or analgesic nephropathy
      (d) Clot—important to find source of bleeding; consideration of renal cell carcinoma, urothelial carcinoma, vascular anomalies
      (e) Stricture
         (i) Primary (congenital UPJ, obstructed megaureter)
         (ii) Secondary (stones, infection, TB, iatrogenic, or traumatic)
   (2) Extrinsic
      (a) Retroperitoneal tumor—lymphoma, sarcoma, metastatic carcinoma
      (b) Inflammatory processes—retroperitoneal fibrosis, abscess
      (c) Endometriosis
c. Diagnosis (Table 8-2.)
   (1) Intravenous pyelography
      (a) Preferred initial study in suspected obstruction in patient with normal renal function.
      (b) Delayed nephrogram, delayed excretion
   (2) Renal ultrasonography
      (a) Pelvocaliectasis suggestive of obstruction
      (b) May have obstruction without pelvocaliectasis or pelvocaliectasis without obstruction
      (c) Useful as screening modality (particularly in acutely azotemic patient)
   (3) Diuretic radionuclide renography
      (a) 99Tc DTPA scan is a useful functional study to assess whether upper tract obstruction exists by monitoring "washout" of radionuclide from renal pelvis after administration of loop diuretic.
      (b) Utility declines in presence of marked azotemia (creatinine >5).
   (4) Retrograde pyelography
      (a) "Gold standard"—excellent anatomic detail
      (b) Invasive—cystoscopy required

    (5) CT

        (a) Particularly useful in assessing extrinsic upper tract obstruction

        (b) Also useful in distinguishing radiolucent stone from tumor, clot, papilla (must have unenhanced as well as enhanced study)

  d. Treatment

    (1) Treatment varies with etiology of obstruction.

    (2) The goal is to relieve obstruction expeditiously to salvage renal function.

    (3) When obstruction is complicated by infection or azotemia, intervention is urgent.

    (4) When possible, retrograde ureteral stenting (JJ stent or ureteral catheter) is preferred.

  e. Indications for percutaneous nephrostomy

    (1) Failed retrograde attempt at relief of obstruction

    (2) High-grade obstruction with inability to achieve retrograde decompression as a result of anatomic factors such as inaccessible ureteral orifices, presence of urinary diversion (ileal loop, Kock pouch, etc.)

    (3) Urosepsis due to upper tract obstruction in patients with prohibitive anesthesia risk

2. Lower tract obstruction

  a. Pathophysiology

    (1) Lower tract obstruction is an anatomic or functional obstruction at, or distal to, bladder neck

    (2) Efficiency of bladder emptying is a result of strength of detrusor contraction relative to bladder neck/urethral resistance.

    (3) Micturition in the neurologically intact patient is a result of detrusor contraction with coordinated sphincter relaxation.

    (4) Chronically elevated bladder neck or urethral resistance results in detrusor hypertrophy, elevated micturitional detrusor pressure with ultimate decompensation resulting in elevated postvoid residual urine, or urinary retention.

        (a) Predisposes to urinary tract infection, bladder calculi, bladder diverticula

        (b) Elevated bladder pressures result in impairment of upper tract drainage with hydronephrosis.

        (c) In severe cases, lower tract obstruction may lead

to acute renal failure with attendent metabolic abnormalities (usually resolve with relief of obstruction).

b. Etiology

(1) Anatomic obstruction

(a) Benign prostatic hyperplasia (most common cause)

(b) Prostatic carcinoma

(i) Present in 50% to 75% of men over age 70

(ii) May also cause upper tract obstruction by local extension into bladder trigone

(c) Bladder neck hypertrophy

(d) Urethral stricture

(e) Miscellaneous causes including bladder/urethral stone, bladder tumor, clot in bladder, fecal impaction, foreign body, meatal stenosis, and phimosis

(2) Functional obstruction

(a) Hypocontractile neuropathic bladder is frequently seen in diabetes, sacral cord injury, spinal shock.

(b) Detrusor/sphincter dyssynergia

(i) Detrusor contraction associated with simultaneous sphincter contraction

(ii) Seen in spinal cord lesions above sacral reflex arch, multiple sclerosis

(iii) Results in incomplete emptying, elevated voiding pressure, and upper tract deterioration

(3) Pharmacologic retention

(a) Anticholinergics, cold preparations, antidepressants

(b) Narcotics

(c) Spinal or general anesthesia

(d) Ethanol

c. Diagnosis

(1) Evaluation is often prompted by obstructive voiding symptoms (hesitancy, decreased force of stream, postvoid dribbling, double voiding, intermittency, nocturia); may have mild urgency component

(2) Occasionally urinary retention or "anuria" is the

presenting sign; often postoperatively or after taking medications with anticholinergic effects.

    (3) Initial diagnostic test should be rectal examination and postvoid residual urine determination

        (a) Obtain urine for analysis and culture.

        (b) Check medications.

    (4) Other helpful diagnostic aids include cystourethroscopy, urodynamics, and retrograde urethrography.

  d. Treatment

    (1) Treatment depends on the etiology of obstruction, severity of obstruction, and presence or absence of infection/azotemia.

    (2) Anatomic obstruction generally at bladder neck is resolved by insertion of a foley catheter.

        (a) Larger catheters (18 to 22F) with coude tips are generally more effective if obstruction is at prostatic level.

        (b) Smaller catheters (12 to 14F) are more effective in urethral stricture disease.

    (3) Prior to manipulation of the infected lower urinary tract, broad-spectrum antibiotics should be administered, and the patient should be observed closely following manipulation for sign of sepsis.

    (4) Watch closely for postobstructive diuresis in the postrenally azotemic patient who has undergone relief of lower urinary tract (or bilateral upper tract) obstruction. Urine output should be replaced ½ ml/ml with D_5 ½ NS while monitoring serum electrolytes until resolution of the diuresis.

IV. PERIOPERATIVE MANAGEMENT OF THE RENAL SYSTEM

A. Established (Chronic) Renal Failure

  1. *Chronic renal failure* is a syndrome that results from the irreversible impairment or destruction of nephrons, regardless of cause, and is assigned when renal insufficiency persists for more than 3 months. Conditions encountered with this syndrome include impaired fluid and electrolyte regulation, suppressed erythropoiesis and immune function, atherosclerosis, hypertension, pericarditis, encephalitis, and distal neuropathy.

2. Perioperative considerations for patients with chronic renal failure.
   a. For elective procedures, dialyze preoperatively and postoperatively.
   b. Due to suppressed immune function, prophylactic antibiotics and careful wound management are essential.
3. Aggressive application of renal replacement therapy (usually hemodialysis or peritoneal dialysis) is essential to minimize complications of chronic renal failure patients in the perioperative setting.

B. Prevention of Acute Renal Failure

1. Maintenance of renal perfusion by aggressive management of hypovolemia, hypoxemia, and low cardiac output are goals in the prevention of ARF.
2. Contrast agents and nephrotoxic drugs should be used only when the benefits outweigh the risk of renal failure.
3. In posttraumatic cases where severe rhabdomyolysis may exist, diuretics, haptoglobin therapy, and alkaline solute diuresis may be protective from myoglobin-induced ARF.
4. Diuretics such as furosemide or mannitol afford renal protection through saluretic effects which clear the tubule of obstruction and prevent back leakage of filtrate.
   a. Mannitol produces an osmotic diuresis and increases renal blood flow to cortical areas.
   b. Loop diuretics such as furosemide and ethacrynic acid have also been tested, although evidence of protection from ARF is inconsistent.
5. Renal-dose dopamine (1 to 3 µg/kg/min) has no demonstrated efficacy in the prevention of ARF.

C. Preoperative Measures

1. Preoperative assessment of renal function includes a careful history and physical, urinalysis, plasma electrolytes, BUN, and creatinine, as well as urine volume. An accurate weight should be measured the night before operation.
2. Administer intravenous fluids the night prior to operation to maintain normal hydration while restricted by NPO orders.

D. Intraoperative Measures

1. Neuromuscular blocking agents such as pancuronium and tubocurarine may cause acidosis and hyperkalemia, and should be avoided in chronic renal failure patients and in those at risk for developing ARF.

2. Aggressive measures should be taken to avoid hypotensive episodes.
3. Maintain an accurate record of fluid balance throughout the operation, including urine output, blood loss, and fluid replacement. Use of vasoactive, inotropic, and diuretic agents should be noted for dose and corresponding response.

E. Postoperative Measures

1. Initial postoperative assessment should begin with careful review of intraoperative fluid balance (urine output, blood loss, and fluid replacement) and hemodynamic course.
2. Vital signs and urine output should be monitored immediately and throughout the postoperative period. Intravascular volume status must be assessed; invasive monitoring of CVP, PCWP, and/or cardiac output must be instituted for patients at risk for ARF, with major cardiac, vascular, or intraabdominal operations and in patients where volume status is difficult to determine. Daily weights are also essential.
3. Hourly urine output should be at least 0.5 to 1 ml/kg/hr. The quality of the urine should also be determined by urinalysis.
4. The presence of glycosuria must be identified and monitored at least q4h. Glucosuria reflects the metabolic control of serum glucose, and surgical stress may lead to glucosuria in up to 50% of surgical patients. Glucose acts as an osmotic diuretic and elevates urine output even if the patient has inadequate preload and renal perfusion.
5. Note deteriorating renal function and correct early. First identify and correct any postrenal etiologies. (See Section III, B.) Then eliminate prerenal etiologies of oliguria (Section V, A, 4b). Figure 8-1. illustrates the management algorithm for acute azotemia and oliguria.

V. MANAGEMENT OF ACUTE RENAL FAILURE (Fig. 8-1)

A. Classification of Acute Renal Failure

1. ARF by definition is an abrupt decrease in kidney function that results in accumulation of nitrogenous solutes (azotemia).
2. Urine output in ARF may be oliguric (urine output less than 400 ml per day) or nonoliguric, in which urine output is normal or increased while solute clearance is markedly

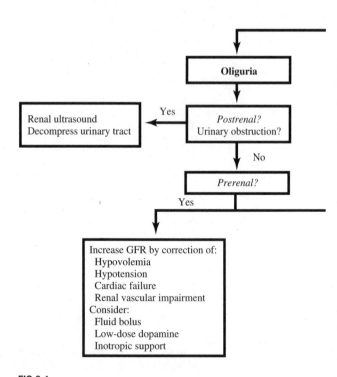

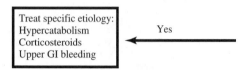

FIG 8-1.
Management algorithm for acute renal failure.

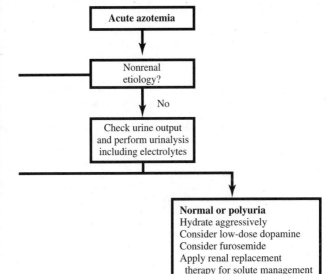

Acute azotemia

↓

Nonrenal etiology?

↓ No

Check urine output
and perform urinalysis
including electrolytes

Normal or polyuria
Hydrate aggressively
Consider low-dose dopamine
Consider furosemide
Apply renal replacement
  therapy for solute management

No

Parenchymal ARF
Discontinue nephrotoxic agent(s)
Treat underlying condition (sepsis, etc.)
Alkalinize urine for pigment nephropathy
Administer low-dose dopamine and furosemide
Apply renal replacement therapy for
solute and fluid management
Provide full protein and caloric support

impaired. Mortality from nonoliguric ARF is significantly less than from oliguric renal failure, although many cases progress to oliguria and have its poor outcome.

3. Regardless of urine output, the sequela of ARF is due to retention of metabolic wastes indicated by a progressive rise in BUN and serum creatinine concentrations. Hypervolemia and electrolyte imbalances further complicate management of oliguric ARF.

4. The pathogenesis of ARF is commonly classified as postrenal, prerenal, or intrinsic parenchymal disease.

   a. Postrenal ARF

      (1) Obstructive uropathy must always be ruled out in the oliguric patient.

      (2) Patients may complain of flank pain due to acute distention of the renal capsule or suprapubic discomfort caused by bladder distention.

      (3) Renal ultrasonography is a quick and simple procedure to evaluate the urinary outflow tract and detect the presence of calculi, tumor, or blood clot. (See Table 8-2.)

      (4) Removal of the obstruction should return renal function to normal.

      (5) Oliguria and uremia are unlikely to result from a unilateral obstruction without pathology in the contralateral kidney (Section III, B).

   b. Prerenal ARF

      (1) The etiology of ARF caused by hypoperfusion of the kidneys is classified as prerenal.

      (2) Surgical patients are at risk for hypovolemia and hypoperfusion, therefore any patient with oliguria should be assumed to be hypovolemic until proven otherwise. Typical circumstances which precipitate prerenal ARF in surgical patients are listed in Table 8-3.

TABLE 8-3.

Causes of Prerenal ARF in Surgical Patients

Volume Changes	Hemodynamic Changes	Vascular Changes
Dehydration	Septic shock	Renal artery stenosis
Blood loss	Cardiogenic shock	Renal vein thrombosis
Third space sequestration	Neurogenic hypotension	Operative vessel occlusion

(3) Evaluation of prerenal etiology of ARF includes the following:
    (a) Review recent fluid balances over the past hours and days. Fluid output significantly greater than input suggests a prerenal etiology of oliguria.
    (b) Review weight changes over the past days. Weight loss in the acute setting is most likely secondary to fluid loss.
    (c) Determine the extent of insensitive losses from diarrhea, sweat, ascites, pleural effusions, and third space sequestration due to SBO. Fluid loss also occurs with large open wounds or burns. Large amounts of intravascular volume may be lost via these routes.
    (d) Assess renal perfusion according to MAP and Do_2
    (e) Identify factors that may increase renal vein pressure and decrease renal perfusion including mean airway pressure, right ventricular failure, and increased intraabdominal pressure.

(4) Results of urinalysis are often helpful in discerning prerenal versus parenchymal etiology of ARF according to Table 8-4.
    (a) In the presence of tubular injury, urine osmolality is close to that of plasma due to lack of tubular concentrating ability. Conversely, a

TABLE 8-4.

Diagnostic Urine Chemistry

Test	Prerenal	Intrinsic (ATN)
Glomerular filtration		
Creatinine clearance (ml/min)	>40	<20
Urine/plasma creatinine	>40	<20
Water reabsorption		
Specific gravity	>1.024	<1.015
Urine osmolarity (mOsm/L)	>400	<350
Urine/plasma osmolarity ratio	>1.5	<1
Sodium Reabsorpton		
Urine sodium (mEq/L)	<20	>30
Fe_{Na} (%)	<1	>1
Urea		
Urine/plasma urea	>8	<3
BUN/creat$_{serum}$	>20	<15

U_{osm} greater than 500 demonstrates excellent concentrating function and is suggestive of prerenal etiology.

(b) In the presence of hypovolemia and hypoperfusion, the renin-angiotensin system is activated and the subsequent release of aldosterone will induce the kidney to reabsorb sodium. Therefore an FE_{Na} less than one is indicative of volume depletion while an elevated FE_{Na} is more consistent with tubular injury or obstruction.

(c) Caution must be taken in interpreting any of these parameters in the presence of a preexisting prerenal state (e.g., CHF, cirrhosis), diuretics, or after the use of contrast dye.

(5) With established oliguria, monitoring CVP, PCWP, and cardiac output is essential to optimize and preserve renal perfusion.

(6) Administration of a fluid challenge (250 to 500 ml in an adult) and restoration of normal renal perfusion will usually result in increased urine output when oliguria is due to prerenal causes.

c. Parenchymal ARF

After excluding prerenal and postrenal causes of oliguria, parenchymal etiologies of ARF must be considered. These include acute tubular necrosis, pigment nephropathy (resulting from circulating myoglobin and hemoglobin), and nephrotoxic agents (various drugs and contrast material). Other causes of parenchymal renal disease such as acute glomerular nephritis and vasculitis are not typically responsible for ARF in the surgical patient.

(1) ATN

(a) ATN results from ischemia to the renal parenchyma and is the most common pathology of ARF.

(b) Under conditions of diminishing renal blood flow, perfusion of the kidneys is first maintained by vasomotor responses which dilate the afferent arteriole and constrict the efferent arteriole. As continued hypotension is detected by the juxtaglomerular apparatus, the renin-angiotensin system is activated in concert with sympathetic release of other vasoactive hormones. These substances produce vasoconstriction of the afferent arteriole and further exacerbate cortical hypoperfusion. As a result, GFR is sharply reduced, and the tubules experience profound ischemia. As a result of damage to the tubular system, casts of cellular debris obstruct the lumen and cellular edema occurs. As tubular cells necrose and slough off, glomerular ultrafiltrate leaks back across the proximal tubular membrane into the interstitium. This "back leakage" of luminal fluid into the peritubular space causes vascular congestion within the renal parenchyma and may prolong ARF.

(2) Pigment nephropathy (myoglobinuria and hemoglobinuria)

    (a) Pigment nephropathy due to hemolysis or rhabdomyolysisis is a common cause of ARF and may occur after trauma, burn, operation, CPB, seizures, alcohol or drug intoxication, prolonged ischemia to muscle groups, or extended coma.

    (b) With ischemia or blunt injury to large muscle masses, myoglobin is released into the circulation. In the kidney it is filtered from blood and reabsorbed by the tubule. Although myoglobin is not a direct nephrotoxin, in the presence of aciduria, myoglobin is converted to ferrihemate which is toxic to renal cells.

    (c) Diagnosis can be made with elevated CPK, serum hemoglobin or myoglobin, and a urine microscopy that shows prominent heme pigment without RBCs in the urine sediment. Hyperkalemia and elevated serum creatinine are also consistent with injury to muscle masses.

    (d) Prevention of myoglobin-induced ARF include generous hydration, use of diuretics, and alkalinization of urine to a pH greater than 6.

(3) Nephrotoxic agents

    (a) Contrast media: Radiographic contrast dye has been documented to cause ARF. The incidence of contrast nephropathy is approximately 1% to 10% and may be predicted according to a number of risk factors. These include contrast load, age, preexisting renal insufficiency, and diabetes. The incidence in patients with normal renal function is significantly lower at 1% to 2%. Contrast nephropathy is usually experienced as an asymptomatic, transient rise in creatinine but may progress to oliguric renal failure requiring hemodialysis. Induced diuresis with fluids and diuretics prior to contrast injection may decrease the incidence and severity of ARF in high-risk patients.

    (b) Nephrotoxic drugs: Drug-induced ARF is responsible for approximately 5% of all cases of ARF. The pathophysiology of drug-induced ARF differs according to the offending agent. The site of damage of several well-documented nephrotoxic drugs is listed in Table 8-5. Through normal reabsorption and secretion, the kidney is exposed to high concentrations of drugs and solutes which may be toxic. This is compounded by hypovolemia, which causes increased reabsorption of water and solutes and exposes the lumen to even higher concentrations of toxins.

B. General Care of ARF Patients

  1. In surgical patients, ARF rarely occurs in an isolated fashion. Rather, ARF is only one component of an MOF syndrome often accompanied by infection. Therefore management of these patients should be focused on treatment of the underlying disease process(es). Development of ARF complicates the care of surgical patients by introducing difficulties to fluid, electrolyte, and nutritional management. The adverse effects of renal replacement therapies further compound these problems. A favorable outcome can be accomplished only through aggressive intervention. This includes surgical drainage of septic foci, excision of necrotic tissue, early implementation of effective renal replacement therapy, and full nutritional support.

    a. Nonoliguric ARF

      (1) Treatment for nonoliguric ARF patients may differ

TABLE 8-5.
Nephrotoxic Drugs

Glomerulus	Renal Arterioles	Proximal Tubule	Distal Tubule	Interstitial
Heroin	Allopurinol	Aminoglycosides	Amphotericin B	Acetaminophen
Hydralazine	Penicillin G	Amphotericin B	Lithium	Aspirin
Penicillamine	Propothiouracil	Cephaloridine	Vitamin D intoxication	Methicillin
Probenecid	Sulfonamides	Polymixin B		Penicillin G
Procainamide	Thiazides			Phenacetin

only slightly from treatment required for identical patients with normal renal function.

   (2) Except for an elevated BUN, management of fluids, solutes, and nutrition is usually unaffected by nonoliguric ARF.

   (3) The extent of renal dysfunction is limited and almost always reversible. Use of renal replacement therapies (and their inherent complications) is rarely necessary.

  b. Oliguric ARF

   (1) Problems of fluid overload can lead to anasarca, pulmonary edema, and CHF.

   (2) The pharmacokinetics of drugs become difficult to predict as a result of decreased elimination and increased volume of distribution. Adjustments of dosages should be made according to Section VI.

   (3) In light of these risks, the volume status of patients with ARF must be carefully monitored. Fluid intake and output must be precisely tabulated and weight measured daily. PA catheterization may be necessary to more closely monitor the fluid status of these patients.

   (4) Treatment options for hypervolemia consist of fluid restriction and/or fluid removal with artificial kidney techniques. However, nutrition and other critical medications are essential to postoperative recovery and should not be limited. Renal replacement should be selected and conducted to allow full nutrition without restriction.

   (5) Dopamine

     (a) The renal circulation contains specific vasodilating dopaminergic receptors that respond to dopamine in low doses (1 to 3 µg/kg/min).

     (b) This dose (commonly referred to as "renal dose") dopamine has been shown to increase renal blood flow, GFR, and urine output.

     (c) In addition, the combination of low-dose dopamine and furosemide have shown synergism in successfully converting oliguric to nonoliguric ARF.

     (d) For these reasons, renal-dose dopamine is

accepted as effective in the treatment of established ARF.

  (e) However, its usefulness in preventing ARF is doubtful. It is also important to note that dopamine will cause renal vasoconstriction when administered in doses above 5 to 10 µg/kg/min.

c. Electrolyte derangements in ARF

  (1) Perform serum electrolyte measurements daily.

  (2) Hyperkalemia (serum potassium > 6.5 mEq/L) is a medical emergency and a frequent electrolyte disorder with ARF.

    (a) Under the conditions of hypercatabolism and tissue necrosis that characterize these patients, large amounts of potassium may be generated and accumulate over a short period of time.

    (b) Acute hyperkalemia decreases cardiac excitability which may ultimately result in asystole. These events are usually preceded by changes in the electrocardiogram that indicate hyperkalemia. These include loss of p waves, widening of the QRS complex, and peaked T waves.

  (3) Hyponatremia, hyperphosphatemia, hypocalcemia, and metabolic acidosis are also common with ARF and must be monitored closely. Treatment consists of appropriate additions or restrictions to intravenous solutions and effective use of the artificial kidney.

d. Hematologic derangements in ARF

  (1) Anemia

    (a) In addition to blood loss because of hemorrhage or operation, erythropoietin production has been shown to decrease in direct proportion with decreasing renal function.

    (b) In the surgical patient with ARF, PRBCs should be transfused to maintain a hematocrit greater than 30%.

  (2) Platelets

    (a) Although poorly understood, platelet dysfunction and coagulopathy are often associated with ARF. A reproducible platelet defect can be demonstrated experimentally with a BUN of 100 mg/dl. However, the cause of this defect has yet to be identified.

(b) Platelets should be transfused to maintain a platelet count greater than 100,000 per high power field.

2. Nutrition and ARF

a. The goal of nutritional support in ARF is to provide optimal amounts of caloric and protein substrates to minimize autocatabolism and allow tissue anabolism, wound healing, and sustained immune function, thereby enhancing chance for recovery.

b. Nutrition for acute versus chronic renal failure patients

(1) In chronic renal failure, patients are generally healthy with energy requirements that differ little from normal individuals. Protein intake is required only for metabolic turnover and is restricted to minimize urea generation and other products of protein metabolism.

(2) By contrast, the metabolic requirements of ARF patients are those of a critically ill hospitalized patient. Actual measurement of resting energy expenditure has shown caloric requirements of MOF patients with an ARF average 50% above normal, healthy individuals. Measured protein requirements are also increased to as much as 2 g/kg in order to provide for anabolic wound healing and sustained immune function. For these patients, protein restriction is counterproductive and potentially detrimental.

3. Special considerations in surgical patients: The mortality rate of ARF in surgical patients is significantly greater than in medical patients.

a. Burns

(1) The burn patient is at risk for developing ARF due to hypovolemia, sepsis, and myoglobinuria.

(2) Effective fluid and electrolyte resuscitation should prevent hypovolemia, and renal failure is rare in burn injury.

(3) When burn or trauma produces muscle necrosis and myoglobinuria, renal failure is common.

(4) The use of daily hemodialysis in massively burned

patients does not improve survival, suggesting that neither nitrogenous wastes nor soluble toxins play a role in burn mortality.

b. CPB

(1) The incidence of ARF after cardiac operation is approximately 1% to 2%.

(2) Blood flow which is nonpulsatile during CPB will only exacerbate renal ischemia if total body oxygen delivery is inadequate.

(3) Some hemolysis always occurs during CPB which may cause ARF if it becomes excessive.

(4) Perioperative low cardiac output is the most important consideration in the development of ARF.

c. Liver failure

(1) The development of ARF secondary to liver dysfunction is referred to as the "hepatorenal syndrome" (HRS).

(2) Clinically, HRS is slowly progressive and characterized by intense sodium chloride retention with absence of sodium chloride in urine.

(3) The ensuing renal dysfunction is unresponsive to volume or hemodynamic maneuvers.

(4) HRS commonly occurs in alcoholic cirrhosis but is also reported in patients with cholestatic jaundice, acute hepatitis, and hepatic malignancy.

(5) Regardless of etiology, patients with HRS are characterized by portal hypertension and tense ascites, although the degree of jaundice may be variable.

(6) Management should focus on the state of the intravascular volume in light of ascites and hypoproteinemia. Sodium and fluid intake is carefully restricted.

(7) In severe cases, a peritoneovenous (LeVeen) shunt may correct the maldistribution of extracellular fluid in HRS and aid management of ARF.

d. Sepsis

(1) Infection is the major cause of death in surgical patients who develop ARF.

(2) Sepsis can also cause ARF through direct and indirect effects which cause both renal injury (ATN) and prerenal azotemia.

(a) Direct effects include endotoxin and prostaglandin damage to the renal microvasculature.

(b) Indirect effects include hypotension, impaired regional Do_2, and metabolic disturbances that may result in ATN.

(c) In addition, management of septicemia often requires the use of nephrotoxic antibiotics which may further exacerbate tubular damage.

(3) Prophylactic antibiotics and aggressive wound management are required to prevent sepsis in ARF patients.

e. Trauma

(1) Like thermal injury, the development of ARF in the posttraumatic patient is multifactorial, and hypovolemia is the major problem. Rapid fluid resuscitation must be instituted to avoid shock, which may lead to ARF if untreated.

(2) If after stabilization and restoration of intravascular volume the patient becomes oliguric, the possibility of traumatic injury to the ureter, bladder, or urethra must be ruled out.

(3) With blunt trauma to large muscle masses, rhabdomyolysis-induced ARF is a significant concern. Microscopic urinalysis for myoglobin and serum CPK measurements will define the extent of muscle injury and risk for developing ARF. Prevention of ARF in this circumstance may be accomplished by prompt induction of an alkaline solute diuresis using intravenous mannitol and sodium bicarbonate.

f. Vascular surgery

(1) The incidence of ARF in vascular surgery is directly related to the position and duration of cross clamping the aorta or renal vessels as well as preexisting renal disease.

(2) Resection of a thoracic aortic aneurysm requires clamping of the aorta proximal to the renal arteries. ARF has been reported to occur in as many as 50% of patients undergoing thoracic aortic aneurysm repair. However, the rate of ARF after resection of abdominal aortic aneurysms (in which renal blood flow is usually maintained) is approximately 7%.

4. Prognosis
   a. Survival of patients with ARF is a function of the successful treatment of the primary disease(s) from which the renal failure was derived. The mortality rate of ischemic ATN without other organ failure is 6%. By contrast, the mortality rate of MOF complicated by ARF ranges from 40% to 80%
   b. Outcome of ARF is related to the number of organ systems failed, the interval from onset of ARF to first dialysis, the maximum serum creatinine prior to dialysis, and the presence of cardiac failure. In patients with ARF, 90% of the deaths can be attributed to sepsis or MOF.
   c. Both survival and recovery of renal function is better in patients with nonoliguric versus oliguric ARF.
   d. In patients who survive the acute phase of illness, recovery of renal function after ARF is dependent on the type and extent of injury to the renal parenchyma.
      (1) Renal replacement therapy may be required for several weeks until urine output and solute excretion return to acceptable levels.
      (2) If renal function has not returned after six weeks, recovery is unlikely and provisions should be made for long-term renal substitution therapy.

VI. RENAL REPLACEMENT THERAPIES
A. General Guidelines

1. The artificial kidney was introduced in the form of hemodialysis by Kolff in 1944 and demonstrated that ARF is potentially reversible. Since that time, hemodialysis has become the standard of care for sustaining the lives of patients who will otherwise die from renal disease.
2. Indications for use of renal replacement therapy include fluid overload (pulmonary edema, CHF), hyperkalemia, metabolic acidosis, uremic encephalopathy, coagulopathy, and acute poisoning. Recent data indicate that initiation of renal replacement early in the course of ARF correlates with improved outcome.
3. Volume (IV fluids, TPN, etc.) should be given as needed for the patient, independent of method of renal replacement. Priority must be placed on treatment of the underlying disease processes, and renal replacement selected and

performed to allow usual treatment of the critically ill surgical patient.

4. Renal replacement therapy should be instituted early in the course of ARF, before hypervolemia, azotemia, or hyperkalemia occur.

5. Currently, three modalities of renal replacement therapy are available for treatment of ARF in the critically ill patient: (1) hemodialysis, (2) peritoneal dialysis, and (3) continuous arteriovenous hemofiltration. The features of these therapies are described and contrasted in Table 8-6.

B. Hemodialysis

1. Description of technique

   a. The patient's blood is pumped via an extracorporeal circuit through a porous hollow–fiber membrane (artificial kidney), which is permeable to solutes of less than two thousand daltons. An isotonic solution surrounds the membrane, which provides a concentration gradient for the selective removal of solutes, such as potassium, urea, and creatinine, while maintaining plasma concentrations of sodium, chloride, and bicarbonate.

   b. Vascular access consists of an arteriovenous shunt or a double lumen venovenous access. Percutaneous venovenous catheters are usually placed in the ICU at the bedside for initial therapy. The catheter and access site should be changed frequently to prevent sepsis. Placement of permanent access (subcutaneous arteriovenous shunt) is indicated if renal replacement is required for more than two weeks with no signs of renal recovery.

   c. Systemic anticoagulation is required for this procedure, although less heparin may be used on patients with a baseline coagulopathy.

   d. Hemodialysis is typically performed every other day for a three to four hour period but will be required more frequently in catabolic patients with a high urea generation rate.

   e. Solute and volume removal is considered very efficient with hemodialysis in comparison to the other methods of renal replacement.

2. Advantages

   a. Hemodialysis is the method of choice for rapid removal of life-threatening electrolyte imbalances, toxins, and poisons.

TABLE 8-6.
Comparison of Renal Replacement Therapies

Description	Therapy		
	Hemodialysis	Peritoneal Dialysis	CAVHD
Assessment	Rapid-intermittent	Slow-intermittent	Slow-continuous
Vascular access	Arteriovenous or venovenous	Abdominal catheter	Arteriovenous or venovenous
Anticoagulation	Usually required	None required	Required
Solute removal	Excellent	Excellent	Excellent
Fluid removal	Excellent	Good	Excellent
Hemodynamic instability	Potentially significant in critically-ill patients	None	None
Risks of procedure	Hypotension	Infection/peritonitis	Hypovolemia
	Hemorrhage	Intraabdominal adhesions	Hemorrhage
	Dysequilibrium syndrome	Respiratory distress	Electrolyte imbalance
Overall appraisal	Useful for urgent removal of solutes or poisons	Contraindicated after recent open abdominal operation	Broad flexibility with fluid and electrolyte balance
	Hemodynamic instability limits use in ICU patients	Useful in burn and cardiac patients and patients with poor vascular access	Solute removal and fluid management of CAVHD equals hemodialysis

b. Hemodialysis may also be applied to hemodynamically stable surgical patients with isolated ARF where contraindication for peritoneal dialysis exists (i.e., postoperative laparotomy).

3. Disadvantages

a. In critically ill surgical patients with ARF, hemodialysis can cause hypotension, hypoxemia, and hemolysis, and can precipitate cardiac arrhythmias. These events limit the application of dialysis in unstable patients.

b. Anticoagulation is also required and may be undesirable in the immediate postoperative or posttrauma setting.

c. Acute CNS disturbances ranging from mild stupor to coma can occur with hemodialysis and are described as the "disequilibrium syndrome." It is attributed to rapid intracellular and extracellular fluid and electrolyte movement across the brain.

C. Peritoneal Dialysis

1. Description of technique

a. Peritoneal dialysis is performed by infusion of several liters of a sterile electrolyte solution with hypertonic dextrose into the abdominal space. Using the peritoneal membrane as a selective barrier, the dialysate solution creates an osmotic pressure gradient that extracts extracellular fluid and solutes out of the mesenteric circulation and into the peritoneal cavity. This fluid is then drained after an equilibration period of 1 to 2 hours.

b. Fluid removal usually ranges from 0.5 to 2 L/hr, although greater fluid and solute clearance can be accomplished by using larger volumes of dialysate, increasing the frequency of exchange cycles, or using a higher dextrose concentration in the dialysate.

c. Tenckhoff catheter placement can be performed in the ICU or the operating room. (See Chapter 5.)

2. Advantages

a. Peritoneal dialysis does not require vascular access or systemic anticoagulation, which makes it useful in patients with peripheral vascular disease or risk of hemorrhage. It is also the treatment of choice for the postcardiothoracic surgical patient with ARF.

b. In addition, the slow rate of equilibrium and fluid extraction with peritoneal dialysis minimizes the problems of disequilibrium and hemodynamic compromise experienced with conventional hemodialysis.

3. Disadvantages
   a. Catheter infection and peritonitis considerations include the following:
      (1) Rigid peritoneal catheters inserted percutaneously in the acute setting become predictably colonized after 48 to 72 hours.
      (2) Subcutaneously-placed silastic catheters are associated with a lower incidence of peritonitis (1.6 episodes per patient-year) and should be implanted with prolonged use of peritoneal dialysis.
      (3) Other access-related complications include visceral injury at the time of catheter placement and formation of intraabdominal adhesions.
   b. Hyperglycemia can occur as a result of the hypertonic glucose of the dialysate.
   c. Respiratory distress may develop from reduced diaphragmatic compliance and increased intraabdominal pressure.
   d. Repeated lavage of the peritoneal cavity causes protein loss of 10 g/day or more and may exacerbate malnutrition in catabolic ARF patients.

D. Continuous Arteriovenous Hemodialysis

1. Description of technique
   a. CAVHD was conceived by Kramer in 1977 and is specifically intended for treatment of ARF in the ICU.
   b. CAVHD is an extracorporeal ultrafiltration technique that removes extracellular fluid across a synthetic membrane via the hydrostatic pressure gradient created between indwelling arterial and venous catheters.
   c. With a systolic BP of 80 mm Hg or more, blood flows through the porous hollow-fiber capillary membrane at a rate of 50 to 150 ml/min, driving plasma water and solutes of up to 10,000 daltons (ultrafiltrate) out of the hemofilter at 500 to 700 ml/hr.
   d. Arteriovenous access is accomplished by percutaneous cannulation of the femoral artery and vein with a low incidence of complications.
   e. Heparinization of the extracorporeal circuit is required, usually at a rate of 500 U/hr.

   f. CAVHD utilizes a dialysate solution that is circulated in the extracapillary space countercurrent to blood flow. This creates a concentration gradient for selective removal of large amounts of solute. The ultrafiltration rate is regulated to achieve desired net fluid balance and no substitution fluid is necessary (Fig. 8-2).

   g. CAVHD is run continuously for as many days as renal replacement is required. Hemofilter performance (as

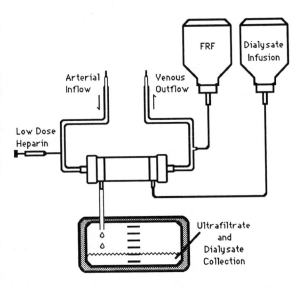

FIG 8-2.

Continuous arteriovenous hemodialysis (CAVHD). CAVHD combines the advantages of continuous hemofiltration with the selective properties and clearance capabilities of hemodialysis. A sterile dialysate solution is infused countercurrent to hemofilter blood flow and provides a concentration gradient for selective removal of large amounts of uremic solutes. (From Mault JR, et al: *Continuous hemofiltration: a reference guide for SCUF, CAVH, and CAVHD,* 1990, University of Michigan Printing.)

monitored by the ultrafiltration rate) decreases over time, requiring replacement with a new hemofilter approximately every two days.

2. Advantages of CAVHD
   a. Little or no incidence of hemodynamic instability is encountered with treatment of unstable critically ill ARF patients. This is attributed to slow and continuous fluid and solute removal in addition to the low blood activating properties of the hemofilter membrane.
   b. CAVHD permits generous flexibility with volume management and eliminates the need for fluid restriction in oliguric ARF. Fluid balance and serum electrolyte concentrations can be titrated to any value, and optimum amounts of nutrition can be provided.
   c. Solute clearance is approximately equal to that which standard hemodialysis can achieve.

3. Disadvantages of CAVHD
   a. Dehydration and electrolyte imbalance may occur as a result of continuous fluid and electrolyte removal.
   b. Hemorrhage may occur as a result of systemic anticoagulation.

4. Management considerations of CAVHD
   a. Ultrafiltration rate
      (1) The ultrafiltration rate is dependent on the patient's BP, the blood flow through the hemofilter, the available free water, and distance between the collection container and the hemofilter.
      (2) In order to prevent excess hemoconcentration of blood at the venous end of the hemofilter (which decreases hemofilter performance and longevity), the maximum ultrafiltration rate (UFR_{max}) should be calculated. First, the hemofilter blood flow rate (BF) is calculated from the circuit time (recorded upon unclamping the hemofilter blood tubing) and the hemofilter circuit volume as follows:

$$BF \ (ml/min) = \frac{circuit \ volume \ (ml)}{circuit \ time \ (sec)} \times \frac{60 \ sec}{min}$$

Next, determine the plasma flow (PF) and UFR_{max}:

$$PF \text{ (ml/min)} = BF \times \frac{(100\% - \text{hematocrit})}{100}$$

$$UFR_{max} \text{ (ml/min)} = 0.2^* \times PF$$

(*For hematocrit less than 40%, use 0.3.)

(3) In CAVHD, both the dialysate and the ultrafiltrate fluids will drain through the ultrafiltrate line into the collection container. To determine the actual UFR, subtract the dialysate infusion rate (DI) from the total fluid collected (TFC) as follows:

$$UFR_{CAVHD} \text{ (ml/min)} = TFC \text{ (ml/min)} - DI \text{ (ml/min)}$$

(4) As described earlier, the clearance capabilities of CAVHD eliminate the need for replacement fluid and limit the use of ultrafiltration to maintenance of a desired fluid balance (DFB). Therefore by using a Hoffman clamp or volumetric control pump on the ultrafiltrate line, the TFC is limited to the sum of the DI plus total IV fluids (TIV) minus all other fluid output (OFO—i.e., urine output, chest tube, and nasogastric drainage), plus or minus the DFB (for a net negative fluid balance, add DFB; for a net positive fluid balance, subtract DFB) as follows:

$$TFC \text{ (ml/hr)} = DI \text{ (ml/hr)} + TIV \text{ (ml/hr)} \\ - OFO \text{ (ml/hr)} + DFB \text{ (ml/hr)}$$

   (a) The minimum TFC allowed equals the rate of DI and must not be restricted below that rate.
   (b) If the calculated TFC is less than the dialysate infusion rate, then a filter replacement fluid (FRF) should be infused to make up the difference.

(5) Thrombus accumulation in the hemofilter will cause decreased blood flow and a subsequent decrease in UFR. If the systolic blood pressure is 80 mm Hg or greater, and the unrestricted UFR is 100 ml/hr or

less, the hemofilter should be discontinued to prevent thrombosis of the vascular access. Increasing the heparin infusion will not reverse clotting that has occurred in the hemofilter and should not be attempted as a means of "saving the filter."

b. Anticoagulation

   (1) The objective of heparinization in continuous hemofiltration is to prevent thrombosis of blood in the hemofilter without necessarily affecting systemic anticoagulation. This objective may or may not be achieved with an individual patient. In most cases, a continuous heparin infusion of approximately 7 to 10 U/kg/hr is administered to patients with normal clotting times; hemofilter longevity averages 48 hours. However, a single hemofilter may last several days with little or no heparin in a patient with a coagulopathy.

   (2) To monitor anticoagulation status, the ACT (normal range 100 to 120 seconds) should be checked frequently. The ACT is a measure of whole blood clotting and is the prefered method for monitoring heparin therapy. (If the ACT is unavailable, TCT or PTT can be effectively substituted.)

c. Fluid and electrolyte balance

   (1) Strict records of all fluids in and out are essential.

   (2) In CAVHD, approximately 8 to 14 L of ultrafiltrate are removed per day according to patient conditions. This ultrafiltrate contains uremic solutes (urea and creatinine) but also essential solutes (Na^+, Cl^-, HCO_3^-, etc.) that must be replaced. The concentrations of these solutes in the ultrafiltrate are identical to those in the patient's plasma. Solute losses can be calculated by multiplying the plasma concentration by the UFR.

d. Drug clearance

   (1) All non–protein-bound drugs will be cleared with the ultrafiltrate. These losses should be compensated by increasing dosages to maintain therapeutic levels.

   (2) The amount of drug clearance (DC) can be estimated from the plasma concentration of the drug

([D]$_p$), the percent of drug-protein binding (%PB), and the UFR as follows:

$$DC \text{ (amount/min)} = [D]_P \times UFR \times (100\% - \%PB)$$

e. Complications
   (1) For severe hypotension, clamp the ultrafiltrate line, but allow the blood flow to continue through the hemofilter. The heparin infusion must also be maintained. With CAVHD, the FRF infusion may be continued if required to expand intravascular volume. With CAVHD, the dialysate infusion must be discontinued when clamping the ultrafiltrate line.
   (2) If any portion of the extracorporeal circuit becomes disconnected, immediately occlude the arterial and venous cannulae, and disconnect the hemofilter circuit.
   (3) Any change in ultrafiltrate color to pink or red indicates rupture of a hemofilter capillary and requires immediate removal and replacement.
f. Discontinuing hemofiltration
   (1) If the maximum unrestricted UFR is 100 ml/hr or less, discontinue hemofiltration.
   (2) If the ultrafiltrate color changes to pink or red, indicating hollow-fiber rupture, discontinue hemofiltration.
   (3) If renal function recovers sufficiently (urine output, decreasing BUN and creatinine) so that all IVs and nutrition can be maintained without fluid restriction, discontinue hemofiltration.
   (4) If renal function is not recovered when all other organ failure(s) have resolved, the patient should be treated with hemodialysis or peritoneal dialysis.

SUGGESTED READING

Abel RM et al: Improved survival from acute renal failure after treatment with intravenous essential 1-amino acids and glucose: results of a prospective double-blind study, *N Engl J Med* 288:695-99, 1973.

Bartlett RH et al: Continuous arteriovenous hemofiltration: improved survival in surgical acute renal failure?, *Surgery* 100:400-408, 1986.

Bennett WM: Guide to drug dosage in renal failure, *Clin Pharmacokinet* 15:326-54, 1988.

Bywaters EGL, Beall D: Crush injuries with impairment of renal function, *Br Med J* 1:427-434, 1941.

Cioffi WG, Taka A, Gamelli RL: Probability of surviving postoperative acute renal failure, *Ann Surg* 200:205-211, 1984.

Graziani G et al: Dopamine and furosemide in oliguric acute renal failure, *Nephron* 37:39-42, 1984.

Kramer P et al: Arteriovenous hemofiltration: a new and simple method for treatment of overhydrated patients resistant to diuretics, *Klin Wochenschr* 55:1121-2, 1977.

Mault JR et al: *Continuous hemofiltration: a reference guide for SCUF, CAVH, and CAVHD,* Ann Arbor, Mich, 1990, University of Michigan Printers.

Schetz M, Lauwers PM, Ferdinande P: Extracorporeal treatment of acute renal failure in the intensive care unit: a critical review, *Intensive Care Med* 15:349-357, 1989.

Schwab SJ et al: Contrast nephrotoxicity: a randomized controlled trail of a nonionic and an ionic radiographic contrast agent, *N Engl J Med* 320:149-53, 1989.

Spurney RF, Fulkerson WJ, Schwab SJ: Acute renal failure in critically ill patients: prognosis for recovery of kidney function after prolonged dialysis support, *Crit Care Med* 19:8-11, 1991.

Vander AJ: *Renal physiology,* ed 4, New York, 1991, McGraw-Hill.

THE GASTROINTESTINAL SYSTEM

9

Ravi S. Chari

I. GASTROINTESTINAL HEMORRHAGE
A. Etiology
1. Upper GI bleeding
   a. Peptic ulceration (either gastric or duodenal)
      (1) Most common cause of upper GI bleeding
      (2) Etiology in 40% to 50% of patients with upper GI bleeding
      (3) Duodenal more common than gastric
   b. Esophageal varices
      (1) 90% to 95% of esophageal varices in the United States result from portal hypertension.
      (2) The mortality rate in patients with cirrhosis is 20% to 80% per bleed.
      (3) Rupture is related to the size of the varix and to wall tension (LaPlace's law).
      (4) 50% of patients with varices bleed from other sources.
      (5) The rate of rebleeding is >70% (usually within 6 weeks).
   c. Mallory-Weiss (mucosal tears at the GE junction)
   d. Erosive gastritis or esophagitis
      (1) Usually slow intermittent bleed causing chronic anemia
      (2) Often results from NSAID use
   e. Dieulafoy arteriovenous malformation
   f. Neoplasms
2. Lower GI bleeding
   a. Common etiologies

   (1) Diverticular disease
   (2) Angiodysplasia
   (3) Neoplasms
   b. Less common etiologies
   (1) Inflammatory bowel disease
   (2) Meckel's diverticulum
   (3) Hemorrhoids

B. Management

1. Resuscitation: Over 80% of all GI bleeding resolves spontaneously and requires only resuscitative care.
   a. Initiate volume replacement.
   (1) Place two large bore (14 or 16 gauge) peripheral IV catheters.
   (2) Infuse crystalloid solution (LR).
   (3) Consider blood transfusion if blood losses >30%.
   b. Perform initial laboratory studies.
   (1) Blood specimens should be obtained and sent for CBC, electrolytes, PT/PTT, type and crossmatch for 6 U of PRBC.
   (2) Hematocrit should be determined every 4 hours during the resuscitation. Hematocrit may not fall for 12 to 36 hours after a bleed; significant blood loss may have occurred despite a normal hematocrit.

2. History and physical examination include the following:
   a. Determine the frequency and duration of the hematemesis or number of melenic stools.
   b. Perform a digital rectal examination.
   (1) The exam may document blood in the GI tract.
   (2) Melena may occur with as little as 50 ml upper GI bleeding.
   c. Use vital signs to help estimate the magnitude of blood loss.
   (1) Loss of 15% to 30% total blood volume: Tachycardia, narrowed pulse pressure, orthostatic hypotension, delayed capillary refill
   (2) Loss of >30% blood volume: Hypotension on recumbency, oliguria

3. A fluid challenge will also help estimate fluid loss. Infuse 2 L lactated Ringer's solution
   a. Vital signs return to normal and stabilize: 15% to 30% blood loss

       b. BP rises but decreases again: 30% to 40% blood loss

       c. Blood pressure continues to fall: >40% blood loss

    4. Monitor volume replacement.

       a. Foley catheter (maintain output > 30 ml/hr)

       b. Hemodynamic monitoring

          (1) CVP measurements

          (2) PA catheter when indicated

    5. Administer blood products.

       a. PRBC

          (1) PRBC use is based on the amount of estimated blood loss and rate of ongoing loss.

          (2) Warmed blood prevents hypothermia and related complications.

       b. Other blood products

          (1) Consider FFP after 6 U PRBC.

          (2) Consider platelet administration after 10 U PRBC.

C.   **Localization of Bleeding Site**

    1. History

       a. Hematemesis implies a bleed proximal to the ligament of Treitz (upper GI bleed).

       b. Violent vomiting prior to onset of hematemesis suggests a Mallory-Weiss tear.

       c. History of alcohol abuse/cirrhosis suggests the following:

          (1) Esophageal varices

          (2) Alcoholic gastritis

       d. History of prior GI bleeding, diverticular disease, ulcers, and NSAID/steroid use also gives clues to etiology.

       e. Unexplained weight loss, supraclavicular adenopathy and new onset hematemesis raise the question of gastric malignancy.

       f. The character of blood in the stool should be considered.

          (1) Melena: Forms due to the effect of gastric acid on Hb and suggests a source proximal to the ligament of Treitz. The action of bacteria and digestive enzymes on the intraluminal blood produces tarry stools. Melena is usually indicative of proximal lesions.

        (2) Hematochezia usually indicates lower GI bleeding, but this is not absolute.

2. NG tube placement
   a. Lavage and aspiration are indicated in *all cases* of GI bleed to evaluate the possibility of an upper GI source.
   b. Chemical testing for occult blood should be carried out on the aspirate even if it appears free of blood.
   c. Lavage is best carried out through a large bore NG or Ewald tube using warm saline to prevent systemic hypothermia.
   d. Lavage of clots from the stomach allows contraction of gastric musculature, decreases gastrin stimulated acid release, and decreases fibrinolysis at the bleeding site.

3. Proctosigmoidoscopy
   a. Allows a rectosigmoid source of bleeding to be evaluated
   b. Indicates if blood is originating above the level of the rectum

4. Upper GI endoscopy
   a. Upper GI endoscopy provides an accurate delineation of bleeding site in >90% of ICU patients.
   b. Endoscopic hemostasis can often be achieved. Recent studies suggest that the incidence of further bleeding, need for surgery, and mortality rates are decreased by endoscopic hemostasis.
   c. Great care should be taken to protect the patient's airway.
   d. If upper endoscopy is unsuccessful in identifying the lesion, angiography may be performed.

5. Colonoscopy indications
   a. Stable hemodynamics
   b. No evidence of active bleeding
   c. Bleeding proximal to the rectum, as identified by proctosigmoidoscopy

6. Radionuclide scintigraphy
   a. Performed using autologous RBCs labelled with technetium: ^{99m}Tc-sulfur colloid or ^{99m}Tc-pertechnetate
      (1) Sulfur colloid scans give high background in

upper abdomen (spleen and liver) and are inaccurate in these regions.
(2) Repeat scanning can be performed over a 24 to 36 hour period after initial scan without having to repeat the labelling process.
(3) These scans can detect bleeding at a rate as low as 0.1 ml/min.
b. May fail to localize bleeding because of pooling
c. Should be followed by arteriography if bleeding continues
7. Arteriography
a. Able to detect bleeding at a rate as low as 0.5 to 1.0 ml/min
b. Therapeutic options using arteriography
(1) Transcatheter embolization
(2) Selective infusion of vasopressin
(a) Start infusion at 0.2 U/min and increase at a rate of 0.1 U/min every hour.
(b) Titrate for stabilization of hematocrit; maximum infusion should be 0.4 to 0.6 U/min.
(c) After bleeding stops, decrease 0.1 U/min q6-12h.

D. Treatment of Upper GI Bleeding
1. Peptic ulceration
a. Histamine receptor antagonists and antacids are used as initial therapy; omeprazole may be added in refractory cases.
b. Endoscopic management of upper GI bleeding includes the following:
(1) Electrocoagulation
(2) Epinephrine injection
c. Operative indications include the following:
(1) Loss of 1500 to 2000 ml of blood acutely
(2) Transfusion requirements of 8 to 10 U PRBCs
(3) Rebleeding that requires more than 1000 mL of blood replacement
(4) Other factors favoring operative intervention
(a) Patients with rare blood types
(b) Patients with advanced age
(c) Patients with significant comorbidity
d. The operative approach for duodenal ulcers is the following:

(1) Ulcer should be oversewn.
(2) Vagotomy is performed.
(3) A drainage procedure (pyloroplasty or gastroen-terostomy) is included.

e. The operative approach for gastric ulcers is the following:

(1) Excise the ulceration.
(2) Alternatively, perform a distal gastrectomy.

2. Esophageal varices

a. Pharmacologic management

(1) Correct coagulopathy with blood products or vitamin K administration.
(2) Attempt to prevent encephalopathy by evacuating blood from GI tract with lavage or cathartics, and administering oral lactulose and neomycin if encephalopathy develops.
(3) Administer vasopressin with a priming bolus of 20 U IV via peripheral vein over 20 minutes, and continue with infusion of 0.2 to 0.6 U/min. With cessation of bleeding, decrease dose 0.1 U/min at 6 to 12 hour intervals. Vasopressin is contraindicated in patients with CAD because of vasoconstrictive effects.
(4) Octreotide has also been used to control variceal hemorrhage. Its effectiveness in controlling bleeding is similar to vasopressin (53% vs. 58%), but it has fewer vasoconstrictive side effects.

b. Endoscopic sclerotherapy

(1) Mainstay of treatment in bleeding varices
(2) Morbidity rate is 2% to 10% and mortality rate is 1% to 3%
(3) Usually successful in initial control of bleeding
(4) Offers survival advantage when used to supplement distal splenorenal shunt

c. Sengstaken-Blakemore tube (See Chapter 5.)

d. Portocaval shunt

(1) Used less with advent of esophageal sclerotherapy
(2) Indications—failure to respond to combined drug infusion, sclerotherapy, or balloon tamponade
(3) Goal is to decompress the splanchnic vasculature; 50% to 80% efficacy

(4) Shunts of choice are side-to-side or H-graft

e. Esophageal transection with reanastomosis with the EEA stapler

(1) Indications: Patient not a transplant candidate, portal anatomy precludes shunting, life-threatening hemorrhage

(2) Mortality rate: Significant

(3) Complications: Anastamotic leakage, stricture

f. Transjugular intrahepatic portosystemic shunt (TIPS) procedure

(1) Treatment of choice in centers where it is available

(2) Affords significant splanchnic decompression, similar to side-to-side shunts

(3) Preserves normal portal vein anatomy

3. Mallory-Weiss tears

a. Bleeding generally responds well to nonoperative therapy.

(1) Use the same approach as for nonoperative peptic ulceration.

(2) Remove the NG tube if at all possible.

(3) Initiate oral alimentation within 24 to 48 hours if possible.

b. Operative control

(1) Indicated if bleeding continues despite nonoperative therapy

(2) Obtained by suture closure of the GE tear through a longitudinal gastrotomy

4. Erosive gastritis

a. Bleeding usually responds to nonoperative measures (as outlined above).

b. Operative therapy includes truncal vagotomy and pyloroplasty, and oversewing of the bleeding erosions.

E. Treatment of Lower GI Bleeding

1. Angiography with intraarterial vasopressin

a. Angiography is initially successful in 80% of cases.

b. Rebleeding will occur in over 50% of cases.

2. Operative intervention

a. Indications for operation

(1) Persistent hemodynamic instability

      (2) Transfusion requirement of >6 to 8 U in a 24 hour period

      (3) Recurrent hemorrhage

   b. Surgical approach

      (1) "Directed" surgical therapy is possible if a site has been identified. Without preoperative localization, a subtotal colectomy is performed, sparing the rectum.

      (2) The mortality rate is 20% to 30% in emergent situations, and is 10% if surgery is elective.

      (3) If the site of bleeding has not been localized preoperatively, the mortality rate is 30% to 50%.

II. MOUTH

A. Parotitis

1. Normal saliva from healthy patients has intrinsic bacteriostatic activity, which makes spontaneous salivary gland infection very unusual in the absence of duct obstruction.

2. Predisposing factors include the following:
   a. Dehydration
   b. Poor oral hygiene
   c. Malnutrition
   d. Avitaminosis
   e. Mucous plug in Stenson's duct
   f. Presence of NG tube

3. Clinical findings include the following:
   a. High fever
   b. Leukocytosis
   c. May find unilateral facial edema (may not be obvious in intubated patients)
   d. Purulent fluid extruded from Stenson's duct on bimanual examination

4. Diagnostic considerations include the following:
   a. Culture fluid from Stenson's duct.
   b. Responsible bacteria are usually staphylococci and streptococci.
   c. Anaerobes may occasionally play a role.

5. Treatment for parotitis includes the following:
   a. Hydration
   b. Appropriate antibiotics

(1) The empiric therapy should cover staphylococci and streptococci.

(2) Therapy should be altered based on culture results.

c. Anticholinergic drug therapy

d. Manual compression of the parotid

e. May require open drainage and debridement in severe cases.

B. Oral Candidiasis

1. Microbiology

   a. *Candida* organisms are normal inhabitants of mucocutaneous body surfaces.

   b. *C. albicans* and *C. tropicalis* are the most virulent.

2. Predisposing factors in patients in the ICU

   a. Diabetes mellitus

   b. Immunosuppression

   c. Broad-spectrum antibiotic therapy

   d. Extensive burns

3. Clinical findings

   a. Lesions appear raised and discrete or as confluent white patches.

   b. Lesions may be asymptomatic or painful.

   c. Patches may have a thick black or brown coating.

   d. Deep fissures in the tongue may be present.

4. Diagnosis

   a. The scraped lesion should leave a hyperemic base.

   b. Budding yeast with pseudohyphae are seen on light microscopy.

5. Treatment

   a. Nystatin irrigation of oropharynx

      (1) 4 to 6 ml (100,000 U/ml) swish and swallow q6h

      (2) Consider for all patients in the ICU on IV antibiotics

   b. IV administration of fluconazole

      (1) May be appropriate for patients receiving prolonged courses of broad-spectrum antibiotics

      (2) 200 mg IV first day followed by 100 mg qd for 2 weeks

6. Complications of oral candidiasis

   a. Colonization of other organs

   b. Indwelling line sepsis

III. ESOPHAGUS

A. Esophagitis

   1. Predisposing factors

      a. Prolonged use of NG tube (allowing reflux)

      b. Lack of appropriate gastric pH monitoring and antiulcer prophylaxis

      c. Therapy with broad-spectrum antibiotics

      d. Compromised immune status

   2. Clinical findings

      a. Patient complains of dysphagia or back pain

      b. NG aspirate

         (1) Low pH (<5)

         (2) Evidence of blood

   3. Endoscopic evaluation (reflux esophagitis graded endoscopically; candidal esophagitis requires endoscopic biopsy for diagnosis)

      a. Grade I: Hyperemic mucosa

      b. Grade II: Superficial ulceration

      c. Grade III: Ulceration, transmural fibrosis, dilatable stricture

      d. Grade IV: Nondilatable stricture

   4. Treatment of reflux esophagitis

      a. Decrease gastric acid (raise pH to 5) using one of the following regimens:

         (1) Omeprazole 20 mg PO qd

         (2) Antacids 15 to 30 ml PO or via NG tube q1-2h

         (3) Oral histamine receptor blockade—one of the following:

            (a) Cimetidine 400 mg PO qid or 800 mg PO bid

            (b) Ranitine 150 mg PO bid

            (c) Famotidine 20 mg PO bid

         (4) IV bolus histamine receptor blockade—one of the following:

            (a) Cimetidine 300 mg IV q6h

            (b) Ranitidine 50 mg IV q8h

            (c) Famotidine 20 mg IV q12h

         (5) Continuous IV infusion histamine receptor blockade—one of the following:

            (a) Cimetidine 300 mg IV bolus, followed with infusion of 37.5 mg/hr; may increase infusion to 50 to 100 mg/hr if necessary

    (b) Ranitidine 50 mg IV loading dose, followed with 0.125 mg/kg/hr

  b. Increase gastric motility and lower esophageal sphincter tone using the following:

   (1) Metoclopramide 10 mg IV q6h

   (2) Erythromycin 250 mg IV q6h

   (3) Cisapride 10 mg PO q6h

 5. Treatment of candidal esophagitis

  a. Nystatin 30 to 60 ml (100,000 U/ml) PO q2-4h

  b. Fluconazole 200 mg PO first day, then 100 mg PO qd for three weeks; IV administration (same dosage schedule) if the patient is NPO

  c. Amphotericin B 10 to 20 mg/kg/day

B. **Tracheoesophageal Fistula**

 1. Predisposing factors

  a. Prolonged ventilatory course, especially with a tracheostomy or an endotracheal tube with a high pressure cuff

  b. Long-term use of NG tube; provides rigid structure that increases the abrasion injury in patients with a tracheostomy or an endotracheal tube

 2. Prevention

  a. Use low pressure cuffs on tracheostomy and endotracheal tubes.

  b. In patients requiring both gastric decompression and ventilator or airway support, consider early placement of gastrostomy tube and tracheostomy.

  c. Remove NG as soon as possible.

 3. Treatment

  a. Utilize operative repair or diversion.

  b. Tracheal stenosis often accompanies repair.

C. **Postesophagectomy Patient Management**

 1. NG tube secured in place

  a. Usually left in place until gastrografin swallow is obtained

  b. May be removed earlier, depending upon surgeon preference

 2. Stress gastritis prophylaxis

 3. Chest tubes (often two are placed)

  a. Anterior tube may be removed on first or second postoperative day.

  b. Posterior tube is left in place until a gastrografin swallow demonstrating no leakage is obtained.

 4. Postoperative fever

  a. A postoperative fever may indicate anastomotic breakdown and leak.

  b. A complete fever workup is indicated with fever, even within the first 24 hours after operation.

 5. Gastrografin swallow (obtained 5 to 7 days postoperatively)

 6. Chest physiotherapy

 7. Complications

  a. Anastamotic leak

   (1) Requires prolonged chest tube drainage

   (2) Requires nutritional support

   (3) Closure documented by a gastrografin swallow

  b. Reflux esophagitis

  c. Aspiration

  d. Pneumothorax

 8. Indications for reoperation

  a. Continued high volume leakage from anastamosis

  b. Sepsis

IV. STOMACH

A. Gastric Ulcers (See Section I.)

B. Stress Gastritis

 1. Overview

  a. Incidence of 60% to 100% in critically ill patients when examined endoscopically

  b. Mortality rate of 50% to 77% when associated with hemorrhage

  c. Ulceration associated with specific entities

   (1) Curling's ulcers: Gastric erosions arising in the extensively burned patient

   (2) Cushing's ulcers: Erosive gastritis and duodenitis encountered in patients with severe head injury

  d. Characteristics of lesions

   (1) Erosions are almost always multiple, shallow and well-demarcated.

   (2) Lesions are primarily situated in the fundus with sparing of the antrum and duodenum.

2. Pathophysiology
   a. Precise factors for gastric mucosal injury remain unidentified.
   b. Two underlying pathological requirements that seem essential are the following:
      (1) Presence of gastric acid
      (2) Hypoperfusion or mucosal ischemia
3. Prophylaxis
   a. Aggressive correction of the shock, regardless of etiology
   b. Correction of coagulopathy
   c. Aggressive treatment of infection
   d. Reduction of gastric luminal acidity (see above); may administer omeprazole in patients with acid production refractory to histamine receptor blockade
   e. Sucralfate 1 g PO q6h; should not be given with antacids or histamine receptor antagonists (the aluminum sucrose octasulfate polymerizes and attaches to the gastric epithelium only in acid medium)
   f. Oral alimentation; considerably decreases the risk of stress bleeding
   g. Misoprostol; may be effective in patients that require NSAID administration
4. Treatment
   a. Gastric lavage will stop established stress gastritis bleeding in more than 80% of patients.
   b. If hemorrhage continues, consider the following:
      (1) Angiography with selective embolization may be performed.
      (2) Surgical options include oversewing of erosions with vagotomy and pyloroplasty subtotal gastrectomy, vagotomy and antrectomy, vagotomy and subtotal gastric resection, or gastric devascularization.

V. LIVER AND GALLBLADDER
A. Portal Hypertension
1. Overview
   a. Complications of chronic liver disease are major causes of morbidity and mortality.

b. Portal hypertension is fourth after cardiovascular disease, cancer, and trauma as a cause of mortality in adults.

c. Alcoholic liver disease is the most common cause in adults.

2. Pathophysiology of portal hypertension

    a. Increased hydrostatic pressure within the portal vein and its tributaries

        (1) The normal portal vein pressure is 5 to 10 mm Hg.

        (2) Portal pressures are elevated by 15 to 40 mm Hg when measured directly.

        (3) Portal pressures are elevated 10 to 30 mm Hg when measured by indirect hepatic wedge technique.

    b. Manifested by the development of portosystemic collaterals

        (1) GE varices

        (2) Hemorrhoidal veins

        (3) Abdominal wall veins via the umbilical vein (caput medusa)

        (4) Retroperitoneal portosystemic shunts

3. Specific complications of portal hypertension

    a. Variceal bleeding (mortality between 20% and 80% per bleed)

    b. Intractable ascites

        (1) Effective extracellular volume is decreased and serum aldosterone is elevated.

        (2) Aldosterone causes a decrease in the glomerular filtration rate and an increase in ADH.

4. Management of specific complications of portal hypertension

    a. Management of variceal bleeding (see above)

    b. Management of ascites

        (1) Sodium and water restriction (central to management plan)

        (2) Diuresis

            (a) Spironolactone (100 to 400 mg/day) counteracts the effect of secondary hyperaldosteronism and conserves potassium.

    (b) Furosemide or bumetanide is used if diuresis remains inadequate (<1 to 2 L/day). Potassium supplementation is often required.

    (c) Diuretics must be temporarily withheld if azotemia supervenes.

   (3) Paracentesis

   (4) Peritoneovenous shunting

B. **Hepatic Failure**

  1. Etiologies of hepatic failure include the following:

   a. Preexisting chronic liver disease with hepatocellular failure

    (1) Variceal hemorrhage most common cause for admission of patients with cirrhosis to ICU

    (2) Insufficient hepatocellular mass to sustain normal liver function

    (3) Causes of acute hepatocellular failure in patients with chronic liver disease

     (a) Infection

     (b) Malignancy

     (c) Toxins (including alcohol)

   b. Fulminant hepatic failure with no evidence of previous liver disease

    (1) Viral hepatitides (most common cause)

    (2) Acetaminophen overdose

    (3) *Amanita* mushroom toxicity

    (4) Fatty liver of pregnancy (third trimester)

    (5) Reye's syndrome

   c. Liver failure arising from other systemic processes; prognosis in this group closely tied to underlying systemic disorder

    (1) Postoperative or posttraumatic

    (2) Sepsis

    (3) Cholestasis

  2. Clinical findings of hepatic failure include the following:

   a. Evidence of liver injury; elevated transaminases

   b. Evidence of hepatic functional insufficiency

    (1) Elevated PT and PTT

    (2) Decreased serum protein levels; albumin and transferrin

    (3) Hypoglycemia

    (4) Hyperbilirubinemia

TABLE 9-1.

Sherlock's Grading Scale for Hepatic Encephalopathy

Grade	Description
1	Confusion or altered mood behavior
2	Drowsiness or inappropriate behavior
3	Inarticulate speech, but obeys simple commands
4	Responsive only to painful stimuli
5	Unresponsive

    c. Evidence of hepatic encephalopathy
      (1) Elevated blood ammonia levels
      (2) Altered mental status
      (3) Changes graded from 1 to 5 (Table 9-1)
      (4) Asterixis
      (5) Increased CSF glutamine
      (6) Other etiologies of altered mental status (always a consideration)
        (a) Infection/sepsis
        (b) Drug intoxication or adverse reaction
        (c) Metabolic abnormalities superimposed on liver disease

3. No specific treatment is available for liver failure. Patients with hepatic insufficiency should receive a 10% glucose IV infusion, and serum blood glucose should be monitored frequently. Treatment is directed toward managing complications of liver failure.
    a. Encephalopathy
      (1) Control of associated complications that may exacerbate hepatic encephalopathy: GI bleeding, renal insufficiency, infection/sepsis, acid-base or electrolyte imbalances
      (2) Ensure adequate nutrition and control excessive dietary protein: 1400 cal/day as carbohydrate and fat as an additional source of calories
      (3) Lactulose therapy increases acid production by bacteria and traps ammonia in the gut lumen in the form of nonabsorbable ammonia ion.
        (a) Begin with 30 to 45 ml PO q1h until diarrhea ensues

        (b) Adjust dose to tid or qid; titrate for production of two to four soft stools per day.

        (c) In obtunded patients, administer via NG tube.

        (d) In patients with ileus, 200 to 300 ml with 700 ml water per rectum q6-12h; retain 40 to 60 minutes.

    (4) Neomycin therapy

        (a) Decreases bacterial flora that generate ammonia and other toxins

        (b) Dose of 1 to 4 g PO or 1 to 2 g in 100 to 200 ml of saline per rectum

    (5) Flumazenil therapy

        (a) A benzodiazepine receptor antagonist

        (b) Reported to have a dramatic but short-lived effect on hepatic encephalopathy

b. Cerebral edema: Second leading cause of neurological impairment in patients with liver disease; found in 25% to 81% of patients with fulminant hepatic failure

    (1) Hyperventilation

    (2) Osmotic diuresis with mannitol (0.5 to 1 g/kg IV)

        (a) Give as rapid infusion when ICP exceed 15 cm H_2O

        (b) May be repeated q6h unless serum osmolality > 320 mOsm

c. Hepatorenal syndrome: Seen in liver failure of all types; characterized by oliguria, low urine sodium concentration (<10 mEq/L), urine-to-plasma creatinine ratio exceeding 30:1, and preserved renal tubular function

    (1) Discontinue diuretics.

    (2) Optimize intravascular volume.

    (3) Adjust sodium and water intake to match output.

d. Coagulopathy: Many proteins involved in coagulation synthesized by normal liver, including protein C, protein S, and vitamin K dependent factors II, VII, IX and X

    (1) Acute factor replacement: FFP for coagulation factor replacement and cryoprecipitate for fibrinogen replacement

(2) Factor synthesis stimulation: Vitamin K 10 to 20 mg IM

e. Infection: Abnormalities in host defense mechanisms in liver failure secondary to impaired neutrophil function or abnormal phagocytic activity of the reticulo-endothelial system

f. Spontaneous bacterial peritonitis

(1) Most common serious infection encountered in the hospitalized cirrhotic; should always be considered when a cirrhotic becomes encephalopathic

(2) Diagnosis by paracentesis; gram-negative bacteria (*Escherichia coli, Klebsiella* organisms) most common etiologic organisms

(3) Treated with appropriate systemic antibiotics (third generation cephalosporin usually adequate)

(4) In-hospital mortality rate for patients with spontaneous bacterial peritonitis >50%

C. Jaundice

1. Etiology

a. Increased bilirubin production (increased serum levels of heme pigment)

(1) Massive transfusions

(2) Hematoma

(3) Crush injury

(4) CPB

(5) Sickle cell anemia

(6) Hemolysis from blood transfusion

b. Decreased bilirubin excretion secondary to hepatocellular dysfunction

(1) Cholestatic jaundice

(2) Hepatitis

(3) Hepatotoxic drugs

(4) TPN

(5) Shock and sepsis

c. Decreased bilirubin excretion secondary to biliary obstruction

2. Laboratory evaluation

a. Direct and indirect bilirubin generally of little clinical value

b. Urinary bilirubin and urobilinogen

    c. Elevated transaminases; indicative of hepatocellular death

    d. Serum amylase to rule out pancreatitis

    e. Serology for hepatitis

    f. PT, PTT, serum albumin, and transferrin to test hepatocellular function

    g. Elevated alkaline phosphatase, GGT, 5′-neucleotidase, and leucine aminopeptidase; suggestive of cholestatic jaundice

3. Radiological evaluation

    a. Ultrasound: 90% to 97% accurate in distinguishing intrahepatic from extrahepatic causes of jaundice; a specific cause can be found in 50% of patients

       (1) Gallstones

       (2) Thickness of gallbladder

       (3) Size of biliary ducts

       (4) Presence of cirrhosis or fatty infiltration

       (5) Masses in head of pancreas

    b. CT: May clarify if level of obstruction not well identified by ultrasound

       (1) More accurate than ultrasound for evaluation of pancreas

       (2) Not hindered by bowel gas, wounds, and dressings

    c. Nuclear scans: Visualization of the gallbladder and biliary tree; variable results at bilirubin concentration greater than 5 mg/dl

    d. Endoscopic retrograde cholangiography (ERCP): >95% success rate of visualizing the biliary tree in experienced hands

       (1) Procedure of choice for evaluation of obstructive jaundice

       (2) Can obtain tumor biopsy or brushing

       (3) Offers therapeutic options including sphincterotomy, stent placement, and basket extraction of stones

    e. Percutaneous transhepatic cholangiography (PTHC): Success rate > 95% in patients with dilated ducts; 70% in patients with nondilated ducts

       (1) Ideal for evaluation of proximal lesions

       (2) Offers therapeutic options including placement

of percutaneous biliary drain or stenting of a proximal biliary tree lesion

D.   Management of Patients Following Hepatic Surgery

1. Hypoglycemia
   a. Liver glycogen stores may be exhausted for several weeks.
   b. Administer 10% dextrose solution for 48 hours or longer if required.
   c. Monitor blood glucose levels closely.
2. Hypoalbuminemia
   a. Albumin synthesis reduced for several weeks
   b. 25 to 50 g albumin per day IV beginning on first postoperative day; continued until no evidence of hepatic insufficiency
3. Hypophosphatemia
   a. Follow serum levels.
   b. Supplement appropriately with potassium phosphate.
4. Hyperbilirubinemia
   a. Hyperbilirubinemia is common after extensive resections because of blood transfusions and transient liver dysfunction.
   b. Important considerations in differential diagnosis of persistent jaundice include injury to the remaining hepatic duct and refractory liver failure.

E.   Postoperative Cholecystitis

1. Acute calculous cholecystitis
   a. Potentially life-threatening complication
   b. Can complicate virtually all surgical procedures
   c. Treatment
      (1) Laparoscopic cholecystectomy in appropriate patients; will only rarely be applied in patients who have recently undergone major procedures
      (2) Open cholecystectomy
      (3) Tube cholecystostomy (see below)
2. Acalculous cholecystitis
   a. Rare, but typically occurs in critically ill patients, especially after trauma and burns; should be considered in all patients with sepsis in ICU setting
   b. Predisposing factors
      (1) Prolonged period of time without enteral nutrition

  (2) Trauma or burn injury

  (3) Diabetes mellitus

  (4) Abdominal arterial insufficiency or vasculitis

  (5) Necrotizing fasciitis

  (6) Allergic granulomatosis, polyarteritis nodosa, and SLE

  (7) AIDS

  (8) Gallbladder hypoperfusion; CHF, hypotensive shock, cardiac arrest

  (9) Hepatic artery chemoinfusions

c. Pathogenesis

  (1) Cystic duct obstruction

  (2) Concentrated bile

  (3) Gallbladder ischemia

  (4) Disease-related risk factors for development of acute acalculous cholecystitis

   (a) Shock

   (b) Respiratory failure

   (c) Renal failure

  (5) Treatment-related risk factors for development of acute acalculous cholecystitis

   (a) Narcotics

   (b) Vasopressors

   (c) Multiple operations

   (d) Multiple blood transfusions (>10 U)

   (e) TPN

d. Diagnosis

  (1) Clinical findings

   (a) Fever

   (b) Right upper quadrant tenderness

  (2) Laboratory abnormalities

   (a) Leukocytosis

   (b) Hyperbilirubinemia, elevated alkaline phosphatase, elevated transaminases

  (3) Ultrasound

   (a) Thickened gallbladder wall (more than 3.5 mm)

   (b) Pericholecystic fluid

   (c) Intramural gas

   (d) Sonolucent intramural layer ("halo" sign) that represents wall edema

    (4) CT
        (a) Equal or superior in sensitivity and specificity to ultrasound
        (b) Allows other causes of sepsis to be identified
    (5) Hepatobiliary scanning
        (a) False negatives occur when there is no obstruction of the cystic duct (as in acalculous cholecystitis).
        (b) False positives in patients receiving TPN or with liver disease.

  e. Treatment
    (1) Cholecystectomy: Mainstay of treatment
    (2) Percutaneous cholecystostomy tube placement: Useful for very critically ill patients
        (a) The tube is placed under radiological guidance (either ultrasound or CT)
        (b) Patients may later undergo elective laparoscopic or open cholecystectomy
        (c) Patients who do not improve after tube cholecystostomy and antibiotic therapy should undergo cholecystectomy.
    (3) Antibiotic therapy: Most common bacteria isolated from bile in acute cholecystitis are *E. coli*, and *Klebsiella* and *Enterococcus* organisms

  f. Gallbladder perforation
    (1) Perforation in postoperative and acalculous cholecystitis is approximately 10%.
    (2) Free perforation is associated with a mortality rate of 22%.
    (3) Localized perforation carries a mortality rate of 6%.
    (4) Overall morbidity rate associated with perforation >70%.

F. Cholangitis and Biliary Sepsis
  1. Pathophysiology
    a. The presence of bacteria in the normal biliary tree does not cause sepsis.
    b. Bacteria in a completely or partially blocked common bile duct causes bilovenous and bilolymphatic reflux and resulting sepsis.
    c. Acute suppurative cholangitis carries a high mortality.

    d. *E. coli* and *Klebsiella* and *Enterococcus* organisms are cultured the most frequently.

    e. Cholangitis is associated with several conditions including the following:

        (1) Choledocholithiasis

        (2) Common bile duct stricture

        (3) Malignant biliary obstruction

        (4) Biliary enteric anastomosis (rare)

        (5) Foreign bodies in biliary tree (stents)

2. Symptoms

    a. Charcot's triad: Fever, jaundice, and right upper quadrant pain; indicative of acute cholangitis

    b. Reynold's pentad: Fever, jaundice, right upper quadrant pain, altered mental status, and hypotension; indicative of acute suppurative cholangitis

3. Laboratory values supportive of diagnosis

    a. Leukocytosis

    b. Hyperbilirubinemia

    c. Elevated alkaline phosphatase levels

    d. Hyperamylasemia

    e. Mild to moderate elevation in liver transaminase levels

4. Ultrasound (confirms suspicion of obstructive jaundice)

5. Treatment

    a. Prophylactic antibiotics in high-risk patients may prevent the development of cholangitis in the following:

        (1) Patients with obstructive jaundice

        (2) Patients suspected of having bacterbilia who are undergoing invasive procedure

        (3) Patients with foreign bodies in the common duct (stent, catheter) who are undergoing invasive procedure

    b. Supportive measures include the following:

        (1) Broad-spectrum antibiotics

        (2) Fluid resuscitation

    c. Decompression

        (1) ERCP or PTHC

        (2) Surgical decompression

            (a) Cholecystectomy alone is not effective in draining an obstructed common duct

        (b) After successful initial drainage, a definitive procedure may be performed electively.
- d. Outcome
    - (1) Mortality rate of untreated suppurative cholangitis is 100%.
    - (2) Mortality rate with surgical intervention is 30%.
    - (3) Mortality rate with surgical intervention in absence of septic shock is 15%.

VI. PANCREAS
A. Acute Pancreatitis
1. Etiology
    - a. Toxic or metabolic factors
        - (1) Alcohol
        - (2) Hyperlipidemia
    - b. Ampullary obstruction
        - (1) Biliary stone
        - (2) Tumor
    - c. Following ERCP
    - d. Infectious causes
        - (1) Mumps
        - (2) Mycoplasma
        - (3) Cocksackie virus
        - (4) *Clinorchis sinensis*
    - e. Ischemia
    - f. Medications
        - (1) Estrogen compounds
        - (2) Thiazide diuretics
2. Pathogenesis
    - a. Pancreatic process
        - (1) Release of pancreatic digestive enzymes
        - (2) Intraparenchymal enzyme activation
        - (3) Tissue destruction and ischemic necrosis
        - (4) Thrombosis of parenchymal vessels secondary to inflammation
    - b. Etiology of shock is multifactorial
        - (1) Sequestration of fluid
        - (2) Kinins, serotonin, trypsin, and vasoactive amines; implicated in diminished peripheral vascular resistance and increased vascular permeability

3. Symptoms
   a. Epigastric pain radiating to the back
   b. Nausea and vomiting
   c. Low-grade fever
4. Physical findings
   a. Palpable abdominal mass
   b. Distended, tender abdomen
   c. Signs suggestive of retroperitoneal hemorrhage
      (1) Cullen's sign: Periumbilical discoloration
      (2) Gray-Turner's sign: Purple discoloration of the flank
5. Laboratory studies
   a. Serum amylase
      (1) Elevated in 95% of cases of gallstone pancreatitis
      (2) May be elevated in up to 30% of alcoholics with underlying chronic pancreatitis
      (3) Generally increases within 2 to 12 hours of onset of symptoms
      (4) Returns to normal over the ensuing 3 to 5 days
      (5) No correlation between degree of serum amylase elevation and the etiology, prognosis, or severity of disease
      (6) Hyperamylasemia (may be seen in patients without acute pancreatitis)
         (a) Following biliary and gastroduodenal abdominal surgery
         (b) Acute and chronic renal failure
         (c) Salivary gland disease
         (d) Liver disease
         (e) Small bowel obstruction
         (f) Diabetic ketoacidosis
         (g) Gynecological disorders (especially ovarian)
         (h) Carbon monoxide poisoning
   b. Elevated serum lipase
   c. Hypocalcemia
   d. Hyperglycemia
   e. Hypoxemia
6. Radiographic studies
   a. Primary role is to rule out other potential cause of symptomatology
   b. Plain abdominal films and CXR
      (1) Obscured psoas margin

      (2) Increased epigastric soft tissue density

      (3) Left pleural effusion

      (4) Pancreatic calcification

  c. Ultrasound

      (1) Abnormal in only 30% to 50% of patients with acute pancreatitis

      (2) Poor visualization of pancreas and retroperitoneum

  d. CT

      (1) Best for overall evaluation of retroperitoneal structures

      (2) May help in defining etiology (cholelithiasis)

      (3) Useful in monitoring later complications of acute pancreatitis, pseudocyst, pancreatic abscess, pancreatic necrosis, or peripancreatic fluid collection

      (4) If normal, does not rule out pancreatitis

7. Differential diagnosis

  a. Peptic ulcer disease

  b. Intestinal obstruction

  c. Mesenteric infarction

  d. Biliary tract disease

8. Supportive therapy

  a. Aggressive fluid resuscitation and correction of electrolyte imbalances

  b. Treatment of hypoxemia

      (1) In patients who survive first 48 hours, 30% to 60% develop pulmonary complications

      (2) Pulmonary dysfunction associated with pancreatitis characterized by early hypoxemia without radiological abnormality

      (3) Respiratory insufficiency with nonspecific radiological abnormalities (diaphragmatic elevation, atelectasis, pulmonary infiltrates, pleural effusions)

      (4) ARDS

  c. Prophylaxis for stress gastritis

  d. Minimization of pancreatic secretion

      (1) NPO

      (2) NG suction (decreases vomiting and aspiration)

  e. Analgesia (meperidine used since it may have less spastic effect on the ampulla of Vater)

  f. Antibiotics

        (1) Generally not indicated

        (2) Used when pancreatic abscess is suspected

    g. Nutritional support

9. Surgical treatment

    a. Gallstone pancreatitis

        (1) 90% of the stones pass spontaneously.

        (2) After acute episode subsides, perform cholecystectomy, intraoperative cholangiogram, and common duct exploration (if indicated).

        (3) Other options include ERCP and sphincterotomy followed by laparoscopic cholecystectomy.

    b. Nonbiliary-associated acute pancreatitis

        (1) Nonoperative treatment is generally successful.

        (2) Operative treatment includes the following:

            (a) Debridement in severe cases of hemorrhagic or necrotizing pancreatitis

            (b) No benefits from peritoneal lavage

10. Ranson's criteria—early prognostic signs in acute pancreatitis

    a. On admission

        (1) Age >55

        (2) WBC >16,000 mm^3

        (3) Serum glucose > 200 mg/dl

        (4) LDH >350 IU/L

        (5) SGOT > 250 SF U %

    b. During initial 48 hours

        (1) Fall in hct >10%

        (2) Calcium < 80 mg/dl

        (3) Pao$_2$ < 60 mm Hg

        (4) Base deficit > 4 mEq/L

        (5) BUN elevation >5 mg/dl

        (6) Third space loss > 6000 ml

    c. Mortality rates

        (1) Fewer than three signs: 1% mortality rate

        (2) Three to four signs: 16% mortality rate

        (3) Five to six signs: 40% mortality rate

        (4) Seven or more signs: 100% mortality rate

11. Prognosis

    a. 75% of patients recover uneventfully.

    b. There is a 10% overall mortality rate.

        (1) Alcohol-induced pancreatitis has the lowest mortality rate (4%).

(2) Postoperative pancreatitis has the highest mortality rate (40%).

12. Sequelae of pancreatitis
   a. Pancreatic pseudocysts
   b. Pancreatic abscess
   c. Splenic vein thrombosis
   d. Gastric varices
   e. Bile duct stricture
   f. Intestinal necrosis
   g. Chronic pain

B. **Postpancreaticoduodenectomy (Whipple Procedure) Management**
   1. Special considerations
      a. Large volume of third space losses are common in the postoperative period secondary to extensive dissection.
      b. Expect prolonged ileus.
   2. Most frequent complications
      a. Bleeding
      b. Infection
      c. Pancreatic fistula
         (1) Routine use of octreotide (100 U SQ q8h) may reduce the incidence of postoperative fistulae.
         (2) Most pancreatic fistulae close without further operation.
         (3) Skin excoriations are not seen in pure pancreatic fistulae, since the enzymes have not come into contact with the intestinal mucosa and therefore are not activated.
   3. Nutritional support—imperative

VII. SMALL INTESTINE
A. **Small Bowel Obstruction**
   1. Pathophysiology
      a. Obstruction of bowel leads to fluid and air accumulation with bowel distention.
      b. Air swallowing is responsible for 75% of the air seen in bowel obstruction.
      c. As the bowel distends, significant third space fluid loss occurs, because of the following:
         (1) Decreased absorption
         (2) Increased luminal secretion

      d. Further distension

         (1) Tissue ischemia occurs.

         (2) Bowel wall necrosis leads to subsequent bacteremia and sepsis.

2. Etiology

    a. Adhesions—responsible for 80% of cases in the U.S.

    b. Hernias—represent the most common cause worldwide

    c. Intussusception—an important cause in children

    d. Neoplasms

    e. Volvulus

3. Clinical findings

    a. Intermittent colicky pain

        (1) Paroxysms of pain occurring every 4 to 5 minutes.

        (2) When succeeded by continuous severe abdominal pain, suspect strangulation with peritonitis.

    b. Nausea and vomiting

    c. Low-grade fever

    d. Abdominal examination

        (1) Distention: Commonly observed but may be absent in proximal obstruction

        (2) Auscultation: High-pitched rushing bowel sounds separated by relatively quiet periods

        (3) Localized tenderness: Suggestive of peritonitis

    e. Rectal examination

        (1) Detection of luminal masses

        (2) Stool for occult blood testing

4. Laboratory evaluation

    a. Mild leukocytosis, hyperamylasemia, azotemia, and hemoconcentration

    b. Electrolyte abnormalities

        (1) Hypochloremia

        (2) Hypokalemia

        (3) Metabolic acidosis in patients with strangulation

5. Radiographic evaluation

    a. Abdominal film

        (1) Air-fluid levels are in a "stepladder" pattern.

        (2) Small bowel loops are centrally located.

        (3) Valvulae conniventes cross the entire lumen ("stack of coins").

        (4) Distended loops (>3 cm) and lack of colonic gas

are seen. (With high small bowel obstruction, dilated loops may not be seen.)

    (5) Signs of strangulation and perforation
        (a) Thickened bowel wall (>3 mm)
        (b) Intramural air (pneumatosis intestinalis)
        (c) Strangulation and free air—suggested by air in the portal system

  b. Barium enema
    (1) A barium enema excludes the colon as a site of obstruction.
    (2) Reflux past the ileocecal valve may confirm diagnosis of small bowel obstruction.

6. Supportive management
  a. Fluid resuscitation: Replace third space losses with isotonic saline or lactated Ringer's solution and follow urine output, CVP, or PA pressures as indicated.
  b. Correction of electrolyte abnormalities: Replace gastric losses with l/2 NS with 30 mEq KCl/L.
  c. Bowel decompression: Use NG suction.

7. Operative intervention
  a. Factors important in the timing of operation
    (1) Duration of obstruction
    (2) Optimization of vital organ function
    (3) Risk of strangulation—presence of one or more of the following mandates early operative intervention:
        (a) Fever
        (b) Tachycardia
        (c) Leukocytosis
        (d) Focal abdominal tenderness
        (e) Evidence of complete small bowel obstruction on upper GI series
        (f) Evidence of colonic obstruction
  b. Mortality rates
    (1) Mortality rate of simple obstruction is 0% to 6%.
    (2) Mortality rate of strangulated obstruction is 15% to 30%.

B. Prolonged Ileus
1. Postoperative ileus may persist for 2 to 5 days.
2. Return of GI motility occurs in the following time frames:

  a. Small bowel (1 to 3 days)
  b. Stomach (3 to 5 days)
  c. Colon (4 to 7 days)
 3. Management in the ICU includes the following:
  a. Rule out peritoneal infection.
  b. Optimize electrolyte levels.
  c. Carefully review medications, especially narcotics and calcium channel blockers.
  d. Perform a primary tube study to differentiate ileus from obstruction.

C. Ischemic Bowel

 1. Etiology
  a. Cardiovascular instability in the critically ill
  b. Activation of procoagulants and other humoral factors
  c. Impaired splanchnic arterial flow or venous return
  d. Anatomic injury from surgery or trauma
  e. Preexisting atherosclerotic disease
 2. Clinical findings
  a. New onset bloody diarrhea
  b. Diffuse abdominal pain and distention
  c. Unexplained metabolic acidosis
  d. Hypovolemia with oliguria and hemoconcentration
  e. Leukocytosis (>14,000), hypocalcemia, hyperphosphatemia
 3. Surgical therapy indicated
  a. Perform an exploration with resection and diversion.
  b. If bowel is ischemic but appears viable, embolectomy or revascularization may be performed.

VIII. COLON

A. Large Bowel Obstruction

 1. Etiology
  a. Colorectal carcinoma (80%)
  b. Diverticulitis
  c. Volvulus
  d. Fecal impaction
 2. Clinical findings
  a. Abdominal pain is invariably present.
  b. Distention is less common if the ileocecal valve is competent.
  c. Vomiting occurs late in the course if at all.

3. Laboratory findings
   a. Fluid and electrolyte disturbances are less common than with small bowel obstruction.
   b. Anemia may be present due to colonic carcinoma.
4. Radiologic findings
   a. Abdominal film: Dilated proximal colon with absence of gas distally
   b. Barium enema: Localizes the lesion
5. Treatment—(Colonic obstruction is a surgical emergency.)
   a. Left-sided lesions: Diverting colostomy with or without resection
   b. Right-sided lesions: Diverting colostomy or ileostomy; may attempt primary anastomosis if soilage minimal and patient stable

B. Intraabdominal Abscess
1. Clinical findings
   a. Symptoms occur 7 to 10 days after operation.
   b. Localized tenderness is present on abdominal, rectal, or pelvic exam.
   c. Spiking fever and leukocytosis are present.
   d. Ultrasound or CT can confirm diagnosis.
2. Treatment
   a. Antibiotic therapy
      (1) Empiric regimens should include coverage of gram-negatives aerobes, enterococcus, and anaerobes.
      (2) Blood and fluid cultures will guide further therapy.
   b. Percutaneous drainage guided by CT or ultrasound
   c. Surgical drainage
      (1) Indications include radiologically inaccessible abscesses or abscesses that do not respond to percutaneous drainage.
      (2) The outcomes of radiological drainage and surgical drainage are comparable.
      (3) Surgical drainage has a higher morbidity rate.

C. Pseudomembranous Colitis
1. Caused by the endotoxin of *Clostridium difficile*
2. Occur after systemic therapy with almost all antibiotics
3. Clinical findings
   a. Acute diarrheal colitis with supervening sepsis

      b. Leukocytosis

      c. May produce septic shock

      d. May observe pseudomembranes on sigmoidoscopy

      e. Diagnosis dependent on demonstration of toxin in stool

   4. Treatment

      a. Vancomycin 125 mg PO q6h for 5 to 10 days, or

      b. Metronidazole 250 mg PO q6h for 5 to 10 days

D.   **Diarrhea**

   1. Differential diagnosis

      a. Osmolar

        (1) Excessive enteral feeding

        (2) Sorbitol and other nonabsorbable medications

        (3) Antacid therapy

        (4) Refeeding after cachexia

      b. Anatomic

        (1) Dumping syndrome

        (2) Blind loop syndrome with bacterial overgrowth

        (3) Fistulae (gastrocolic, enteroenteric, enterocolic)

        (4) Partial bowel obstruction

      c. Secretory—endocrine

        (1) Hyperthyroidism

        (2) Zollinger-Ellison syndrome

        (3) Watery diarrhea hypophosphatemia acidosis (WDHA) syndrome

      d. Secretory—exocrine

        (1) Pancreatic insufficiency

        (2) Impaired bile reabsorption

      e. Infection

        (1) *Salmonella* organisms

        (2) *Shigella* organisms

        (3) *C. difficile*

   2. Evaluation

      a. Rectal examination

      b. Stool sample evaluation

        (1) Ova and parasites

        (2) Fat, blood, and mucous

        (3) *C. difficile* toxin

        (4) Reducing substances

      c. Review of medication and nutritional therapy

      d. Radiologic contrast studies to define GI tract anatomic abnormalities

3. Treatment
   a. Therapy is based upon diagnosis.
   b. Therapy with antidiarrheals is usually contraindicated.

SUGGESTED READING

Barie PS: *Acalculous and postoperative cholecystitis.* In Barie PS, Shires TG, editors: *Surgical intensive care,* Boston, 1993, Little, Brown and Co.

Geus WP, Lamers CB: Prevention of stress ulcer bleeding: a review, *Scand J Gastroenterol* 178 (Suppl):32-41, 1990.

Kurland B, Brandt LJ, Delany HM: Diagnostic tests for intestinal ischemia, *Surg Clin NA* 72A:143-55, 1992.

Miller TA, Reed RL III, Moody FG: *Gastrointestinal hemorrhage.* In Barie PS, Shires TG, editors: *Surgical intensive care,* Boston, 1993, Little, Brown and Co.

Shires TG, Bush HL, Barie PS: *Portal hypertension.* In Barie PS, Shires TG, editors: *Surgical intensive care,* Boston, 1993, Little, Brown and Co.

Williams R, Gimson AE: Intensive care and management of acute hepatic failure, *Dig Dis Sci* 36F:820-6, 1991.

THE VASCULAR SYSTEM   *10*

Lewis B. Schwartz

I. INTRODUCTION

Vascular disease is one of the most common diagnoses in patients on admission to the ICU, and successful care is dependent on a thorough understanding of vascular anatomy and pathophysiology. This chapter addresses the general management of the vascular patient (including fundamental vascular principles and guidelines for preoperative and postoperative care) and describes specific manifestations of vascular disease. Vascular problems found less frequently in the ICU setting (including upper extremity disease, thoracic outlet syndrome, popliteal aneurysms, portal hypertension, and venous insufficiency) are not specifically addressed, and the interested reader is referred to the many available surgical textbooks for further information.

II. GENERAL CARE OF THE VASCULAR SURGICAL PATIENT

A. The Vascular Evaluation

The initial vascular examination at the time of hospital admission is often incomplete; documentation at the time of ICU admission is mandatory.

    1. History

        a. Symptoms of vascular disease vary with the anatomic location of the vascular bed.

        b. The symptoms of chronic vascular disease and acute vascular insufficiency are usually easily distinguished.

    2. Inspection

        a. Adequately perfused extremities are light pink.

        b. Pallor or bluish discoloration indicates poor perfusion.

        c. Dark blue or black discoloration usually indicates irreversible tissue loss.

3. Palpation
   a. Pulses are examined in the carotid, brachial, radial, ulnar, femoral, dorsalis pedis, and posterior tibial positions (Fig. 10-1) as well as in any vascular grafts that have been implanted.
   b. Pulses are designated as *present, absent,* or *aneurysmal.* Pulse grading as 1+, 2+, 3+, or 4+ is unreliable and should be discouraged.

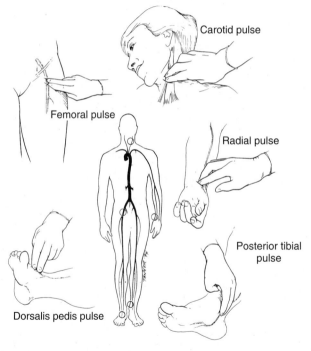

FIG 10-1.
Examination of the carotid, radial, femoral, posterior tibial, and dorsalis pedis pulses.

     c. Capillary refill is examined by gently squeezing and blanching the patient's digit between the examiner's thumb and first proximal phalanx; the color should return in the time it takes to say "capillary refill". Slow capillary refill is indicative of poor tissue perfusion.

     d. The abdomen is palpated for the presence of pulsatile masses.

  4. Auscultation

     a. The carotid, abdominal, and femoral arteries are auscultated with the stethoscope for the presence of bruits.

     b. Any peripheral pulses that are not palpable are tested with the Doppler ultrasound instrument. It is more sensitive than the examining finger and can detect a blood flow velocity as low as 5 cm/sec. Doppler signals are classified as audible or inaudible.

     c. A useful measure of the degree of peripheral vascular insufficiency is the ankle-brachial index (ABI). First, systolic brachial artery pressure is measured with a blood pressure cuff and Doppler. Then, cuffs applied to the calf and systolic BPs are measured in the posterior tibial and dorsalis pedis arteries. The highest systolic pressure in the foot is divided by the systolic brachial pressure, which usually results in a number between 0 and 1 (the ABI). In young patients, the ABI may actually exceed 1 because of the slightly higher systemic pressure in the legs compared to the upper body. Figure 10-2 demonstrates an example of an ABI calculation in a patient with left superficial femoral artery obstruction. An ABI of less than 0.6 is usually found in claudication; an ABI of less than 0.3 accompanies rest pain. The ABI is useful for preoperative evaluation as well as demonstration of postoperative improvement.

  5. Documentation

     a. The most convenient way to represent the vascular status is by a simple table of peripheral pulses.

     b. Figure 10-3 shows an example of this type of table.

B. Preoperative Evaluation

  1. History and physical examination

  2. Laboratory evaluation

     a. CBC

     b. Serum electrolytes

     c. BUN

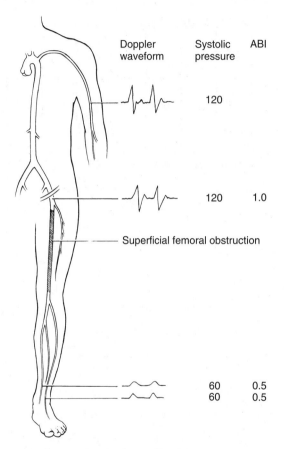

Doppler waveform	Systolic pressure	ABI
	120	
	120	1.0
Superficial femoral obstruction		
	60	0.5
	60	0.5

FIG 10-2.

Measurement of segmental arterial pressure and ABI in a patient with left superficial femoral artery obstruction and calf claudication. The systolic pressure measured with the hand-held Doppler probe in either the posterior tibial or dorsalis pedis artery is divided by the systolic brachial pressure. In this case, the ABI is 0.5, indicating moderate vascular insufficiency.

	Carotid	Brachial	Radial	Fem	PT	DP	ABI
Right	✔ₐ	✔	✔	✔	✔	✔	1
Left	✔	✔	✔	✔ₐ	✔_Dop	—	0.5

FIG 10-3.

Documentation of the pulse examination in an ICU patient with left superficial femoral artery obstruction and a right carotid bruit. ✔ = palpable pulse; ✔ₐ = palpable pulse and audible bruit; ✔_Dop = pulse absent, audible Doppler signed; — = pulse absent, no audible Doppler signal.

    d. Creatinine
    e. PT
    f. PTT
    g. Urinalysis
    h. ECG
    i. Posteroanterior and lateral CXR
3. Blood crossmatching
    a. Aortic reconstruction: 4 U
    b. Infrainguinal reconstruction: 2 U
    c. Renal or mesenteric artery reconstruction: 4 U
    d. Carotid endarterectomy: Type & screen
4. Bowel preparation
    a. Cathartics are helpful in the preparation for intraabdominal procedures.
    b. Low-volume enemas may also be used.
5. Assessment of cardiac risk
    a. Risk of fatal MI, heart failure, or significant dysrhythmia in vascular surgical patients: 3% to 6%
    b. Percentage of early deaths in vascular surgical patients attributable to cardiac complications: 50%
    c. Incidence of hemodynamically significant stenosis in at least one coronary vessel in patients undergoing aortic reconstruction: 80%

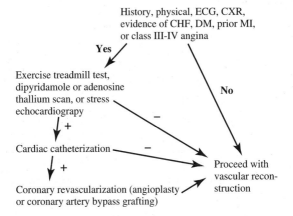

FIG 10-4.
Evaluation of cardiac risk in vascular surgery patients.

    d. Incidence of hemodynamically significant stenosis in at least one coronary vessel in asymptomatic patients undergoing aortic reconstruction: 40%

    e. Incidence of left main or three vessel CAD in asymptomatic patients undergoing aortic reconstruction: 15%

    f. Significant cardiac risk factors: Prior CHF, angina, prior MI, diabetes

    g. Risk of cardiac morbidity in patients without risk factors (*a* through *f*): 1%

    h. Patients with any risk factors (*a* through *f*): Should undergo further evaluation, such as exercise treadmill testing, stress echocardiography, or dipyridamole (or adenosine) thallium imaging to identify areas of inadequate myocardial perfusion

    i. Patients with positive stress testing: Should be considered for coronary arteriography and coronary revascularization prior to elective vascular surgery (treatment algorithm in Figure 10-4)

6. Assessment of pulmonary risk
   a. Risk factors for pulmonary complications include smoking, prior episodes of respiratory failure, asthma, and shortness of breath during activity.
   b. Patients who have significant shortness of breath with activity or have evidence of severe lung disease on examination should undergo pulmonary function testing and ABG analysis.
   c. Findings which may predict postoperative pulmonary complications include the following:
      (1) Pulmonary function test: FEV_1 < 1000 ml (<50% of predicted)
      (2) ABG analysis: Pao_2 < 60 mm Hg, or $Paco_2$ > 50 mm Hg
   d. Pulmonary function may be optimized by cessation of smoking, treatment of bronchitis, use of bronchodilators, and encouragement of deep breathing postoperatively.
7. Assessment of infectious risk
   a. Risk factors for postoperative infection include obesity, diabetes mellitus, leukocytosis, urinary tract infection, skin rash, malnutrition, uremia, advanced malignancy, immunosuppression (including steroid use), and immunodeficiency.
   b. Underlying conditions should be corrected prior to elective surgery, especially if use of prosthetic material is planned.
8. Nutritional assessment
   a. Patients who are malnourished (>10% body weight loss in 30 days) may benefit from preoperative enteral or parenteral nutritional supplementation. This is especially important in mesenteric occlusive disease in which significant weight loss is common.
   b. Obesity is a major risk factor in vascular surgical patients. Patients who are morbidly obese (100 pounds overweight) or moderately obese (15 to 40 pounds overweight) should be encouraged to lose weight prior to elective operation.
9. Diabetes mellitus
   a. Approximately 7% of diabetics have clinically evident peripheral vascular disease, and 2% will develop symptoms. Foot ulceration with secondary infection

is responsible for 25% of hospitalizations of diabetics.

b. Glucose control is often difficult postoperatively as a result of diet alterations, fluid shifts, and operative stress.

10. Assessment of renal function

a. The mortality rate in patients with postoperative ARF is 50%.

b. Preoperative studies include BUN, creatinine, and urinalysis.

c. The most effective strategy for avoiding postoperative renal failure is adequate hydration.

C. Postoperative Care

1. On admission to the ICU, the history and operative and anesthetic records are reviewed. A notation of intraoperative blood loss and fluid replacement is made.

2. An admission physical examination is performed as outlined above. Special attention is paid to the appearance of wound dressings and the presence of pulses and Doppler signals in fresh vascular grafts.

3. A routine laboratory evaluation is performed, which includes CBC, serum electrolytes, BUN, creatinine, calcium, magnesium, PT, PTT, ECG, and portable CXR.

4. Evaluation of intravascular volume status includes the following:

a. Preservation of adequate intravascular volume is essential in maintaining tissue perfusion and preventing distal limb ischemia, renal failure, myocardial ischemia, CVA, and gastric stress ulceration.

b. In general, intravenous fluid should be delivered in order to maintain a urine output of at least 0.5 ml/kg/hr (about 30 ml/hr in adults).

c. If the intravascular volume status is in question, a PA catheter should be inserted for measurement of PCWP, cardiac output, and Svo_2.

d. In general, oliguria during the first 36 postoperative hours (in the absence of renovascular disease) is considered to be hypovolemia and is treated with intravenous fluid resuscitation.

e. In general, oliguria after the first 36 hours is generally a result of volume overload and may be treated with diuretics.

5. Strategies for controlling hypertension include the following:
   a. Hypertension may cause serious complications in the early postoperative period including bleeding, graft disruption, myocardial ischemia, and stroke.
   b. Intraarterial BP monitoring should be routine for most vascular procedures, especially carotid, aortic, or renal reconstruction.
   c. Systolic BP should be maintained within 10% of the patient's preoperative systolic BP; if the patient was hypertensive preoperatively, systolic BP should not exceed 150 mm Hg.
   d. In many instances, specific pharmacologic control of hypertension may be unnecessary if pain control is adequate.
   e. If required, the most effective agent for rapid BP control is sodium nitroprusside (50 mg in 250 ml D_5W) as an IV drip, titrated to the desired effect. Because of the potential for overdose and hypotension, sodium nitroprusside should only be delivered in an ICU setting with continuous intraarterial pressure monitoring.
   f. Other effective intravenous agents include labetolol (initial dose of 2.5 to 5.0 mg), nitroglycerin (initial rate of 5 µg/min), and hydralazine (initial dose of 5 to 10 mg).
   g. If hypertension persists in the postoperative period, the patient's preoperative antihypertensive regimen should be reinstituted as soon as bowel function returns. If additional agents are required, control may be enhanced with nifedipine (10 to 20 mg SL q3h), nitroglycerin 2% ointment (1″ q6h), prazosin (1 to 2 mg PO q6h), or clonidine (0.1 mg PO q12h).
6. Myocardial ischemia should be prevented.
   a. Perhaps the best method of prophylaxis against myocardial ischemia is an adequate preoperative evaluation combined with an expeditious operation and strict intravascular volume management.
   b. Cardiac work is proportional to SV, HR, and BP, thus control of these elements may prevent a myocardial event. Control of SV and BP are addressed above. If tachycardia (>110 beats/min) is a significant problem, labetolol may administered.

    c. Any sudden change in cardiac status should be investigated with a 12-lead ECG, repeat physical and laboratory examination, and cardiac isoenzymes.

7. Strategies for preventing renal failure include the following:

    a. The single most effective strategy for the prevention of renal dysfunction is maintenance of adequate intravascular volume.

    b. Many clinicians advocate low dose dopamine for prevention of renal failure. In the vascular surgical patient, low dose dopamine (2 to 5 µg/kg/min) has the effect of increasing renal blood flow, redistributing blood flow to the renal cortex, increasing glomerular filtration rate and sodium excretion, and facilitating diuresis when intravascular volume is adequate. However, its effectiveness in the prevention of acute renal failure has not been established.

8. Prophylaxis to prevent stress ulceration (acute stress gastritis) should be utilized.

    a. Although it is generally agreed that prophylaxis will prevent acute stress gastritis following vascular surgery, opinions vary as to the optimal medical regimen for effective prevention.

    b. Accepted treatment options include antacids, histamine antagonists, or sucralfate. Regardless of the agent chosen, prophylaxis should continue until the patient is taking a clear liquid diet.

9. Strategies for preventing infection include the following:

    a. In general, routine perioperative antibiotics should be given as a single dose preoperatively, repeated doses intraoperatively, and continued for 24 to 48 hours following vascular surgical procedures. A first or second generation cephalosporin is acceptable. For patients with penicillin allergy, vancomycin is preferred.

    b. Wound dressings placed in the operating room may be left in place for 2 to 3 days if they remain dry. If the dressings become saturated, they should be changed promptly.

10. Prophylaxis to prevent DVT and PE should be utilized.

    a. Early mobilization, encouragement of leg exercises in bed, and proper recumbent patient positioning (ankles higher than knees, knees higher than heart) should routinely be employed.

b. Most vascular surgical patients do not require pharmacologic prophylaxis against DVT and PE because systemic anticoagulation is used during most procedures.

c. Pharmacologic prophylaxis should be considered for patients at high risk for DVT and PE (patients with prior history of thrombosis, malignancy, or disorders of coagulation).

III. SPECIFIC VASCULAR DISEASES

A. Abdominal Aortic Aneurysm

1. Abdominal aortic aneurysm is among the most common vascular problems encountered in the ICU. Usually, patients are admitted following elective repair. Infrequently, patients will be admitted to the ICU for preoperative evaluation or following exploration for abdominal aortic aneurysm rupture.

2. Controversy exists regarding the size of an abdominal aortic aneurysm that should be repaired surgically. A recent report recommended repair if the aneurysm was ≥4 cm in diameter and there were no relative contraindications (MI within 6 months, CHF, severe angina, renal dysfunction, poor mental status, or markedly advanced age).

3. The mortality rate for elective aneurysm repair should not exceed 2%.

4. Most patients with aneurysm rupture expire before arrival at a hospital. For patients that undergo surgery for rupture, a mortality rate of 50% and a major morbidity rate of 80% can be expected. The poor expected outcome for abdominal aortic aneurysm rupture has remained constant over the past 30 years.

5. Special considerations in the postoperative patient should be addressed.

a. The ICU admission physical exam is critically important, especially with regard to abdominal girth, the character of the flanks, the presence of femoral and distal pulses, and the status of peripheral perfusion.

b. Hypertension should be strictly controlled.

c. Gastrointestinal decompression by nasogastric suction will be required regardless of the surgical approach (transperitoneal vs. retroperitoneal).

d. Vigilance for ongoing blood loss must be maintained with regular assessment of cardiac filling pressures, urine output, and hematocrit. The patient's coagulation status should be checked, including PT, PTT, fibrinogen, platelet count, and serum calcium. If the admission PTT is abnormal, reversal of heparin with protamine may be helpful. If hemostasis proves inadequate, the patient should be promptly returned to the operating room.

e. It is not uncommon for patients to arrive in the ICU hypothermic after aortic reconstruction. Hypothermia is detrimental to perfusion and coagulation; fluid warmers, overhead warmers, and blankets should be used to warm the patient. A simple maneuver such as increasing the room temperature may help to alleviate hypothermia.

f. Because the incidence of renal dysfunction in elective and emergent repair is as high as 10% and 60% respectively, many strategies for renal preservation have been suggested. Some clinicians administer intravenous mannitol, furosemide, or dopamine prior to aortic clamping or in the early postoperative period. However, these interventions have not been shown to be efficacious in randomized trials; adequate fluid administration remains the most effective method for prevention of renal dysfunction.

g. Intestinal ischemia remains a serious complication of aortic replacement, occurring in approximately 5% of cases. It occurs as a result of routine sacrifice of the inferior mesenteric artery (IMA) during dissection. The diagnosis may be made intraoperatively by inspection of the bowel; if its viability is in question, the IMA should be reimplanted. More commonly however, the diagnosis is suspected postoperatively with the occurrence of abdominal pain, diarrhea, and hematochezia. The diagnosis of ischemic colon is confirmed by flexible sigmoidoscopy or colonoscopy. If transmural ischemia is present, reoperation and colon resection is necessary.

B. Aortoiliac Occlusive Disease

1. AIOD (also known as Leriche's syndrome) typically has symptoms of fatigue or claudication of the buttocks and

thighs, symmetric atrophy of the limbs, pallor of the legs and feet, and in males, impotence. Another less frequent presentation of AIOD is the sudden appearance of painful, punctate, purple lesions on the toes and heel referred to as *trash foot* or *blue toes syndrome,* which is caused by atheroembolism from aortic plaque.

2. The traditional operative approach to AIOD is aortobi-femoral bypass grafting, usually with a bifurcated woven Dacron graft. The mortality for aortic replacement should not exceed 2%, and the reported 5-year patency is approximately 90%.

3. Other approaches to AIOD, depending on the lesions involved, include iliac angioplasty and femoro-femoral bypass grafting.

4. Special considerations in the postoperative patient include the following:

   a. Postoperative care is similar to care for patients with aortic replacement for AAA. One difference is the presence of three incisions (midline and bilateral groin) in patients with aortobifemoral grafting. After AAA repair, many patients will have only a midline incision if a straight or aortoiliac graft was utilized.

   b. Pulse examination and documentation is critical after aortobifemoral grafting, and any loss of groin or distal pulsations should prompt immediate reexploration.

   c. Early complications of aortobifemoral grafting include hemorrhage, wound infection, MI, respiratory insuffi-ciency, renal failure, and distal extremity ischemia.

   d. Late complications can be devastating and include pseudoaneurysm formation, graft infection, and aor-toduodenal fistula. In general, late complications of aortic grafting carry a mortality rate exceeding 30%.

C. **Infrainguinal Occlusive Disease**

1. Atherosclerotic disease below the inguinal ligament is manifested as claudication of the calf, rest pain of the foot, foot ulcers, or gangrene.

2. These patients are difficult to treat since they often have serious comorbidity including advanced age, hypertension, COPD, heart disease, and diabetes mellitus.

3. Surgical strategy depends on the location of lesions and specific symptoms, but usually includes femoro-popliteal or femoro-distal bypass grafting (i.e., to the anterior tibial,

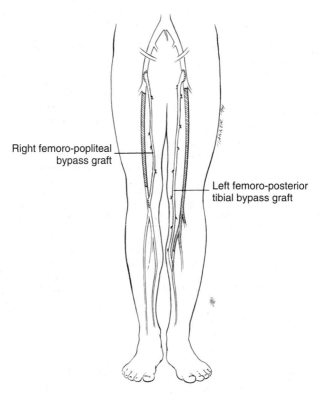

Right femoro-popliteal
bypass graft

Left femoro-posterior
tibial bypass graft

FIG 10-5.
Patient with right femoro-popliteal graft and left femoro-posterior tibial graft.

posterior tibial, peroneal, or dorsalis pedis arteries; Fig.
10-5). Commonly used conduits include the reversed
greater saphenous vein, the in-situ greater saphenous vein,
and Gore-tex (PTFE).
4. Results of bypass grafting are strongly dependent on
preoperative symptoms and the site of distal anastomosis.

Five-year patency rates range from 80% for femoro-popliteal bypass for claudication to 40% for femoro-distal bypass for limb salvage.

5. Special considerations in the postoperative patient include the following:

   a. One of the most important functions of the ICU physician is close observation for graft occlusion. The diagnosis should be suspected if the extremity becomes pallorous, exquisitely painful, or if there is any change in the pulses or Doppler signals in the graft or foot. Many occluded grafts can be salvaged if the diagnosis is made in a timely manner.

   b. Careful fluid, metabolic, and cardiac management is critical due to the frequent presence of underlying disease.

   c. The mortality for below-knee and above-knee amputations is approximately 15% and 40%, respectively, emphasizing the importance of the associated medical problems in these patients.

   d. Postoperative anticoagulation should be considered in patients with distal prosthetic grafts, axillo-femoral grafts, hypercoagulable states, or repeated graft failures.

D. Acute Arterial Insufficiency

1. The symptom complex usually contains one or more of the *five P's:* pain, pallor, pulselessness, paresthesia, and paralysis. The pain of acute ischemia is sudden and unrelenting. Acute vascular obstruction due to embolus or thrombus should be suspected in any patient complaining of the sudden appearance of a painful, cool extremity. The absence of distal Doppler signals combined with pain usually indicates that some form of surgical intervention will be required.

2. When a diagnosis of acute arterial insufficiency or a "threatened limb" is suspected, timing is crucial. Depending of the preexistence of collateral circulation, a "golden period" of 4 to 8 hours exists during which time intervention must be made or tissue loss may be irreversible.

3. The patient should promptly be systemically anticoagulated.

4. The definitive treatment largely depends on the duration of symptoms and the physical findings. If several hours have elapsed, there is no femoral pulse, and the diagnosis is certain, the patient should promptly be taken to the operating room for femoral artery exploration and thromboembolectomy. If the femoral pulse is present, and the diagnosis is uncertain, an arteriogram may be obtained to guide therapy.

5. The choice of therapy depends on the anatomic location of the occlusion. Femoral thromboembolism may be treated with thromboembolectomy and less commonly, with bypass grafting. Acute vascular graft occlusion usually will require graft revision. In selected cases, thrombolytic therapy with urokinase or streptokinase may be employed, although this strategy must still be considered experimental. If thrombolytic therapy is successful, some form of anatomic reconstruction will be necessary to ensure patency.

6. Distal thrombosis carries a poor prognosis. Thrombolytic therapy may be successful in some cases, but eventual limb loss is common.

7. Special considerations in the postoperative patient include the following:
   a. Reperfusion of an ischemic extremity often results in washout of ischemic byproducts into the systemic circulation. These byproducts include lactic acid, potassium, myoglobin, CPK, and LDH.
   b. Acidosis, hyperkalemia, and myoglobinemia may be life-threatening.
      (1) Acidosis may be treated with sodium bicarbonate.
      (2) Hyperkalemia may be managed with insulin and glucose, furosemide and saline, sodium bicarbonate, calcium gluconate, sodium polystyrene sulfonate (Kayexalate), or hemodialysis.
      (3) Myoglobinuria may be treated with aggressive volume resuscitation, osmotic diuresis with mannitol, and urine alkalinization. The goal of therapy is to induce euvolemic diuresis and maintain a urine output of 100 ml/hr.
   c. Reperfusion may also be complicated by compartment syndrome, which is elevation of pressure within the

limited spaces of the anterior, lateral, superficial posterior, and deep posterior compartments of the lower leg, secondary to edema. If compartment pressure exceeds 30 mm Hg, arterial compromise ensues. The initial symptom may be pain, preceding motor or sensory loss. The treatment for compartment syndrome is immediate operative fasciotomy.

E. Cerebrovascular Disease

1. CVA, or stroke, is the third leading cause of death in the United States. There are approximately 400,000 new strokes annually.

2. It is estimated that 50% of strokes are due to atheroembolism from the extracranial carotid arteries.

3. Carotid atheroembolism may cause one of three syndromes: TIA, RIND, or stroke.

   a. Symptoms: Hemiparesis, unilateral extremity sensory loss or paresthesias, unilateral facial droop, aphasia, monocular loss of vision (amaurosis fugax)

   b. Duration: TIA < 24 hours, RIND < 7 days, Stroke > 7 days

4. Approximately 75% of strokes will be heralded by TIA.

5. The results of randomized clinical trials now indicate that patients with cortical TIA and internal carotid artery stenosis of 70% to 99% treated with maximal medical therapy have a stroke rate of approximately 25% in two years. The risk of stroke in this same group of patients can be decreased to 9% with the performance of carotid endarterectomy.

6. Carotid endarterectomy is also recommended for patients with completed stroke and appropriate carotid lesions.

7. The beneficial effect of carotid endarterectomy in patients with TIA and lesser degrees of stenosis or plaque or in asymptomatic patients has not been firmly established, although clinical trials are ongoing.

8. Special considerations in the postoperative patient include the following:

   a. The initial examination should include a review of the operative and anesthesia record, examination of the neck, and a complete neurologic evaluation. The drain (if present) should be examined carefully and its adequacy assessed.

    b. Control of blood pressure is critical. Hypotension may cause cerebral hypoperfusion and hypertension may lead to bleeding complications.

    c. If new neurologic deficits are present or subsequently develop, immediate radiologic evaluation and/or reexploration are indicated.

    d. Postoperative bleeding into the neck may cause tracheal compromise and respiratory failure necessitating immediate endotracheal intubation, removal of the sutures or staples, and reexploration.

F. Renovascular Hypertension

    1. Approximately 2% to 5% of patients with hypertension have renovascular hypertension as the etiology.

    2. Renovascular hypertension is caused by a stenotic lesion in one or both renal arteries. The renal artery stenosis is a stimulus for increased renin release by the juxtaglomerular apparatus of the renal cortex. Renin converts angiotensinogen to angiotensin I, which is then converted in the lung to angiotensin II by ACE. Angiotensin II has a variety of physiologic effects, including effects on the sympathetic nervous system, the adrenal cortex (production of aldosterone), the renal tubules, the renal arterioles, and stimulation of vascular smooth muscle. The net effect of these processes is hypertension resulting from increasing arteriolar constriction, cardiac output, and sodium and water retention (Fig. 10-6).

    3. The diagnosis of renovascular hypertension should be suspected in patients with onset of hypertension at a relatively young age, the absence of family history, or hypertension which is severe and difficult to control pharmacologically.

    4. Diagnosis includes the following:

        a. Radioisotope renography

        b. Renal vein renin assays

        c. Renal function studies

        d. Arteriography

    5. Surgical intervention is indicated for control of hypertension and in some cases for preservation of renal function. A number of therapeutic approaches are available including aortorenal bypass grafting, hepatorenal bypass grafting, splenorenal bypass grafting, percutaneous balloon angioplasty, and nephrectomy.

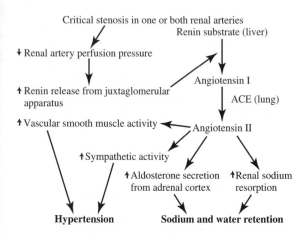

FIG 10-6.
The pathogenesis of renovascular hypertension.

6. Results of surgery are excellent, and improvement or resolution in hypertension and preservation of renal function is achieved in 80% of patients.
7. Special considerations in the postoperative patient include the following:
    a. Postoperative care is similar to the care described for aortic reconstruction.
    b. BP control is important. No attempt should be made to wean hypertensive medications in the early postoperative period since adequate BP control is necessary to avoid bleeding and cardiac complications.
    c. Fluid management is often difficult because of the tendency toward preoperative fluid overload from chronic aldosterone oversecretion. Pulmonary arterial pressure and cardiac output measurements are helpful.
    d. Sudden, uncontrollable hypertension or a decrement in renal function may indicate graft failure and should be further evaluated with renal scanning or arteriography.

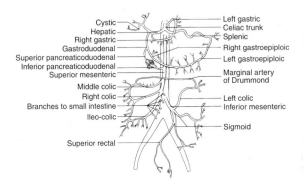

FIG 10-7.
The mesenteric circulation.

G. Acute Mesenteric Ischemia

1. Acute mesenteric ischemia is caused by compromise of the blood supply to the bowel secondary to stenosis or occlusion of the celiac axis, superior mesenteric artery (SMA), or IMA (Fig. 10-7).

2. The most common etiologies of acute mesenteric ischemia are embolism and thrombosis; less common causes include low cardiac output syndrome, shock, vasopressor administration, and aortic dissection.

3. Abdominal pain is universally present. The pain is often sudden in onset, crampy in nature, and may be associated with sudden bowel evacuation (often bloody and massive).

4. The classic symptom is abdominal pain out of proportion to the physical examination. Other signs occur later and include distention, rigidity, and hypotension.

5. Laboratory values are nonspecific and include hemoconcentration, hyperamylasemia, metabolic acidosis, and hyperphosphatemia.

6. The classic radiographic finding is pneumatosis intestinalis, but this occurs late and usually indicates gangrene.

7. Angiography confirms the diagnosis but should not delay therapy. It is reserved for stable patients in whom the diagnosis is uncertain.

8. Acute mesenteric ischemia is a surgical emergency. The treatment is immediate abdominal exploration with bowel resection and possibly aorto-mesenteric bypass, depending on the intraoperative findings. The decision to perform a "second look" operation in 48 hours to reexamine the bowel is made intraoperatively.

9. Results generally are quite poor; mortality rate from acute mesenteric ischemia exceeds 50%.

10. Special considerations in the postoperative patient include the following:
    a. Ongoing fluid loss should be expected since acute mesenteric ischemia is accompanied by intestinal edema and massive fluid sequestration.
    b. TPN should be initiated 48 hours after exploration, since prolonged ileus may also be expected and these patients are often malnourished.
    c. Persistent acidosis usually indicates ongoing intestinal ischemia and should prompt reexploration.
    d. Postoperative anticoagulation should be considered.

H. Chronic Mesenteric Ischemia

1. Atherosclerotic disease of the mesenteric vessels may lead to inadequate perfusion during times of increased oxygen demand, leading to postprandial abdominal pain, "food fear," and weight loss.

2. Abundant collateral circulation of the intestine exists via the marginal artery of Drummond (Fig. 10-7). Vascular compromise usually occurs only when two of the three major vessels are affected.

3. Abdominal pain is the *sine qua non,* and there is usually a postprandial pattern (intestinal angina). Pain rarely lasts more than one hour following meals and often correlates with the amount of food ingested.

4. Angiography is essential for the diagnosis and allows for the planning of revascularization.

5. The treatment of choice is mesenteric revascularization. Revascularization of all stenotic or occluded arteries (when feasible) produces the best results. The preferred conduit is the autogenous vein, although synthetic prostheses are also acceptable.

6. Since many patients with chronic intestinal ischemia are malnourished, preoperative TPN should be considered if the patient has lost ≥10% body weight in the last 30 days.

I. **Vascular Trauma**

1. Vascular trauma may occur as a result of penetrating or blunt injuries. Either mechanism can produce partial or complete arterial transection, vessel wall injury resulting in thrombosis, or combined arterial and venous disruption resulting in arteriovenous fistula formation.

2. Indications for immediate surgical exploration include arterial bleeding, an expanding or pulsatile hematoma, frank limb ischemia, pulse deficit, or the presence of a bruit.

3. Indications for arteriography in suspected vascular injury are controversial and include a stable hematoma, adjacent nerve or muscle injury, proximity of the injury to major vascular structures, and the presence of persistent shock.

4. Special considerations in the traumatized or postoperative patient include the following:

   a. Occult vascular injuries may be missed during evaluation in the emergency department. Trauma patients admitted to the ICU must be carefully examined and monitored for signs and symptoms of ongoing bleeding and ischemia.

   b. Volume resuscitation is critical to maintain adequate tissue perfusion and avoid the complications of shock including MI, ARDS, renal failure, and sepsis.

   c. 60% of patients with vascular trauma will have associated major injuries.

   d. Certain orthopedic injuries have a very high rate of associated vascular trauma including posterior dislocation of the knee (popliteal artery), supracondylar fracture of the humerus (brachial artery), shoulder dislocation (axillary artery), pelvic fracture (hypogastric artery and vein), or fractures of the shaft of the radius, ulna, or tibia (compartment syndrome).

   e. Traumatized limbs must be carefully monitored for compartment syndrome, since irreversible tissue damage can occur rapidly, sometimes in as little as four hours after compartment pressures rise. As mentioned above, symptoms include pain out of proportion to injury, sensory loss, or paresthesias. Motor dysfunction occurs later and may indicate tissue loss. Compartment pressures should be measured promptly, and fasciotomy performed if pressure exceeds 30 mm Hg.

J. Deep Venous Thrombosis and Pulmonary Embolism

1. DVT occurs in up to 20% patients following major abdominal surgery and in up to 70% of patients following major lower extremity orthopedic surgery.

2. DVT may occur in any deep venous system, although the most common vessels involved are the iliac vein, common femoral vein, deep femoral vein, popliteal vein, and deep veins of the calf.

3. Many patients with DVT are asymptomatic. When symptoms do occur, patients may complain of dull unilateral leg pain which is worse with movement.

4. Clinical signs are unreliable, although the most constant is unilateral leg swelling. Calf pain on dorsiflexion of the ankle (Homan's sign), the presence of a palpable "cord" (a thrombosed superficial vein), and calf or thigh tenderness can sometimes be elicited, but these signs are nonspecific.

5. Even when the clinical history, complaints, and physical findings are suggestive of DVT, the diagnosis is eventually confirmed in only about 50% of cases.

6. DVT may be diagnosed by duplex ultrasonography or MRI, but contrast venography remains the gold standard.

7. The treatment for established DVT in the iliofemoral or axillary/subclavian vein is anticoagulation.

8. Anticoagulation is usually initiated with heparin, which promotes the activation of antithrombin III, a naturally occurring plasma protein that neutralizes factors IX, X, XI, and XII. The recommended heparin dose is a bolus of 70 to 100 U/kg followed by a continuous infusion of 15 to 25 U/kg/hr. Monitoring of anticoagulation is accomplished using the PTT, which should be kept in the range of 1.5 to 2.0 times control. The platelet count must be monitored judiciously, since heparin therapy may induce thrombocytopenia in up to 5% of patients. In rare cases, the complication of heparin-associated thrombocytopenia and thrombosis (HATT) may develop, characterized by paradoxical arterial thrombosis. Treatment is immediate discontinuation of the heparin infusion.

9. Following initial treatment with heparin, therapy may be continued with warfarin (Coumadin), an oral inhibitor of the vitamin K-dependent clotting factors II, VII, IX, and X. Warfarin therapy may be begun as soon as the patient is fully anticoagulated with heparin, but the overlap of heparin and warfarin should be at least 4 days in duration, since one of the initial effects of warfarin is inhibition of protein C (a powerful natural anticoagulant). The dose of warfarin is usually 7.5 to 10 mg daily for 2 to 3 days and titrated thereafter to achieve a PT of 1.5 to 2 times control. In general, anticoagulation for uncomplicated DVT should be continued for 3 to 6 months.

10. In some cases for reasons that are unclear, thromboses from the deep venous system may embolize to the lungs (PE). Approximately 95% of PE have their origin in the deep veins of the pelvis and thigh.

11. The effects of embolization on pulmonary function depend on the size of the embolus, but they usually include increased pulmonary vascular resistance, V/Q mismatch with increased dead space and hypoxemia, and decreased pulmonary compliance.

12. The diagnosis of PE, like the diagnosis of DVT, requires a high index of clinical suspicion. PE is a great imitator; the classic triad of dyspnea, chest pain, and hemoptysis occurs in less than 15% of cases. As many as 20% of patients are entirely asymptomatic. When symptoms do occur, the patient may complain of dyspnea, chest or pleuritic pain, or confusion. Clinical signs are also unreliable, although tachypnea and tachycardia may be observed.

13. Laboratory tests are nonspecific. Approximately 90% of patients with PE are hypoxemic. The ECG is abnormal in 10% to 40% of cases but usually only reveals nonspecific ST segment or T wave changes. The plain chest radiograph is abnormal in 70% to 80% of patients and virtually diagnostic if Westermark's sign (diminished pulmonary markings) is present. In most cases, however, CXR findings are nonspecific and may include parenchymal infiltrates, atelectasis, and pleural effusion.

14. The ventilation-perfusion scintiscan (V/Q scan), which utilizes a combination of the techniques of lung perfusion scanning and ventilation scanning, is performed to establish the diagnosis of PE. Perfusion scanning is performed

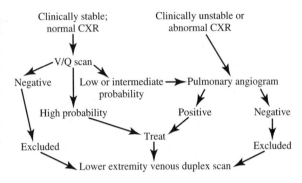

FIG 10-8.
The diagnosis of pulmonary embolism.

by the injection of ^{99m}Tc-labeled microspheres or albumin macroaggregates into the venous circulation, which by scintillation counting demonstrates the distribution of pulmonary blood flow. The study is compared to the ventilation scan, in which ^{133}Xe gas is inspired, and a serial image of the ventilated pulmonary segments is obtained. The sequentially obtained V/Q scans are compared in order to identify segments that are ventilated but not perfused and hence, may represent areas of embolization. A normal V/Q scan essentially rules out PE, and a positive scan establishes the diagnosis with 90% certainty. About 70% of scans however, will be interpreted as "low" or "intermediate probability," and depending on the clinical scenario, pulmonary arteriography may be required to establish the diagnosis with certainty. A diagnostic algorithm for PE is given in Figure 10-8.

15. PE can be clinically classified as minor, major, or massive, although much overlap within categories occurs. If the pulmonary arterial occlusion is estimated at 20% to 30%, and the patient is clinically stable, then anticoagulation with heparin is indicated as outlined in the treatment algorithm in Figure 10-9. Anticoagulation is

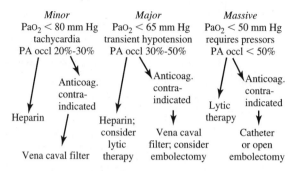

FIG 10-9.
The treatment of pulmonary embolism.

continued with warfarin over a 6 to 12 month period. If there is a major contraindication to anticoagulation (recent major surgery, GI bleeding, recent hemorrhagic stroke, HATT), the placement of a vena caval filter should be considered.

16. Vena caval filters are devices which are placed percutaneously into the vena cava for the purpose of trapping blood clots and preventing embolization from the lower extremities. The techniques of filter placement have been refined; currently the risk of misplacement or failure of insertion is less than 4%, vena caval occlusion is about 5%, and recurrent PE is about 4%. Nonetheless, placement of a vena caval filter should be reserved for patients who have a serious complication from or contraindication to anticoagulation therapy.

17. For patients with major or massive PE or failure to respond to anticoagulation, the use of thrombolytic or surgical therapy should be considered. Open surgical embolectomy is currently performed using cardiopulmonary bypass techniques, with a survival rate of approximately 60% among those patients stable enough to undergo exploration.

K. Arterial Access

1. Arterial cannulation for hemodynamic monitoring

    a. Continuous BP monitoring may be indicated for major vascular procedures, hemodynamic instability, cardiac dysfunction, sepsis, shock, or positive-pressure ventilation.

    b. The benefits of continuous on-line blood pressure monitoring must be weighed against the infrequent occurrence of vascular complications, including thrombosis, hemorrhage, infection, pseudoaneurysm formation, and arteriovenous fistula formation.

    c. The preferred sites for intraarterial pressure measurement in the ICU include the radial, brachial, dorsalis pedis, common femoral, and axillary arteries.

    d. Sites that do not have a strong palpable pulse should not be considered for cannulation.

    e. Sterile technique should be rigidly applied and catheters routinely changed every 3 to 5 days for the prevention of infection.

2. Complications of angiography via the femoral artery (incidence of 0% to 5%)

    a. Risk factors for the development of complications include female gender, advanced age, preexisting lower extremity peripheral vascular disease, presence of an aortobifemoral bypass graft, obesity, extremely low body weight, large catheter size, the use of multiple catheters, multiple punctures, prolonged procedure time, limited operator experience, presence of CHF or hypertension, failure of adequate anticoagulation, concomitant performance of percutaneous angioplasty or valvuloplasty, and puncture of the external iliac or superficial femoral artery (as opposed to the common femoral artery)

    b. Hemorrhage and pseudoaneurysm formation occur as a result of inadequate hemostasis.

        (1) Patients with significant ongoing blood loss or hematoma expansion should be taken to the operating room for control.

        (2) When blood loss is controlled, but the femoral artery puncture site fails to heal, a perivascular hematoma forms; this is termed a *pseudoaneurysm* (false aneurysm) since there is no true aneurysm

wall. The classic physical finding is a pulsatile groin mass. While an uncomplicated hematoma may transmit a pulse, a pseudoaneurysm is pulsatile in a radial direction on palpation of the lateral edges of the mass. The clinical impression can be easily and accurately confirmed by duplex ultrasound examination, and angiography is usually not required.

(3) The treatment of pseudoaneurysms should be individualized according to the morphology of the lesion and the overall status of the patient. Many pseudoaneurysms will seal spontaneously shortly after catheterization or with the aid of ultrasound-guided compression. If the lesion does not close within 3 to 4 days, continued observation may be complicated by frank rupture or pressure necrosis of the skin, and an attempt at closure is warranted.

c. Femoral artery thrombosis (1%)

(1) Thromboembolism may occur as a result of local thrombosis at the puncture site or from distal embolization from the puncture site or indwelling catheter.

(2) The signs and symptoms classically include pain, pallor, pulselessness, paresthesias, and paralysis; paresthesias and paralysis are late signs and suggest tissue loss.

(3) Immediate groin exploration and revascularization offers the best chance for limb salvage. Thromboembolectomy followed by repair is sufficient in most cases. More extensive vascular reconstruction including local endarterectomy, patch angioplasty, short segment resection, or formal bypass is required in 10% to 20% of operations.

d. Arteriovenous fistula formation

(1) Arteriovenous fistula formation occurs as a result of simultaneous puncture of the femoral artery and vein, which creates a passage for blood from the high pressure arterial system to the venous circulation.

(2) Arteriovenous fistulae may present as an asymptomatic thrill or bruit in the early post-catheterization period, or later with congestive

heart failure, increasing angina, claudication, or leg swelling.

(3) The diagnosis is usually suspected because of the presence of a thrill or bruit and confirmation may be sought by duplex Doppler ultrasonography.

(4) Many arteriovenous fistulae will close spontaneously, and therefore lesions diagnosed in the early postcatheterization period without arterial, venous, or cardiac insufficiency may be observed. If the fistula has not resolved after a period of about six weeks however, spontaneous resolution is unlikely, and repair may be considered to obviate hemodynamic and infectious sequelae.

3. Complications of angiography via the brachial artery

a. Although the risk of brachial artery thrombosis is estimated to be as high as 20% to 30%, more recent series quote rates of 1% to 5%.

b. Most clinicians recommend cut-down and brachial arteriotomy, although acceptable preliminary results have also been reported using percutaneous access.

c. Brachial artery thrombosis

(1) Brachial artery thrombosis accounts for more than 90% of complications using this approach.

(2) The small size of the brachial artery is responsible for its poor tolerance of indwelling catheters and arteriorrhaphy.

(3) Because of the abundant collateral circulation about the elbow, brachial artery thrombosis seldom produces severe or limb threatening symptoms. Complaints of hand coolness, paresthesias, or ischemic pain are likely to lead to recognition of brachial artery thrombosis. Loss of pulses should never be attributed to arterial spasm; the deficit is due to thrombosis until proven otherwise.

(4) The treatment of choice is thrombectomy. Brachial artery thrombosis managed expectantly may lead to the development of distal embolization, late arm claudication, and tissue loss in a significant percentage of cases. A significant delay in surgery results in poor operative outcome with increased likelihood of rethrombosis and persistent neurological deficit.

(5) Repair can often be performed by thrombectomy alone or thrombectomy followed by resection of the affected arterial segment and primary reanastomosis. Results of surgery are generally excellent, with long-term secondary patency and good clinical outcome exceeding 90%.

(6) The single most important factor affecting patency and the need for subsequent reexploration is the expediency of diagnosis and repair.

SUGGESTED READING

Eagle KA, Singer et al: Dipyridamole-thallium scanning in patients undergoing vascular surgery: optimizing preoperative evaluation of cardiac risk, *JAMA* 257:2185, 1987.

Ernst CB, Stanley JC, editors: *Current therapy in vascular surgery,* ed 2, Philadelphia, 1991, BC Decker.

Greenfield LJ, et al, editors: *Surgery: scientific principles and practice,* Philadelphia, 1993, JB Lippincott.

Hollier LH, Taylor LM, Ochsner J: Recommended indications for operative treatment of abdominal aortic aneurysms. Report of a subcommittee of the Joint Council of the Society for Vascular Surgery and the North American Chapter of the International Society for Cardiovascular Surgery, *J Vasc Surg* 15:1046, 1992.

McCann RL, Schwartz LB, Georgiade GS: Management of abdominal aortic graft complications, *Ann Surg* 217:729, 1993.

McCann RL, Schwartz LB, Pieper KS: Vascular complications of cardiac catheterization, *J Vasc Surg* 14:375, 1991.

North American Symptomatic Carotid Endarterectomy Trial Collaborators: Beneficial effect of carotid endarterectomy in symptomatic patients with high-grade carotid stenosis, *N Engl J Med* 325:445, 1991.

Sabiston DC Jr, editor: *Textbook of surgery: the biological basis of modern surgical practice*, ed 14, Philadelphia, 1991, WB Saunders.

THE ENDOCRINE SYSTEM   *11*

Paul M. Ahearne

I. THE STRESS RESPONSE TO SURGERY OR TRAUMA

A. Adrenergic Response

1. Primary purpose is to increase blood flow to the brain and heart.
2. Hormones of the adrenal medulla are the following:
   a. Epinephrine
   b. Norepinephrine
3. Physiologic changes include the following:
   a. Increased peripheral vascular resistance
   b. Increased HR, cardiac output
   c. Increased BP
   d. Increased blood flow to the muscles
   e. Splanchnic vasoconstriction, decreasing blood flow to the GI tract
   f. Increased metabolic rate
   g. Increased gluconeogenesis and glycolysis
   h. Increased minute ventilation
   i. CNS stimulation

B. Pituitary Hormonal Response

1. ADH
   a. Release from the posterior pituitary increases proportionately with severity of stress
      (1) Duration of increase is usually several days following cessation of the inciting stress.
      (2) Response is blocked by high-dose morphine, fentanyl, and epidural anesthesia.
   b. Stimulates renal tubular water reabsorption
      (1) Regulates osmotic pressure of extracellular fluid
      (2) Regulates blood volume

        c. Potent vasopressor

        d. Direct sympathetic effect on pancreatic islets

          (1) Increased glucagon release

          (2) Decreased insulin release

  2. ACTH

        a. Increased release with general anesthesia

        b. Rise is not proportional to the severity of the surgery or trauma

        c. Causes release of cortisol from the adrenal cortex, which has several effects

          (1) Gluconeogenesis

          (2) Protein mobilization

          (3) Fat mobilization

          (4) Antiinflammatory actions

  3. GH

        a. Secretion controlled by hypothalamic growth hormone releasing factor (GHRF) and growth hormone inhibiting factor (GHIF)

        b. Release following surgery or trauma proportional to the severity of the inciting event

        c. Normalization of levels after approximately 7 days

        d. Effects of GH

          (1) Decreases glucose utilization for energy (inhibits action of insulin)

          (2) Enhances amino acid uptake and protein synthesis

          (3) Reduces protein catabolism

          (4) Increases release of fatty acids from adipose tissue and promotes conversion to acetyl-CoA

  4. TSH

        a. Usually unchanged by surgery

        b. T_4 unchanged

        c. Normalization of decreased T_3 levels in approximately 3 to 7 days

C. Renin-Angiotensin System Response

  1. Renin

        a. Synthesized in the juxtaglomerular apparatus of the kidney

        b. Released in response to hypovolemia and decreased BP

        c. Converts angiotensinogen (synthesized in the liver) to angiotensin I

  2. Angiotensin II

a. Formed from angiotensin I by the action of ACE present in lung
b. Actions of angiotensin II
    (1) Vasoconstrictive effects on arteriolar and venous smooth muscle
        (a) Increases BP
        (b) Increases venous return
    (2) Direct effect on kidney to cause sodium and water retention
    (3) Increases ADH and catecholamine secretion
    (4) Stimulates secretion of aldosterone by the adrenal cortex
    (5) Increases renal tubular reabsorption of sodium and therefore of water
    (6) Increases excretion of potassium

II. HYPOTHALAMIC AND PITUITARY DISORDERS
A. Anterior Pituitary Failure

1. Etiology includes the following:
    a. Destruction of nerve tissue
        (1) Neurosurgery
        (2) Trauma
        (3) Radiation
    b. Tumor
    c. Infection
2. Panhypopituitarism can cause deficiencies in all six anterior pituitary hormones.
3. Symptoms are primarily manifested by ACTH and TSH insufficiency.
    a. Signs and symptoms of ACTH deficiency in the critically ill patient
        (1) Fatigue and weakness
        (2) Hypoglycemia
        (3) Postural hypotension
    b. Signs and symptoms of TSH deficiency (Section VII, B)
    c. Laboratory evaluation
        (1) Serum ACTH and TSH levels reduced
        (2) Cortisol, T_4, and T_3 are also low
        (3) CT/MRI scan to detect pituitary pathology
        (4) Cosyntropin stimulation test (Section IV)

        d. Treatment

           (1) ACTH deficiency (Section IV)

           (2) TSH deficiency (Section VII)

B. Posterior Pituitary Failure

  1. Etiology

     a. 50% of cases are caused by damage to hypothalamus, pituitary stalk, or posterior pituitary gland.

       (1) Head trauma

       (2) Surgical procedures in the area of the hypothalamus

       (3) Radiation

     b. 25% of cases are idiopathic.

  2. Leads to diabetes insipidus

     a. Loss of more than 85% to 90% of the neurons is necessary for diabetes insipidus to become clinically evident.

     b. Diabetes insipidus as a result of trauma or surgical procedures is often transient.

       (1) Occurs within several days of the inciting event

       (2) Resolves over several days

     c. Pathophysiology of diabetes insipidus includes the following:

       (1) Impaired ability to synthesize or release ADH in response to normal stimuli

       (2) Failure of the kidney to respond to ADH

          (a) Renal disease

          (b) Potassium deficiency

          (c) Hypercalcemia

          (d) Drug induced; lithium, methoxyflurane

     d. Signs and symptoms include the following:

       (1) Polyuria; as little as 3 to 4 L/day to as much as 25 L/day

       (2) Polydipsia

       (3) Severe thirst

     e. Laboratory abnormalities for diabetes insipidus include the following:

       (1) Increased serum sodium, BUN, creatinine

       (2) Urine specific gravity < 1.005

       (3) P_{osm} > 290 mOsm/kg

       (4) U_{osm} < 200 mOsm/kg

       (5) Water deprivation test if patient is stable enough to undergo fluid restriction

f. Treatment is the following:
(1) DDAVP (a synthetic analogue of ADH)
(a) 5 to 20 µg intranasal q12h
(b) 1 to 2 µg subcutaneous qd
(2) Pitressin tannate in oil 5 U IM q24-72h
(3) Lypressin 10 to 20 U intranasal q4-6h

III. DIABETES MELLITUS
A. Major Effects
1. Decreased utilization of glucose by the body cells causing increased serum glucose levels
2. Increased mobilization of fats with deposition in vascular walls
3. Depletion of body tissue proteins promoting decreased healing capacity

B. Routine Preoperative and Postoperative Care
1. Preoperative recommendations
a. Blood glucose measurement q6h
b. NPO after midnight and one-half normal PM insulin dose
c. Maintenance IV fluids
(1) Normal renal function: D_5 0.9% saline + 20 mEq/ KCl/L at 75 to 100 ml/hr
(2) Renal insufficiency or failure: IV fluids titrated according to renal function
d. One-half normal insulin dose morning of surgery (all as regular insulin)
e. Sliding scale insulin orders (Table 11-1)

TABLE 11-1.

Serum Glucose (mg %)	Humulin Dose (U SC)
<90	If symptomatic, orange juice PO or 25-50 ml D_{50} IV
	Reassess basal insulin
90-200	0
201-250	4
251-300	8
301-350	12
351-400	16
>400	20
	Reassess basal insulin

2. Postoperative orders
    a. Maintenance IV fluids
        (1) D_5 LR at 30 to 150 ml/hour
        (2) Fluids initiated according to length and type of procedure as well as according to renal function
    b. Insulin
        (1) Basal insulin 5 to 10 U SC q6h
        (2) Blood glucose measurements q6h with sliding scale insulin as above
        (3) For poorly controlled diabetes
            (a) Insulin drip
                (i) Administer 50 U regular insulin in 500 ml 0.9% saline.
                (ii) Start infusion at 30 ml/hr (3 U/hr).
            (b) Blood glucose measurements q1-4h and titrate insulin drip titrated to keep blood glucose between 90 and 200 mg%.

C. **Hypoglycemia**
    1. Most often caused by excess insulin administration
        a. Many patients do not follow their diets well, and their home insulin requirements are higher than in the hospital.
        b. Therefore insulin requirements in patients receiving IV fluids or on a controlled diet are often much less than their home regimen.
    2. Signs and symptoms
        a. Weakness, nervousness, tremor
        b. Tachycardia, palpitations
        c. Sweating
        d. Headache
        e. Hypothermia
        f. Mental dullness, confusion
    3. Diagnosis
        a. A blood sugar can be obtained.
        b. It is often prudent to treat the patient based on symptoms alone.
    4. Treatment
        a. D_{50} 50 ml IV
        b. Orange juice PO if the patient is alert and taking PO fluids
        c. Dramatic and immediate recovery after treatment if diagnosis of hypoglycemia is correct

D. Diabetic Ketoacidosis
1. Develops in the setting of absolute or relative insulin deficiency
2. Precipitating factors
   a. Coexistent medical illness
   b. Severe stress
      (1) Trauma
      (2) Major surgery
3. Pathophysiology
   a. The release of regulatory hormones (catecholamines, cortisol, glucagon, and GH) counteracts the effects of insulin.
   b. Decreased use and increased production of glucose and ketoacids produce hyperglycemia and ketoacidosis.
   c. Glucose levels are often between 500 and 700 mg% but may be less than 350 mg%.
      (1) Diabetic ketoacidosis in pregnancy or active alcoholism is associated with lower glucose levels.
      (2) Water, sodium, potassium, magnesium, and phosphorus deficits are all commonly seen.
4. Signs and symptoms
   a. Polyuria, polydipsia
   b. Weakness, lethargy, myalgia
   c. Headache
   d. Abdominal pain, nausea, vomiting
   e. Hypothermia (hyperthermia if associated with infection)
   f. Hyporeflexia
   g. Acetone breath
   h. Uncoordinated movements, coma, or stupor in later stages
   i. Hyperpnea
5. Laboratory abnormalities
   a. Glucosuria
   b. Hyperglycemia
   c. Ketonemia
   d. Decreased serum bicarbonate and pH
   e. Leukocytosis
6. Treatment
   a. Insulin
      (1) 10 U regular insulin IV loading dose

(2) Insulin drip; 50 U regular insulin/500 ml 0.9% saline at 5 to 10 U/hr (0.1 U/kg/hr) until both blood glucose < 300 mg% and pH $\geq$ 7.3

b. IV fluids

    (1) Administer 0.9% saline 1 to 2 L/hr $\times$ 1 hour then 1 L/hr $\times$ 2 to 4 hours.

    (2) Adjust rate based on patient volume status.

    (3) When blood glucose reaches 250 to 300 mg%, add D_5 0.9% saline at 50 to 200 ml/hr to infusion.

    (4) Accurately record inputs and outputs.

c. Potassium

    (1) 50% to 80% of potassium given is lost in the urine, therefore patients with oliguria or anuria require reduced amounts for replacement.

    (2) Monitor potassium every hour until stable.

d. Magnesium and phosphorus deficits—occur but seldom require therapy

e. Usually not necessary to use bicarbonate supplementation

7. Complications

  a. Cerebral edema

    (1) Manifested by drowsiness, lethargy, and headache occuring during successful therapy

    (2) Treated with mannitol and glucocorticoids

  b. Hyperchloremic nonanion gap metabolic acidosis normalization in 2 to 4 days as kidneys restore chloride and bicarbonate balance

E. Hyperosmolar Hyperglycemic Nonketotic Diabetes

1. Occurs mostly in older patients who often have mild diabetes mellitus or no diabetic history

2. Etiology

  a. Hypokalemia

  b. Medications

    (1) Phenytoin

    (2) β-Blockers

    (3) Diuretics

    (4) Glucocorticoids

  c. Stress

    (1) Infection

    (2) Burns, trauma, surgery

    (3) Pancreatitis

    (4) Hemodialysis

3. Signs and symptoms
   a. Polyuria, polydipsia
   b. Lethargy
   c. Altered mental status
4. Laboratory abnormalities
   a. Hyperglycemia (usually >800 mg%)
   b. Normal pH and HCO_3^-; possible mild lactic acidosis
   c. Serum osmolality > 450 mOsm/kg
   d. Absence of ketonemia
   e. Otherwise, similar to diabetic ketoacidosis
5. Similar treatment to diabetic ketoacidosis except that fluid and potassium requirements are often higher
6. Complications
   a. Cerebral edema
   b. ATN
   c. MI
   d. Cerebral hemorrhage

IV. ADRENAL GLAND
A. Adrenal Gland
1. The adrenal gland is divided into the cortex and the medulla.
2. The medulla is responsible for secretion of catecholamines; primarily epinephrine and norepinephrine.
3. The cortex is responsible for the secretion of cortisol.
   a. Stimulates gluconeogenesis
   b. Has protein catabolic effects
      (1) Increased amino acid utilization for glucose
      (2) Decreased utilization for protein synthesis
   c. Mobilizes fat from adipose tissue
   d. Has immunosuppressive effects
   e. Decreases production and action of insulin and thyroxine

B. Acute Adrenal Insufficiency
1. Most often seen in patients who are (or recently have been) taking exogenous corticosteroids
2. Signs and symptoms
   a. Weakness, lethargy, fatigue
   b. Myalgia, arthralgia
   c. Anorexia, nausea, vomiting, abdominal pain
   d. Orthostatic hypotension

3. Laboratory abnormalities
   a. Hyponatremia
   b. Hyperkalemia
   c. Acidosis
   d. Lymphocytosis
   e. Hypoglycemia
   f. Cortisol level < 20 µg/dl in the setting of severe stress
      (1) Normal value at 7 to 8 AM = 5 to 25 µg/dl
      (2) Normal value at 10 to 11 PM = 5 to 10 µg/dl
   g. ACTH stimulation test
      (1) Cosyntropin (synthetic ACTH) 250 µg IM
      (2) Serum cortisol evaluations at 0, 30, and 60 minutes after administration of cosyntropin
      (3) Normal response
         (a) Increase in serum cortisol level of at least 7 µg/dl over baseline
         (b) Serum cortisol ≥ 20 µg/dl

4. Treatment
   a. Hydrocortisone 100 mg IV q6h
   b. Hydrocortisone tapering when clinically stable
      (1) Rate of taper depends on the duration of treatment
      (2) Longer the steroid therapy, slower the taper

C. Chronic Adrenal Insufficiency

1. Patients receiving chronic corticosteroid therapy will be unable to mount a stress response.
2. Perioperative therapy for major surgery includes the following:
   a. Preoperative: Hydrocortisone 100 mg IV the night prior to surgery
   b. Postoperative: Hydrocortisone 100 mg IV q6-8h × 24 hours; then hydrocortisone 100 mg IV q12h × 24 hours; then hydrocortisone 50 mg IV q12h × 24 hours; then hydrocortisone 50 mg IV qAM or maintenance dose
   c. May use equivalent doses of prednisone once patient is tolerating a regular diet
3. May need 2 to 3 days of double or triple maintenance doses for minor stress

D. Pheochromocytoma

1. Arise from the enterochromaffin system
   a. Most tumors are active, secreting epinephrine and/or norepinephrine.

    b. These tumors are particularly lethal in pregnant women.

      (1) Mortality rate of 17% for mother

      (2) Mortality rate of 26% for fetus

2. Signs and symptoms

    a. Hypertension, either sustained or paroxysmal

    b. Sweating, cutaneous flushing

    c. Hypermetabolism (fever, weight loss, glucose intolerance)

    d. Headaches

    e. Tachycardia, palpitations, cardiac dysrhythmias, angina

    f. Mental status changes or irregularities, anxiety or panic attacks

3. Diagnosis

    a. 24 hour urine collection showing elevated levels of the following:

      (1) Vanillylmandelic acid

      (2) Metanephrine/normetanephrine

      (3) Free catecholamines

    b. Elevated plasma catecholamine levels

      (1) Normal < 600 ng/L

      (2) Normal patients with hypertension < 1400 ng/L

    c. Clonidine suppression test

      (1) Plasma

        (a) Administer clonidine 0.3 mg PO.

        (b) Measure serum catecholamine level at 0 and 3 hours.

        (c) A normal response is a decrease in catecholamines.

      (2) Urine

        (a) Clonidine 0.3 mg PO at 9 AM

        (b) 10 hour urine collection from 9PM to 7AM

        (c) Normal response

          (i) Urine epinephrine < 20 nMol/nmol creatinine

          (ii) Urine norepinephrine < 60 nMol/nmol creatinine

    d. Anatomic localization

      (1) CT or MRI to look primarily at the adrenal glands

      (2) ^{131}I-MIBG scan

        (a) Radiolabeled guanethidine analogue is actively taken up by pheochromocytoma cells.

        (b) Thyroidal iodine uptake is blocked by administration of potassium iodide.

        (c) This scan detects extraadrenal, small, residual, or recurrent tumors.

    4. Treatment

      a. Perioperative management

        (1) Prevention of complications associated with excessive catecholamine secretion

          (a) Do not perform invasive studies. (They can provoke catecholamine crises.)

          (b) Minimize intraoperative manipulation.

        (2) Preoperative pharmacologic blockade of catecholamine response

          (a) Prevents immediate complications upon surgical removal of catecholamine source

          (b) Allows preoperative volume reexpansion

          (c) α-Adrenergic blockade—phenoxybenzamine 10 to 20 mg PO tid-qid × 7 to 11 days; or prazosin 2 to 5 mg PO bid × 7 to 11 days

          (d) β-Adrenergic blockade using propranolol 10 to 40 mg PO q6-8h

      b. Acute hypertensive crisis—nitroprusside 1 mg/250 ml $D_5W = 4$ μg/ml, titrated to effect; or phentolamine 5 mg/500 ml $D_5W = 10$ μg/ml, titrated to effect

V. THYROID

A. Thyrotoxicosis

    1. An acute exacerbation of an underlying hyperthyroid condition

    2. Etiology

      a. Graves' disease is the most common etiologic factor.

      b. Other thyroid diseases may also precipitate a thyroid crisis.

    3. Precipitating factors

      a. Surgery

      b. Radioactive iodine treatment

      c. Parturition

      d. Stressful illness or infection

    4. Signs and symptoms

      a. Heat intolerance, hyperthermia, sweating, cutaneous flushing

      b. Diarrhea, nausea, vomiting

    c. Weakness, weight loss

    d. Dyspnea

    e. Nervousness, agitation, restlessness, delirium

    f. Hyperkinesis, hyperreflexia

    g. Tachycardia, atrial fibrillation

5. Laboratory abnormalities

    a. TSH usually undetectable in serum

    b. Increased serum T_4 and T_3.

6. Treatment

    a. Inhibition of hormone synthesis—propylthiouracil 800 to 1200 mg PO loading dose, then 200 to 300 mg PO q6h; or methimazole 25 mg PO q6h

    b. Inhibition of thyroid hormone release using one of the following:

      (1) Sodium iodide 0.5 g IV q12h

      (2) Saturated solution of potassium iodide (SSKI) 1 to 10 drops PO tid

    c. Block conversion of T_4 to T_3—dexamethasone 2 mg PO/IV q6h; or hydrocortisone 50 to 100 mg IV q8h

    d. Symptomatic treatment of excess T_4

      (1) Propranolol 40 to 60 mg PO or 1 to 2 mg IV q6h

      (2) Reserpine 1 mg PO/IM/IV q6-12h in patients with heart failure or asthma that cannot tolerate β-blockade

B. Hypothyroidism

1. Contributing factors

    a. Previous radioactive iodine treatment

    b. Prior neck surgery

    c. Prior exogenous thyroxine therapy

2. Signs and symptoms

    a. Cold intolerance

    b. Constipation

    c. Dry, scaly skin

    d. Lethargy, weakness

    e. Bradycardia

    f. Delayed deep tendon reflexes

    g. Peripheral and periorbital edema

    h. Decreased hypoxic and hypercapnic ventilatory drives

3. Laboratory abnormalities

    a. Elevated TSH

    b. Low free thyroxine index

4. Treatment: Thyroxine 100 to 200 μg PO qd

5. Myxedema coma
   a. Caused by a severe deficit in circulating thyroid hormones
   b. Usually seen in individuals with a long history of hypothyroidism
   c. As many as 50% of the cases have occurred after hospitalization
   d. Common precipitating factors
      (1) Pulmonary infection (most common) or other infection
      (2) Surgery or trauma
      (3) Hypoglycemia, hypovolemia
      (4) CVA
      (5) CHF
   e. Diagnosis is made on the clinical grounds of a precipitating event followed by:
      (1) Altered mental status
      (2) Profound hypothermia
   f. Treatment
      (1) Treat the precipitating cause.
      (2) Passively warm the patient.
      (3) Administer crystalloid fluid if the patient is hypovolemic.
      (4) Administer hydrocortisone 100 mg IV q6h.
      (5) Administer T_4 300 to 500 µg IV loading dose then 100 µg IV qid.
6. Euthyroid sick syndrome
   a. Most common thyroid abnormality seen in critically ill patients
   b. Thought to be due to a deficiency in the enzyme which converts T_4 to T_3
      (1) T_4 is preferentially degraded into reverse T_3 (rT_3) which is physiologically inactive.
      (2) Diminished active T_3 production limits the utilization of protein and oxygen.
   c. Signs and symptoms consistent with hypothyroidism
   d. Laboratory abnormalities
      (1) TSH is undetectable.
      (2) Free thyroxine index is low.
      (3) Serum T_4 and T_3 are low.
      (4) rT_3 is elevated.
   e. Treatment: Not indicated and may be deleterious

SUGGESTED READING

Civetta JM, Taylor RW, Kirby RR, editors: *Critical care,* ed 2, Philadelphia, 1992, JB Lippincott.

Freisen SR, Thompson NW, editors: *Surgical endocrinology,* ed 2, Philadelphia, 1990, JB Lippincott.

Hershman JM, editor: *Endocrine pathophysiology: a patient oriented approach,* ed 3, Philadelphia, 1988, Lea & Febiger.

Watkins J, Salo M editors: *Trauma, stress, and immunity in anesthesia and surgery,* Boston, 1982, Butterworth.

THE HEMATOLOGIC SYSTEM

12

Carmelo A. Milano

I. PATIENT EVALUATION
A. Laboratory Tests
1. PT
   a. Tissue thromboplastin (a factor VII activator) and calcium are added to platelet-poor plasma and the clotting time is determined. The PT is most sensitive to deficiencies in factor VII (extrinsic coagulation pathway) and factor X but may also be prolonged with deficiencies in factor V, prothrombin, and fibrinogen.
   b. Prolongation is seen with liver insufficiency, vitamin K deficiency, and warfarin ingestion.
2. APTT
   a. Platelet-poor plasma is incubated with a platelet membrane substitute (phospholipid) and a factor XII activator, and then recalcified. All factors except VII and XIII are measured by this assay.
   b. APTT evaluates the intrinsic coagulation pathway.
   c. APTT is prolonged with congenital factor VIII or IX deficiency or heparin therapy.
3. TCT
   a. A standard concentration of thrombin is added to plasma and the clotting time is measured, assessing fibrinogen level and conversion to fibrin.
   b. TCT is prolonged by hypofibrinogenemia, dysfibrinogenemia, and heparin.
4. Fibrinogen assay
   a. Fibrinogen is measured employing a modified TCT (normal 160 to 360 mg/dl).

b. Fibrinogen decreases with DIC, fibrinolysis, liver insufficiency, and massive transfusion.

5. FDP assay

a. Plasma is mixed with latex beads coated with an antibody to the fragment D-dimer domain of fibrin. The fragment D-dimer domain is a fibrin-specific region that occurs through factor XIIIa cross-linking of fibrin polymers. Fragment D-dimer appears in the blood after plasmin degrades cross-linked fibrin. Unlike the fibrinogen degradation products latex agglutination assay, the D-dimer assay does not cross react with fibrinogen and therefore distinguishes fibrinolytic from fibrinogenolytic processes.

b. Titers are elevated with DIC, primary fibrinolysis, liver disease, and thromboembolism.

6. Specific factor assay

a. Specific factor-deficient substrate plasma is incubated with the patient's plasma.

b. Failure of clotting time to correct indicates a specific factor deficiency (available for factors II, V, VII, VIII, IX, X, XI, XII).

7. von Willebrand factor (vWF): Ristocetin cofactor assay

a. Fixed platelets are mixed with ristocetin (normally triggers vWF-induced platelet activation), and plasma is added. Platelet agglutination is monitored by measuring changes in light transmission. The time required for agglutination is prolonged when a vWF deficiency is present.

b. This test is a sensitive and a specific test for von Willebrand's disease (vWD).

8. Bleeding time

a. A blood pressure cuff is placed on the arm and inflated to 40 mm Hg. A commercial instrument is then used to perform a small skin incision on the anterior surface of the forearm. The incision is dabbed with filter paper every 30 seconds, and the bleeding time is determined as the time required for bleeding to stop. The normal range is 3 to 10 minutes, but considerable variability exists.

b. Prolonged bleeding time occurs with abnormal platelet function. Platelet counts < 50,000 may induce prolonged bleeding time, therefore the test is most useful in assessing platelet function in patients with normal counts.

9. Lupus anticoagulant panel

a. Initial studies include PT, APTT, incubated mix test, and TCT. With the incubated mix test, the test plasma is incubated with normal plasma containing appropriate coagulation factors; correction of clotting times indicates specific factor deficiencies, and failure of clotting times to correct suggests the presence of inhibitors. TCT is performed to exclude heparin therapy as the possible inhibitor. In patients whose clotting times fail to correct with mix and who have a normal TCT, more sensitive assays (such as the Russell viper venom time) are performed to confirm the presence of inhibitors. While some inhibitors impede normal coagulation and predispose to bleeding, the lupus-like anticoagulant has been associated with increased risk of thrombosis.

b. Lupus anticoagulant panel is often obtained to help explain an unexpected, elevated PT or APTT. It should also be obtained on patients suspected of having a hypercoagulable state.

10. Activated whole blood clotting time

a. ACT is used to monitor heparin anticoagulation during cardiac surgery.

b. The ACT correlates with heparin dose in a linear manner.

11. Indirect and direct antiglobulin (Coombs') tests

a. Detect the presence of RBC antibodies in the patient's serum (indirect Coombs') or on the patient's antiRBCs (direct Coombs')

b. Useful in evaluating delayed transfusion reactions, autoimmune hemolytic anemia, and hemolytic disease of the newborn

B. Routine Preoperative Evaluation

1. History

a. Unusual bleeding with prior trauma or surgery, including dental procedures

b. History of epistaxis, easy bruising, DVT/PE, unusual menstrual bleeding, liver disease, malignancy, or renal disease

c. Family history of bleeding

d. Medications (warfarin, aspirin, NSAIDs)

2. Physical examination: Contusion, telangiectasia, jaundice, hepatomegaly, splenomegaly, hemarthrosis
3. Laboratory data: Decision to obtain additional laboratory tests depends on the history, physical examination, and the nature of the planned procedure; patients grouped into the following three categories:
   a. Category I: Negative history and physical examination, minor procedure—no additional lab tests
   b. Category II: Negative history and physical examination, major procedure—CBC to evaluate hematocrit and platelet count; may obtain additional tests such as PT and APTT, although in the setting of an unremarkable history and physical examination, the benefit of these tests is unproved, and they are probably not cost effective.
   c. Category III: Positive history, physical examination, procedures which cause alteration of coagulation (CPB or liver resection), or procedures in which the consequences of unexpected bleeding may be catastrophic (neurosurgical or ophthalmologic procedures)—additional tests warranted including platelet count, PT, APTT, and bleeding time
4. Considerations for patients on chronic warfarin anticoagulation who present for elective surgery
   a. Some minor procedures can be performed without significant risk, even with the PT prolonged to 1.3 to 1.5 × control.
   b. Warfarin treatment for DVT can be substituted with pneumatic compression devices, subcutaneous heparin, or placement of a vena caval filter.
   c. Bioprosthetic valves are less prone to thrombosis than mechanical valves; valves in the aortic position are less prone than those in the mitral position.
   d. Treatment
      (1) Hold warfarin (do not reverse with vitamin K).
      (2) When PT < 1.2 to 1.5 × control, start heparin infusion.
      (3) Hold heparin 4 to 6 hours prior to surgery.
      (4) Resume heparin infusion immediately after procedure (do not bolus).
      (5) Resume warfarin several days postoperatively.

C. **Evaluation of Bleeding in the Postoperative Patient**
The first and most important question is whether or not a mechanical source of bleeding is present that could be corrected surgically. Bleeding from a single region of an incision implies a mechanical source. Alternatively, multiple bleeding sites such as needle punctures, IV sites, the endotracheal tube, or hematuria imply a nonmechanical systemic disorder of coagulation.

1. History
   a. Consider any preoperative or intraoperative use of anticoagulants.
   b. A preoperative history of liver or renal disease may also be significant.
   c. Certain procedures such as liver resection or those involving CPB also result in distinct coagulation deficits.

2. Physical examination
   a. Evaluation of all potential sites of bleeding: All wounds, mucosal surfaces, and intravascular catheters
   b. Body temperature: Normal coagulation impeded by hypothermia (particularly common in trauma or CPB patients)
   c. Elevated BP: May contribute to bleeding in patients after vascular surgery

3. Laboratory data
   a. Hematocrit: Losses replaced with PRBCs and isotonic saline
   b. Platelet count
      (1) If the platelet count < 50,000/mm^3, platelet transfusion in an actively bleeding patient is warranted.
      (2) Abnormal platelet function can be assessed with bleeding time; patients actively bleeding with a prolonged bleeding time may require platelet transfusion even if the platelet count > 50,000/mm^3. Patients with renal failure, vWD, and who have recently ingested aspirin may have normal platelet counts but impaired platelet function.
   c. Coagulation system
      (1) Obtain PT, APTT, fibrinogen level, and FDP assay.
      (2) If the PT is prolonged and the APTT normal, consider hepatic insufficiency, vitamin K deficiency,

and malnutrition as possible etiologies. Treat with FFP, 2 U initially, and vitamin K 10 to 15 mg IM/IV q12h. Follow serial PT to monitor correction.

(3) If the APTT is prolonged and the PT normal, consider heparin administration or congenital factor VIII or IX deficiency as possible etiologies. Heparin effect may be reversed with protamine sulfate 25 to 50 mg IV over 10 minutes (doses greater than 50 mg are seldom required); repeat the APTT or ACT to assess complete reversal. A specific factor deficiency is treated with either cryoprecipitate or factor concentrate.

(4) If both the PT and APTT are prolonged, obtain fibrinogen level and FDP assay

  (a) If there is a low fibrinogen level (<100 mg/dl), consider DIC, primary fibrinolysis, massive transfusion, recent fibrinolytic therapy, or severe liver disease as possible etiologies.

  (b) A positive assay for FDPs signifies increased degradation of fibrin seen with DIC and primary fibrinolysis. Treatment for both DIC and primary fibrinolysis involves addressing the primary cause of these conditions. Administration of FFP or cryoprecipitate replaces fibrinogen and other factor losses. Epsilon-aminocaproic acid (5 g IV load, 1 g/hr IV maintenance) may also play a role in the treatment of primary fibrinolysis.

II. SPECIFIC HEMATOLOGICAL CONDITIONS
A. Sickle Cell Disease and Sickle Cell Trait

1. Sickle cell trait affects approximately 8% of black Americans, and 0.15% suffer from sickle cell disease.

2. A diagnosis can be made by demonstrating sickling of patient's RBCs under conditions of reduced oxygen tension. If this screening test is positive, hemoglobin electrophoresis can be conducted, which definitively distinguishes sickle cell trait from sickle cell disease.

3. Patients with sickle cell trait are generally asymptomatic and their overall life expectancy and frequency of hospitalization are unchanged. Patients with sickle cell disease have

impaired development and a severe hemolytic anemia; they have a variety of serious clinical problems which begin as early as 6 months of age.

   a. Acute infections: There is an increased risk for overwhelming infection by encapsulated organisms such as *Streptococcus pneumoniae* and *Haemophilus influenzae.* Sickle cell patients should receive the pneumococcal and influenza vaccines.

   b. Aplastic crisis: This occurs when decreased RBC production, usually following a viral or bacterial infection, is superimposed on the preexisting shortened RBC survival. Treatment is supportive and includes PRBC transfusions as needed. It is important to exclude a concomitant folate deficiency which may develop in these patients.

   c. Sequestration: Large volumes of blood rapidly accumulate in the sinusoids of the spleen, which produces hypovolemia, shock, and if not reversed, death.

      (1) Sequestration usually occurs in patients under the age of 5 years; older patients generally develop autoinfarction of the spleen and are functionally asplenic.

      (2) Symptoms include pallor, listlessness, abdominal fullness, and abdominal pain.

      (3) Physical examination reveals a large, tender spleen.

      (4) Treatment includes hemodynamic support with IV fluids and PRBC transfusions. Since recurrence is common, splenectomy is recommended after a second episode.

   d. Painful crisis: Microvascular occlusion secondary to RBC sludging causes painful crisis.

      (1) Painful crisis usually involves the extremities, but abdominal pain and abdominal distention are common and often difficult to distinguish from an acute abdomen.

      (2) Treatment includes IV hydration, supplemental O_2 therapy, analgesics, and correction of any acid-base disorder.

4. Preoperative care for sickle cell disease patients includes the following:

   a. For major surgery, preoperative transfusion to hematocrit 30% to 35% is indicated; many sickle cell disease patients may have developed alloantibodies to RBCs making it difficult to obtain compatible blood.

b. Hydrate liberally with 1.5 × maintenance throughout the perioperative period, since dehydration is a major predisposing factor for RBC sickling and sludging.

c. Avoid hypoxia; supplemental O_2 may be helpful.

B. Hemolysis

1. Hemolysis may occur in severe burn patients, in patients with electrical injuries, or may accompany sepsis and DIC.

2. Any intravascular prosthesis or device in contact with blood may induce hemolysis (cardiac valve prostheses, ventricular assist devices, IABP, or ECMO circuits)

3. Diagnostic signs of hemolysis include the following:
   a. Falling hematocrit
   b. Low serum haptoglobin
   c. Elevated serum and urine-free hemoglobin
   d. Elevated LDH

4. Treatment involves addressing the underlying cause and avoiding hemoglobin-induced renal failure.
   a. Urine output should be maintained at a level greater than 1 ml/kg/hr with saline infusion.
   b. Diuretics may be used as needed.
   c. Sodium bicarbonate may be added to the IV fluids to maintain the urinary pH at a level greater than 6 and which facilitates excretion of the hemoglobin.

C. Congenital Disorders of Coagulation

1. Hemophilia A
   a. Hemophilia A is a result of a deficiency or absence of normal factor VIII activity secondary to a molecular defect in the coagulant portion of factor VIII.
   b. Symptoms depend on the level of functional factor VIII present.
      (1) Patients with levels > 25% have normal hemostasis.
      (2) Patients with levels that are 5% to 25% normal do not suffer spontaneous bleeding but develop serious problems after surgery or trauma.
      (3) The majority of patients have levels < 5% and suffer recurrent spontaneous bleeds including intracranial, intraarticular, and urinary tract hemorrhage.
   c. Diagnosis often can be made based on personal or family history. Elevated PTT occurs with factor VIII levels <

30%. Definitive diagnosis requires measurement of factor VIII levels.

d. Treatment for hemophilia A includes the following:

(1) Spontaneous hemarthrosis or retroperitoneal bleeding requires transfusion several times per day or continuous transfusion of factor VIII to maintain levels of 25% to 50% for at least 72 hours.

(2) Patients undergoing elective surgical procedures should be screened for circulating inhibitors (present in approximately 6% of severe hemophiliacs) which prevent the correction of factor VIII levels necessary for surgery. In the absence of inhibitors, factor VIII levels are corrected with a factor VIII concentrate (25 U/ml). Prior to surgery, levels are corrected to 100% and maintained postoperatively above 40%.

(3) The following formula estimates the number of units required to raise levels:

$$\text{Dose (U)} = (\text{desired \% activity} - \text{initial \% activity}) \times \text{weight (kg)}/2$$

(4) Since the half-life of factor VIII is 8 to 12 hours, two thirds of the initial replacement dose should be repeated every 12 hours to maintain the desired level.

2. Hemophilia B

a. Hemophilia B results from the deficiency or absence of factor IX activity.

b. Symptoms are similar to but less severe than hemophilia A. Prolongation of APTT is an initial finding, and the diagnosis is confirmed with measurement of factor IX levels.

c. Replacement therapy is required for factor IX deficient patients undergoing surgery. Either FFP or a plasma fraction enriched in the prothrombin complex proteins may be used. FFP is the preferred source since it lacks possible thrombotic side effects described with prothrombin complex proteins. Preoperative replacement to 60% and postoperative maintenance of > 20% to 30% of normal beats for 10 to 14 days are adequate. The half-life and dosing interval of factor IX is 16 to 24 hours.

D. Acquired Disorders of Coagulation

1. Vitamin K deficiency

    a. Vitamin K serves as a cofactor in the hepatic synthesis of factors II, VII, IX, and X, as well as protein C and protein S. Most of the vitamin K that is utilized by the body is produced by the microbial flora of the gut and is absorbed as fat in the ileum. Vitamin K deficiency is suggested by the clinical history and a prolonged PT. Deficiency of vitamin K can result from obstructive jaundice, hepatic insufficiency, use of antibiotics that suppress gut flora, prolonged inanition, short gut syndrome, and any other causes of fat malabsorption.

    b. Treatment for Vitamin K deficiency includes the following:

        (1) Correct underlying disorder whenever possible.

        (2) Administer vitamin K 10 mg IM/IV daily × 3 days; failure of the PT to correct suggests causes other than vitamin K deficiency.

        (3) For emergent surgery, begin factor replacement with FFP, monitor correction of PT, and continue infusion as needed to maintain complete correction.

2. Liver disease

    a. The liver plays a complex role in the maintenance of normal hemostasis. With hepatic insufficiency, there is a decrease in the synthesis of prothrombin, fibrinogen and other coagulation factors. Liver disease may cause reduced vitamin K absorption, which further complicates the problem of decreased synthesis. The liver is also a major site of clearance of activated clotting factors, and the reduced clearance that results with liver failure may trigger uncontrolled fibrinolysis and DIC. Platelet number may also be reduced in cirrhotics with portal hypertension and splenomegaly, while platelet function is impaired by liver failure and alcohol. Finally, it is important to realize that the liver is the site of production for endogenous anticoagulants—plasminogen, antithrombin III, and protein C—therefore liver insufficiency may result in both hemostatic and hypercoagulable disorders.

    b. Management of the bleeding patient with liver disease includes the following:

    (1) Directed, specific treatment is indicated if an isolated bleeding point can be identified.

    (2) Obtain PT, PTT, fibrinogen level, bleeding time, and platelet count; obtaining factor VIII level may be helpful diagnostically to distinguish DIC from a primary problem with hepatic synthesis. (Since factor VIII is not synthesized in the liver, its level would be normal for hepatic synthesis defect but decreased for DIC.)

    (3) Administer vitamin K 10 mg IM/IV daily × 3 days; a response to vitamin K should be evident within 1 to 2 days. Failure of PT to correct after vitamin K suggests severe hepatic synthetic impairment.

    (4) Transfuse platelets for counts < 50,000 to 75,000/mm^3. If bleeding time is prolonged, a platelet transfusion may be indicated, even with normal counts.

    (5) FFP is the best factor replacement; care should be taken to avoid volume overload.

    (6) Severely depressed fibrinogen levels with marked elevation of the FDPs implies DIC or primary fibrinolysis. Sources of sepsis should be evaluated. Fibrinogen should be replaced with cryoprecipitate, and epsilon-aminocaproic acid may help inhibit ongoing fibrinolysis.

3. Hemostatic disorder of uremia

  a. Patients with uremia usually have normal factor levels and normal platelet counts. The defect lies in platelet adhesion and aggregation; transfused platelets rapidly become dysfunctional. It is also important to consider the possibility of residual heparin from dialysis.

  b. Management includes the following:

    (1) Preoperatively, obtain a PT, APTT, bleeding time, and platelet count.

    (2) Perform dialysis immediately preoperatively, since dialysis has a beneficial effect on platelet dysfunction.

    (3) If the bleeding time is prolonged, infuse 0.3 to 0.4 µg/kg DDAVP 1 hour prior to surgery.

    (4) If unexpected bleeding develops intraoperatively or postoperatively, repeat DDAVP infusion and start infusion of cryoprecipitate.

4. Massive transfusion
   a. Definition: A massive transfusion is the replacement of greater than one blood volume (5000 ml for a 70-kg patient) in a 24 hour period. The majority of these patients will demonstrate laboratory evidence of coagulopathy, and at least half demonstrate clinical evidence of a hemostatic defect.
   b. Platelet loss: This is perhaps the most significant consideration. PRBCs fail to replace the loss of platelets that occur with bleeding; furthermore, there may be loss of platelet hemostatic function resulting from acidosis, hypothermia, or drug infusions. Generally, transfuse 8 U of platelets for every 10 to 12 U of PRBCs.
   c. Factor deficiencies: Factor levels are much less labile during massive transfusion because of endogenous stores. Nevertheless, serial PT/APTT should be obtained during massive transfusions. Generally, 2 U FFP should be administered for every 10 U PRBCs transfused.
   d. Hypothermia: Patient exposure, hypoperfusion, and the administration of unwarmed intravenous fluids all contribute to the development of hypothermia, which may itself inhibit normal hemostasis. All fluids and blood products must be warmed prior to infusion, and in addition, overhead lamps and warming blankets should be used.
   e. Citrate toxicity: PRBCs contain citrate, which is added as an anticoagulant. Rapid infusion of PRBCs (several units over less than 1 hour) may result in reduced ionized calcium secondary to calcium complexing with citrate. Therefore calcium gluconate (10%) 10 ml IV may be administered during massive transfusion and ionized calcium levels monitored.
   f. Acidosis may occur initially during massive transfusion secondary to citrate but rarely requires treatment. The citric acid is rapidly converted to pyruvate and bicarbonate, which may produce metabolic alkalosis. Acidosis in this patient group is more likely secondary to hypoperfusion.
   g. Transfused RBCs have depleted amounts of 2,3-diphosphoglycerate, which normally enhances release of oxygen at the tissues. Therefore during massive transfusion, oxygen delivery may be reduced and a

higher hematocrit may be required to provide adequate Do_2.

5. DIC
   a. Definition: DIC is unregulated activation of the coagulation cascade by tissue thromboplastin or other agents (endotoxin) with subsequent consumption of both platelets and coagulation factors. Clinical manifestations may be either bleeding or thrombosis.
   b. Common causes among surgical patients: These include sepsis, massive trauma, pancreatitis, liver disease, peritoneovenous shunts, disseminated malignancy, and obstetrical catastrophes.
   c. Diagnosis: Laboratory manifestations include thrombocytopenia, presence of schistocytes on peripheral smear, prolongation of both the PT and APTT, diminished fibrinogen levels, and increased FDPs. The amount of fibrinogen decrease may be the best gauge of the clinical severity of DIC.
   d. Treatment for DIC includes the following:
      (1) When possible, correct underlying cause (sepsis, shock, trauma, retained fetal products).
      (2) In bleeding patient, administer FFP (2 U initially) for general factor replacement, and follow PT/APTT.
      (3) Severe depletion of fibrinogen < 100 mg/dl in actively bleeding patient warrants replacement with cryoprecipitate.
      (4) Perform a platelets transfusion for bleeding if platelet count < 50,000/mm^3.
      (5) Epsilon-aminocaproic acid is only indicated for life-threatening hemorrhage with evidence of marked fibrinolysis (elevated FDPs).
6. Primary fibrinolysis
   a. Clinical manifestations and laboratory data are very similar to DIC. There may be a relatively greater decrease in fibrinogen and increase in FDPs, with more normal PT/APTT and platelet counts.
   b. Causes include liver disease, inherited disorders (such as alpha-2 plasmin inhibitor deficiency), and metastatic prostate cancer.
   c. Fibrinogen replacement with cryoprecipitate and administration of epsilon-aminocaproic acid should be

considered as part of the treatment when bleeding develops.

7. Coagulopathy after CPB

   a. Coagulation defects that may arise during CPB are diverse and include DIC and primary fibrinolysis.

   b. As with bleeding after any type of surgery, the most important question to ask is whether there is a surgical site which could account for the bleeding and could be addressed with reoperation.

   c. It is important to determine whether heparin administered prior to CPB has been fully reversed. Considering the short half-life of heparin, bleeding that occurs several hours after completion of the procedure is unlikely to be due to residual heparinization.

   d. Most patients have mild hypothermia following CPB, which contributes to coagulation defects; body temperature can be normalized with heating lamps, heating blankets, and infusion of warmed IV fluids.

   e. Systemic hypertension can aggravate mediastinal bleeding and should be addressed with afterload-reducing agents.

   f. Platelet destruction and impairment are more common following CPB than defects in coagulation factors. The platelet count does not reflect platelet function, and platelet transfusion may be appropriate even when counts are greater than 50,000/mm^3.

E. Platelet Disorders

Normal platelet counts range from 150,000 to 450,000/mm^3, and normal surgical hemostasis requires between 60,000/mm^3 and 100,000/mm^3. Thrombocytopenia results from decreased production (marrow failure), platelet sequestration (hypersplenism), or increased platelet destruction (autoantibody, prosthetic valves, DIC). Rapid decreases in platelet count (>25% in 24 hours) suggests destruction rather than decreased production. Deficient platelet production is confirmed by bone marrow aspiration demonstrating decreased numbers of megakaryocytes.

1. ITP

   a. ITP is a result of platelet destruction due to autoantibodies. The disease is self limiting in children, with near total recovery seen within 6 months. Adults suffer a more chronic form.

    b. The medical treatment is prednisone 1 to 3 mg/kg/day; the majority of patients, however, will relapse on medical treatment and will require splenectomy.

    c. Preoperative preparation for splenectomy in ITP includes the following:

        (1) Administer pneumococcal vaccine preoperatively.

        (2) Transfuse platelets intraoperatively to obtain a platelet count > 50,000/mm^3.

        (3) Continue steroids postoperatively until platelet counts return to normal, then taper gradually.

    d. Accessory spleens are a cause of recurrence after splenectomy.

2. TTP

    a. TTP is a rare syndrome caused by inappropriate, unregulated aggregation of platelets.

    b. Characteristic findings include microvascular deposition of hyaline thrombi, microangiopathic hemolytic anemia, thrombocytopenia, fever, renal failure, fluctuating levels of consciousness, and focal neurologic deficits.

    c. Treatment involves the use of exchange transfusion and intensive plasmapheresis; only half of the patients recover.

3. Drug-induced thrombocytopenia

    a. Any patient with unexplained thrombocytopenia should have all medications carefully reviewed.

    b. Certain medications inhibit platelet production, while others trigger an immune response in which the platelets are innocent bystanders.

    c. Common agents which cause thrombocytopenia include most chemotherapeutic agents, alcohol, thiazide diuretics, diphenylhydantoin, numerous antibiotics, cimetidine, ranitidine, quinidine, and estrogens.

4. Splenic sequestration

    a. Splenic enlargement from any cause results in a greater fraction of total platelets residing in the spleen.

    b. Therefore the absolute number of circulating platelets declines.

5. Heparin-induced thrombocytopenia

    a. Heparin-induced thrombocytopenia is thought to be caused by an IgG-heparin immune complex, which causes platelet activation and aggregation.

b. Although most cases have occurred with patients receiving large doses of heparin, small doses (such as line flushes) may induce thrombocytopenia.

c. Thrombocytopenia usually begins between 3 and 15 days after heparin therapy and is more common with heparin derived from bovine lung than from porcine gut.

d. Although patients remain asymptomatic in most cases, the syndrome of HATT may develop, which is characterized by diffuse arterial thrombosis (0.4% in patients receiving therapeutic doses of porcine heparin).

e. Management of HATT includes the following:
   (1) Daily platelet counts should be performed on patients receiving heparin.
   (2) If the platelet count falls below 100,000/mm^3 or has an abrupt decline, heparin should be discontinued, and warfarin therapy begun.

6. Decreased platelet function
   a. Aspirin and NSAIDs inhibit the platelet enzyme cyclo-oxygenase and reduce the production of thromboxane A_2, which mediates platelet secretion and aggregation.
   b. Aspirin irreversibly acetylates cyclooxygenase; a single dose impairs hemostasis for 5 to 7 days.
   c. NSAIDs inhibit in a competitive, reversible fashion and the effect is more transient.

7. von Willebrand's disease (vWD)
   a. vWD is the most common inherited bleeding disorder. It is an autosomal dominant disorder in which there is a deficiency of vWF, which normally facilitates platelet adhesion and acts as a carrier for coagulant factor VIII.
   b. Classifications include types I, IIa, IIb, and III. Types I, IIa, and III represent progressively more severe deficiencies of vWF function. Type IIb represents a form in which there is an excess of abnormal vWF, which results in increased platelet aggregation and may result in thrombocytopenia.
   c. Clinical manifestations are heterogeneous, ranging from abnormal bleeding only after surgery or trauma to spontaneous bleeding.
   d. Laboratory diagnosis includes prolonged bleeding time, reduced vWF, reduction in ristocetin cofactor activity, and reduced factor VIII activity.

e. Prior to surgery or after major trauma, patients should be treated with cryoprecipitate. After minor trauma or in patients with mild vWD, DDAVP 0.3 μg/kg IV may be sufficient. DDAVP is contraindicated in patients with type IIb vWF.

8. Thrombocytosis

   a. Thrombocytosis is classified as primary (myeloproliferative disorders) or secondary (in response to inflammation, acute bleeding, iron deficiency, splenectomy, or neoplasm).

   b. In primary thrombocytosis, platelet function is invariably impaired and patients may develop bleeding or thrombotic complications. Hydroxyurea or alkylating agents can be used to reduce platelet counts in symptomatic patients with primary thrombocytosis.

F. Hypercoagulable States

Hypercoagulable states are a result of congenital or acquired defects in the biochemical mechanisms that normally inhibit thrombus formation. As many as 10% to 20% of patients with recurrent thromboembolism, DVT, or PE have a hypercoagulable state. Any patient with recurrent arterial or venous thrombosis or any thromboembolism in the first or second decade of life should be evaluated for the presence of a hypercoagulable state.

1. Antithrombin III deficiency

   a. This defect is an inherited deficiency of antithrombin III, which normally complexes with the serine protease coagulation factors, reducing their rate of activation.

   b. Patients with mildly decreased antithrombin III levels can be anticoagulated with heparin. Patients with a severe deficiency cannot be anticoagulated with heparin unless antithrombin III (in the form of FFP) is first administered. These patients should be maintained chronically on warfarin.

2. Protein C deficiency

   a. Protein C is a vitamin K-dependent factor synthesized in the liver, which is normally activated by thrombin and inactivates factors Va and VIIIa.

   b. Patients may be heterozygous or homozygous for the defect, with the latter representing a much less common, more severe form of the disease. Patients who are heterozygous may be anticoagulated with heparin or warfarin; those who have experienced recurrent thrombotic episodes should remain on warfarin for life.

   c. Warfarin therapy however, may further decrease protein C levels and must be approached with caution; some of these patients may be resistant to warfarin anticoagulation and may develop warfarin-induced skin necrosis.

3. Protein S deficiency

   a. Protein S, like protein C, inhibits thrombosis by participating in the inactivation of activated factors V and VIII.

   b. Patients with protein S deficiency may be homozygous or heterozygous for the defect. Although protein S deficiency is less common than protein C deficiency, the symptoms, diagnosis, and treatment are similar.

4. Lupus-like anticoagulants

   a. This disorder is a result of heterogenous antiphospholipid antibodies which prolong phospholipid-dependent coagulation assays and can be detected in various pathologic conditions other than SLE.

   b. Despite the term *anticoagulant* and the characteristic prolongation of the APTT with this disorder, clinically, these patients experience increased episodes of thrombosis.

   c. Any patient with recurrent thrombosis should be evaluated for lupus-like anticoagulants; patients with lupus-like anticoagulants and venous thrombosis should be maintained on warfarin.

III. BLOOD COMPONENT THERAPY
A. Whole Blood

1. Whole blood contains RBCs and plasma components; it is anticoagulated with any one of several anticoagulant solutions including citrate phosphate dextrose.

2. Whole blood is indicated in patients with impaired oxygen carrying capacity and hypovolemia, such as trauma patients with massive blood loss.

3. If ABO group and Rh type are not known, transfuse O-negative blood.

4. If ABO group and Rh type are known, transfuse type-specific blood.

B. Packed Red Blood Cells

1. PRBCs are prepared by removing supernatant plasma from whole blood. The hematocrit is 65% to 70% and the volume is about 300 ml/U.

2. PRBCs are the product of choice for improving of oxygen carrying capacity without extensive blood volume expansion.

3. The indications for transfusion are not absolute and depend on individual patients; an asymptomatic young patient recovering from uncomplicated surgery may tolerate a hematocrit < 20% without the need for transfusion. Conversely, an elderly patient with cardiopulmonary insufficiency and a complicated postoperative course may show improved Vo_2 and Do_2 following transfusion, even if the hematocrit is as high as 35% to 40%.

4. In an adult, 1 U PRBCs should raise the hemoglobin 1 g/dl or the hematocrit by 3%.

C. Frozen (Deglycerolized) Red Blood Cells

1. Frozen RBCs are prepared by suspension in glycerol and freezing. Frozen RBCs are thawed and washed of glycerol prior to transfusion.

2. Advantages of frozen RBCs include the preservation of rare RBC types, improved RBC viability, maintenance of ATP and 2,3-DPG concentrations, and a reduction in leukocytes and donor plasma.

3. Disadvantages of frozen RBCs include the high cost and the need for transfusion within 24 hours of thawing.

D. Fresh Frozen Plasma

1. FFP is separated from whole blood by centrifugation; it is frozen within 8 hours and stored frozen until used. The activity of labile factors (V and VIII) rapidly declines after thawing, therefore it should be used as soon as possible.

2. FFP contains factors II, V, VII, VIII, vWF, IX, X, XI, and XII in concentrations similar to those in normal plasma. While FFP provides a broad spectrum of coagulation components, rather large volumes are required to raise levels appreciably in recipients.

3. FFP is indicated in the management of patients with multiple coagulation defects, such as hepatic insufficiency, coagulopathy associated with massive transfusion, or DIC.

4. FFP contains anti-A, anti-B and anti-Rh antibodies; type- and Rh-specific plasma should be used.

5. Since FFP is a single-donor product, 1 U carries the same risk of virally transmitted disease as 1 U of whole blood.

E. Cryoprecipitate

1. Cryoprecipitate is prepared by thawing FFP to 1° to 6° C and recovering the precipitate, which is then refrozen and stored. Cryoprecipitate from several different donors may be pooled prior to refreezing.

2. After thawing, it should remain at room temperature and never be refrozen.

3. Contains 150 mg fibrinogen per bag, 80 U coagulant factor VIII per bag and large amounts of vWF

4. Indications include hemophilia A, vWD, primary fibrinolysis, or DIC when fibrinogen levels are markedly depressed (<100 mg/dl).

F. Factor VIII Concentrate

1. Very high concentration of factor VIII (25 U/ml) without fibrinogen and with variable amounts of vWF

2. Pooled from a large population of donors

3. Indicated primarily for hemophilia A

4. Viral hepatitis and HIV transmission (previously very serious complications), now reduced by new methods of controlled heating and viral screening of blood

G. Prothrombin Complex Concentrate

1. Contains factors II, VII, IX, and X in concentrations higher than FFP

2. Pooled product from multiple donors; viral transmission reduced by controlled heating

3. Indicated in hemophilia B

H. Platelets

1. A concentrate of platelets is separated from a single unit of whole blood and suspended in a small amount of the original plasma; units are generally pooled prior to transfusion.

2. Since some donor plasma is present, the platelets must be ABO compatible.

3. Each unit of platelets can be expected to raise the platelet count of the normal 70-kg adult 5,000 to 10,000/mm^3 and that of an 18-kg child by 20,000/mm^3.

4. Active bleeding in a patient with a platelet count < 50,000/mm^3 is the primary indication for transfusion. Platelet transfusion may be indicated for patients with higher counts who are bleeding if they have abnormal platelet function.

I. Autotransfusion

1. Autologous blood may be donated one month prior to elective surgery, which allows the patient time to regenerate red cells. This blood is processed and stored similarly to standard blood products.

2. Intraoperative collection of shed blood with immediate reinfusion is commonly employed with cardiac surgery. With noncardiac surgery, shed blood usually is treated with citrate or heparin prior to reinfusion. Such recovery systems may result in activation of the clotting system with subsequent reinfusion of FDPs, which may actually have a negative effect on normal coagulation.

J. Complications of Transfusions

1. Acute hemolytic transfusion reaction

   a. This particular reaction occurs when donor's RBCs and recipient's plasma are incompatible. Undetected serologic incompatibilities can cause these reactions; however, most are due to ABO mismatches secondary to clerical error.

   b. Manifestations include shock, chills, fever, dyspnea, chest pain, back pain, headache, or abnormal bleeding. In an anesthetized patient, fever, tachycardia, or hypotension may be signs of transfusion reactions. DIC and renal failure may ensue.

   c. Treatment for acute hemolytic transfusion reaction includes the following:

      (1) Stop the transfusion.

      (2) Send both patient blood and donor blood for typing.

      (3) Support the circulation; pressors may be initially required, but crystalloid or colloid infusion should be the primary treatment.

      (4) Maintain a high urine output with saline infusions or diuretics. Saline may be supplemented with sodium bicarbonate to maintain urine at a $pH > 6$ and facilitate excretion of hemoglobin.

      (5) Treat DIC and bleeding with factor or platelet replacement.

2. Delayed hemolytic reaction

   a. A delayed hemolytic reactions rarely occurs and is usually a result of recipient antibodies undetected at the time of transfusion.

   b. Signs may occur 4 to 14 days after the transfusion and
      include a progressive fall in the hematocrit, fever,
      hemoglobinuria, hyperbilirubinemia, and renal failure.
   c. Treatment is similar to treatment for an acute hemolytic
      reaction.
3. Transmission of viral disease
   a. Viral hepatitis
      (1) Viral hepatitis is the most important infectious
          complication of blood product transfusions.
      (2) Serological tests to screen donors are now available
          for both hepatitis B and hepatitis C; however, donors
          may have very low but infective levels of these
          viruses which are not detected.
      (3) The incidence of contamination is estimated to be
          less than 1 in 100 U for hepatitis B and less than 1
          in 200 U for hepatitis C. The incidence of post-
          transfusion hepatitis (all types) in patients who have
          received multiple transfusions is approximately 7%.
      (4) A small fraction of patients who become infected
          with either hepatitis B or C will develop chronic
          hepatitis, cirrhosis, and liver failure.
      (5) Concentrated factor products such as factor VIII
          concentrate are currently treated with controlled
          heating, which inactivates viruses and further re-
          duces the risk of infection with hepatitis B, hepatitis
          C, or HIV. FFP and cryoprecipitate cannot be heat
          treated.
   b. HIV I and HIV II
      (1) An antibody test is currently employed to help
          screen out infected donors; however, donors may
          be infectious for a period of time prior to serocon-
          version.
      (2) The incidence of contaminated units is approxi-
          mately 1 in 40,000 to 100,000 U, and not all patients
          who receive contaminated units will become in-
          fected.
   c. CMV
      (1) Transmission of this pathogen is significant only in
          CMV-negative, immunosuppressed patients (such
          as transplant recipients).
      (2) Since CMV is predominantly intracellular, trans-
          mission with noncellular products is not a concern.

Furthermore, leukofiltration of PRBCs and platelet products markedly reduces transmission and should be employed in seronegative immunosuppressed patients.

4. Bacterial contamination of blood products
   a. Contamination is rare and usually occurs with older, stored products.
   b. When contamination occurs however, the organisms are often gram-negative bacilli, and recipients may develop severe endotoxin reactions. Manifestations include a sudden, high fever, chills, and hypotension.
   c. If contamination is suspected, discontinue transfusion, culture the product being transfused, and start broad-spectrum antibiotics.

5. Febrile reactions
   a. Febrile reactions occur in about 1% of transfusions and are a result of antibodies that agglutinate leukocytes.
   b. Patients with these reactions should be examined to rule out a more serious complication, but in most instances the fever may be treated symptomatically (Tylenol) and the transfusion completed.
   c. Patients with recurrent febrile reactions will benefit from leukocyte-reduced products.

6. Allergic reactions
   a. Allergic reactions are manifested as hives or pruritus and occur with 1% of transfusions.
   b. These reactions are triggered by plasma proteins in the transfusion.
   c. Antihistamines (Benadryl 25 to 50 mg PO/IM) may ameliorate symptoms and usually the transfusion may be completed.

7. Citrate toxicity
   a. Immediately after the transfusion, citrate anticoagulants may result in a small acidosis, but the ultimate effect is a metabolic alkalosis as citrate is metabolized.
   b. In addition, citrate binds serum calcium and may result in a transient hypocalcemia. Although not a concern with small transfusions, the development of sudden tetany, hypotension, and decreased cardiac output in a patient receiving a massive transfusion may signal hypocalcemia. Calcium gluconate (10%) 10 ml IV should be administered to massively transfused pa-

tients to avoid hypocalcemia; if transfusion continues, periodic measurement of ionized calcium is recommended.

8. Pulmonary edema
   a. The majority of infused blood products remain intravascular and therefore may rapidly expand intravascular volume.
   b. Elderly patients with impaired cardiac function are at risk of developing cardiopulmonary edema; in these patients, slower infusion is indicated when possible, and concomitant administration of a diuretic may be indicated.
   c. Noncardiogenic pulmonary edema may also occur with a massive transfusion.

IV. PHARMACOLOGIC THERAPY
A. Heparin
1. Heparin is a glycosaminoglycan which complexes with AT III, accelerating the inhibition of thrombin, factor Xa, and factor IXa. By this mechanism, heparin inhibits thrombus formation and permits the endogenous fibrinolytic system to take effect.
2. Indications include PE, DVT, peripheral arterial thrombus or embolus, and acute coronary thrombosis.
3. Intravenous heparin considerations include the following:
   a. The onset of action is virtually immediate. The biological half-life varies between 30 and 90 minutes.
   b. The average 70-kg patient should be loaded with 5000 to 10,000 U IV bolus and continued on an infusion of 1000 U/hr. A convenient preparation consists of 25,000 U in 250 ml of either D_5W or normal saline (10 U/ml).
   c. The APTT should be obtained in 6 hours; a value of 1.5 to 2.5 times control has been shown to inhibit thrombus formation in DVT models. If the APTT is higher than desired, decrease the infusion to approximately 800 U/hr; if it is less than desired, increase to approximately 1200 U/hr. An APTT should be repeated every 6 hours until stable and then daily.
   d. Subcutaneous heparin 5000 U SQ q8h is effective DVT prophylaxis.
4. In general, all patients should be adequately anticoagulated with heparin prior to beginning warfarin. Warfarin therapy

may result in an initial hypercoagulable state secondary to inhibition of protein C and S synthesis.

5. Side effects of heparin include the following:

   a. Bleeding: Minor bleeding may be managed by temporarily holding the infusion or reducing the dose. Major bleeding requires that the heparin be stopped. In addition, protamine sulfate 25 to 50 mg IV may be used to reverse heparin. The protamine dose should be given slowly over at least 5 to 10 minutes.

   b. Heparin-induced thrombocytopenia: Daily platelet counts should be obtained on all patients receiving heparin; an absolute platelet count less than 100,000/mm^3 or a rapid decline in platelet count warrants discontinuation of heparin.

   c. Osteoporosis: This side effect can develop in patients receiving moderate doses of heparin for several months

B. Warfarin

1. Warfarin inhibits hepatic conversion of vitamin K to an active form, and therefore prevents its function as a cofactor for the modification of protein C, protein S, and factors II, VII, IX, and X. Without this modification these factors are inactive, and the net result is an inhibition of thrombus formation. Like heparin, warfarin does not dissolve clots that have already formed.

2. Warfarin produces an anticoagulant effect in 24 to 48 hours, resulting from a reduction of factor VII (half-life 6 hours). Several more days of therapy may be required for full anticoagulation. Depletion of protein C and S occur even before factor VII, therefore a brief hypercoagulable state may precede warfarin-induced anticoagulation. The initial warfarin dose is 5 to 10 mg PO daily × 2 days; subsequent daily doses should be approximately half the initial dose and as indicated by the PT.

3. Methods for monitoring warfarin therapy include the following:

   a. Warfarin anticoagulation is monitored with the PT. Because institutions use different thromboplastin reagents, the same PT value at different institutions may represent different degrees of anticoagulation.

   b. An international normalized ratio (INR) has been developed to standardize measurements:

$$INR = [\text{patient's PT/control PT}] \times C,$$

where the power value C, unique for each institution's thromboplastin reagent, reflects the international sensitivity index (ISI). The ISI is a measure of the responsiveness of a given thromboplastin to reduction of vitamin K-dependent factors relative to an international standardized thromboplastin. In North America, the ISI ranges from 1.8 to 2.8.

c. The recommended INR for prophylaxis of DVT, treatment of DVT/PE, and prevention of systemic emboli from tissue heart valves or chronic atrial fibrillation is 2 to 3; assuming a median North American ISI of 2.3, this would mean a PT ratio of 1.4 to 1.6.

d. In patients with a mechanical heart valve, an INR of 2.5 to 3.5 is recommended (PT ratio of approximately 1.5 to 1.7).

4. Reversal considerations include the following:

a. After stopping warfarin, a change in the PT ratio does not occur for at least 2 days, and normalization requires approximately 1 week.

b. High-dose vitamin K (10 to 15 mg IV q12h) will result in a reversal of the PT ratio in as rapidly as 6 hours; however, patients who have received such doses become refractory to warfarin anticoagulation for at least 1 week.

c. Low-dose vitamin K (0.5 to 1 mg IV daily) will result in a slower reversal of warfarin anticoagulation (over 24 hours) but without subsequent warfarin resistance.

d. FFP rapidly reverses warfarin anticoagulation.

5. Side effects of warfarin include the following:

a. Bleeding

(1) Bleeding is affected by the intensity of anticoagulation (much higher risk of bleeding with an INR of 3 to 4 as compared to an INR of 2 to 3).

(2) Patients who have a high risk for bleeding while receiving warfarin therapy include those with renal insufficiency, atrial fibrillation, previous stroke, previous GI bleed, and advanced age.

(3) Concomitant use of antiplatelet agents (particularly aspirin) increases the risk of bleeding.

(4) For minor bleeding, temporarily withholding or reducing the warfarin dose may be acceptable. For major bleeds, reversal of warfarin is indicated.

   b. Skin necrosis
      (1) Skin necrosis is a rare complication which develops during the first week of therapy, as a result of thrombosis of the microvasculature within the subcutaneous fat.
      (2) Treatment involves discontinuing warfarin and heparinizing the patient.
   c. Pregnancy
      (1) Warfarin crosses the placenta, is teratogenic, and may produce fetal death.
      (2) Heparin is an acceptable anticoagulant during pregnancy.

C. Aspirin
   1. Aspirin irreversibly inhibits the enzyme cyclooxygenase, blocking of platelet generation of thromboxane A_2, which normally induces platelet aggregation and vasoconstriction. Patients treated with aspirin have dysfunctional platelets and increased bleeding times.
   2. The dosage is 160 to 325 mg PO daily. The effect of a single dose is for the life span of the platelets (7 to 10 days), with platelet replacement occurring at 10% per day.
   3. Indications include stable angina, unstable angina, acute MI, TIA, thrombotic stroke, peripheral arterial disease, pregnancy-induced hypertension, and placental insufficiency. It has also been shown to help prevent MI in asymptomatic men and women over the age of 50 years. In addition, patients who develop thrombotic complications while on warfarin therapy may benefit from the addition of aspirin. Finally, there is also evidence that aspirin may inhibit thrombosis of coronary artery bypass grafts.
   4. Side effects of aspirin include the following:
      a. Allergic reactions occasionally necessitate the discontinuation of aspirin.
      b. GI complications result from the ability of aspirin to inhibit prostaglandin synthesis by the gastric mucosa, with a subsequent increase in acid-induced mucosal injury, erosion, and potential bleeding. This complication is dose-dependent and is significantly reduced when the dose is lowered to 160 mg/day.

D. Fibrinolytic Agents
   1. Activate plasminogen to plasmin, which dissolves fibrin; unlike heparin and warfarin, fibrinolytic agents are able to dissolve clot that has already formed.

    a. rt-PA activates plasminogen associated with thrombus and causes fibrin degradation.

    b. Urokinase and streptokinase are not fibrin-specific. They affect the degradation of fibrinogen and several other plasma proteins in addition to fibrin, with subsequent large rises in FDP titers.

2. Indications for fibrinolytic agents include the following:

    a. Acute MI (resulted in a reduction of the in-hospital and 1-year mortality rates)

    b. Life-threatening DVT/PE (See Chapters 7 and 10.)

    c. Acute peripheral arterial occlusion (See Chapters 7 and 10.)

3. Absolute contraindications include the presence of aortic dissection, acute pericarditis, and active bleeding; any hemostatic wound (surgical incision, IV, arterial line site, trauma, or organ biopsy site) may potentially rehemorrhage with fibrinolytic therapy.

4. Complications of fibrinolytic agents include the following:

    a. Bleeding

        (1) The most devastating complication is intracranial hemorrhage; in patients with MI treated with fibrinolytics the incidence is approximately 1%.

        (2) Management for severe bleeds includes discontinuing infusion, fibrinogen replacement with cryoprecipitate and epsilon-aminocaproic acid.

    b. Allergic reactions

        (1) Most patients have antibodies to streptokinase, which occurs naturally as a foreign protein produced by type B streptococci; following treatment with streptokinase, titers rise significantly and may neutralize repeat treatments.

        (2) Allergic manifestations (fever, rash, rigor, or bronchospasm) occur in approximately 5% of patients being treated with streptokinase. Anaphylactic shock occurs in <0.5%.

        (3) No serious allergic reactions occur with urokinase or rt-PA.

5. Methods for monitoring fibrinolytic therapy include the following:

    a. The systemic fibrinolytic state induced by urokinase or streptokinase is manifested by prolongation of the APTT and TCT, marked rises in the FDPs, and a decrease in the fibrinogen level.

   b. These measures indicate induction of fibrinolytic activity with streptokinase or urokinase; rt-PA induces much more modest alterations. However, the risk of bleeding in individual patients does not clearly relate to any of these parameters, and the dose is not titrated according to these values. Concomitant heparin therapy is monitored with the APTT.

E. Epsilon-Aminocaproic Acid

1. Epsilon-aminocaproic acid inhibits fibrinolysis.
2. Dose 5 g IV load (given over 30 minutes), then 1 g/hr IV; may also be given orally.
3. Indications are unclear and limited by the incidence of complicating thrombotic events; may be administered in severe DIC, postCPB coagulopathy, or with bleeding complicating fibrinolytic therapy. In these situations, uncontrolled fibrinolysis is suggested by increased FDPs.

F. DDAVP (1-Deamino, 8-D-Arginine Vasopressin)

1. DDAVP is a synthetic analog of ADH which stimulates the release of endogenous vWF from endothelial stores.
2. The dose is 0.3 µg/kg IV; this may be repeated at 12 to 24 hour intervals, but tachyphylaxis may occur.
3. Indications include minor hemophilia A, vWD, and minor bleeding in patients with uremia.

G. Ancrod

1. Ancrod is used for systemic anticoagulation of patients with heparin-induced thrombocytopenia.
2. It is a thrombin-like enzyme which depletes the α-fibrinopeptides from fibrinogen, rendering subsequent fibrin polymers more susceptible to degradation.
3. The initial dose is 2 U/kg IV over 6 hours, with subsequent dosing based on the fibrinogen level.

H. Dextran

1. A high molecular weight polysaccharide which functions as a volume expander and thereby decreases blood viscosity; may also reduce platelet adhesiveness and reduce factor VIII activity
2. May improve early patency rates in some types of lower extremity arterial bypass procedures
3. The dosage is two 500-ml bottles on the day of surgery and

then one bottle on each of the succeeding 3 postoperative days at 75 ml/hr.

SUGGESTED READING

American Red Cross 1751, Circular of Information, August 1, 1992.

Collins JA: *Blood transfusions and disorders of surgical bleeding.* In Sabiston DC Jr, editor: *Textbook of surgery,* ed 14, Philadelphia, 1991, WB Saunders.

Dyke C, Sobel M: The management of coagulation problems in the surgical patient, *Advances in surgery* 24:229, 1991.

Greenfield LJ: Lupus-like anticoagulant and thrombosis, *J Vasc Surg* 7:818, 1988.

THE CENTRAL NERVOUS SYSTEM

13

William N. Peugh

I. THE NEUROLOGIC EVALUATION
A. History

1. Aim: To define global and focal deficits with particular attention to causes of impairment treatable by medical or surgical means
2. Past medical history
   a. Review of current and recent pharmacologic therapies and chemical abuse history
      (1) Benzodiazepines
      (2) Anticonvulsants
      (3) Narcotics
      (4) Antihypertensives with potential for rebound hypertension
      (5) Thyroid replacement
      (6) Steroids
      (7) Methyl xanthines
      (8) Digoxin
      (9) Drugs of abuse: Cocaine, ethanol, PCP, narcotics, benzodiazepines, and barbiturates
   b. Systemic illnesses: Endocrine, renal, pulmonary, cardiac
   c. Prior CNS events
   d. Prior trauma
   e. Past surgery
   f. Drug and alcohol abuse
   g. Tobacco abuse
3. Acute traumatic injury
   a. Mechanism

    b. Function and level of consciousness at scene and during transport

    c. Time course of changes

    d. Adequacy of oxygenation during transport and resuscitation

    e. Hemodynamics, shock

  4. Interventions: Focus on factors altering physical examination

    a. Drugs administered

       (1) Narcotics

       (2) Benzodiazepines and barbiturates

       (3) Anticonvulsants

       (4) Depolarizing and nondepolarizing muscle relaxants

       (5) Antipsychotics

       (6) Antihistamines

       (7) Antagonists: Naloxone and flumazenil

       (8) Atropine

       (9) Drugs of abuse: Cocaine, ethanol, PCP, narcotics, benzodiazepines, and barbiturates

    b. Airway management

    c. Procedures

B. Physical Exam

  1. ABCs of initial examination and stabilization

  2. Signs of injuries and prior surgery

  3. Level of consciousness

  4. Mental status: Orientation, memory, cooperation, calculation

  5. Cranial nerves

  6. Sensory: Attempting to define radiculopathy, plexopathy or individual neuropathy vs. spinal cord level

  7. Motor: Strength and coordination

  8. Reflexes: Deep tendon reflexes at all cord levels including assessment of rectal tone, anal wink, and bulbocavernosus reflexes

  9. Response to pain: Decorticate (arm flexion, leg extension; implies forebrain dysfunction) and decerebrate (arm and leg extension; implies midbrain dysfunction) posturing

  10. Fundus: Delayed papillary response to increased intracranial pressure

  11. Respiratory pattern and hemodynamics: Especially Cheyne-Stokes respiration (seen early in herniation) and elevated systolic BP (Cushing's reflex resulting from raised intracranial pressure)

C. **Acute Systemic Illness**
Thoroughly assess the patient for signs of the following systemic conditions which may directly impair CNS function:
1. Shock
   a. Examination of peripheral perfusion, pulses, vital signs, venous filling; helpful to have invasive monitoring
   b. Cardiogenic: Low cardiac output and poor peripheral perfusion in spite of adequate preload
   c. Septic: High cardiac output, warm extremities, and low SVR
   d. Hypovolemic: Trauma with exsanguination/inadequate volume resuscitation
   e. Spinal: Spinal cord trauma with loss of sympathetic tone and resultant intravascular hypovolemia
2. Respiratory failure
   a. Examination of periphery for cyanosis; pulse oximetry and ABG analysis
   b. Hypoxemia, with resultant acute confusion
   c. Hypercarbia, with depressed mental status

D. **Radiologic Imaging**
1. CT
   a. Noncontrasted in trauma
   b. Contrasted for neoplasm or infection
2. MRI
   a. Especially for suspected posterior fossa lesions
   b. Some patients ineligible because of pacemakers, recently implanted orthopedic devices, or some surgical clips

II. SPECIFIC PATTERNS OF DYSFUNCTION
A. **Delirium and ICU Psychosis**
1. Diagnosis of exclusion: Must differentiate from seizures, psychotic disorders, effects of systemic disease, and anatomic CNS pathology
2. Delirium: Defined as a global, transient impairment of cognition; a common disorder occurring in 10% to 15% of all surgical patients
3. Clinical features
   a. Confusion, disorientation
   b. Agitation, anxiety
   c. Combativeness
   d. Hallucinations, delusions
   e. Paranoia

    f. Irritability, hyperexcitability

    g. May have increased or decreased motor behavior

    h. Incoherent speech

    i. Insomnia

    j. Decreased level of consciousness/alertness

    k. Inappropriate behavior, disinhibition

    l. Varying symptoms from one time to another; often worse at night

4. Predisposing factors

    a. Over 50 years of age

    b. Baseline impairment: CVA, dementia, blindness, deafness, malnutrition, underlying psychotic or depressive disorder

    c. Renal or liver disease resulting in metabolic derangement

    d. Recent episodes of hypoperfusion or hypoxemia

5. Etiology

    a. Drugs and drug interactions which affect metabolism of CNS active agents: Common agents—lidocaine, digoxin, aminophylline, and H_2 blockers

    b. Period for ethanol or benzodiazepine withdrawal: 24 to 72 hours; often corresponds to the acute postoperative period

    c. Hyperthyroid or hypothyroid states

    d. Corticosteroid insufficiency or excess

    e. Abnormalities in glucose metabolism

    f. Respiratory disturbances including hypoxemia, poor oxygen carrying capacity, and hypercarbia

    g. Toxins related to acute renal or hepatic failure

    h. Sepsis, with or without fever

    i. Nutritional/cofactor deficiencies (thiamin, vitamin B_{12}, nicotinic acid)

    j. Environmental displacement, noise, sleep deprivation (or sleep pattern disruption)

6. Therapy

    a. Withdrawal of nonessential medications and simplification of regimen

    b. Correction of all abnormal metabolic and endocrine findings

    c. Empiric: Folate 1 mg and thiamin 100 mg qd for 3 days

    d. Treatment of hypoxemia, acid-base disorders, anemia, and shock

    e. Treatment of sepsis with appropriate definitive therapy

directed at primary source of infection in addition to systemic antibiotics

  f. Environmental changes

    (1) Provide outdoor sources of light (patient's bed placed near or facing a window).

    (2) Obtain familiar personal objects for the patient's room.

    (3) Keep a clock in the patient's range of view.

    (4) Minimize invasive lines and procedures.

  g. Pharmacotherapy

    (1) Administer diphenhydramine 50 mg PO or 25 to 50 mg IV to help normalize sleep-wake cycles.

    (2) Haloperidol is the agent of choice for refractory delirium. If extrapyramidal side effects develop, use diphenhydramine.

      (a) Administer 2 to 5 mg IV or IM; this dose may be repeated in 10 minutes.

      (b) Double the dose and administer q20min until therapeutic effect obtained.

      (c) Use on a scheduled (not PRN) basis to prevent therapeutic escape.

      (d) Doses as high as a 150-mg single dose and 975 mg over 24 hours have been documented without adverse sequelae.

  h. Ethanol withdrawal therapy

    (1) Multivitamins, thiamin 100 mg, and folate 1 mg qd for 3 days

    (2) Magnesium and potassium supplementation

    (3) Benzodiazepines titrated to obtain adequate sedation using short-acting agents (midazolam or lorazepam); tapered over 4 to 5 days

    (4) May use clonidine to control tachycardia and hypertension; clonidine 0.2 mg PO initially and placement of transdermal patches—patches removed on third and fourth days to obtain taper effect

B. Seizures

  1. Considered a symptom of another underlying process

  2. Etiology: Varies with age

    a. Infants: Perinatal injury, congenital (metabolic and anatomic) defects, and infection

    b. Children: Infection, inherited diseases, and trauma

    c. Adults: Tumor, traumatic mass lesions, infarcts, drug

TABLE 13-1.

Associations of Focal CNS Lesions

Site	Findings
Anterior frontal lobe	Contralateral head and eye deviation
Motor cortex	Contralateral tonic-clonic movements of a single body part
Sensory cortex	Focal paresthesias
Occipital cortex	Spots of light or transient contralateral visual field deficits
Temporal cortex	Hallucinations—auditory, olfactory, visceral

withdrawal, hyponatremia, and vascular lesions

3. Classification (Table 13-1)
   a. Focal seizures are always caused by a focal cortical lesion, with the anatomic site of the lesion determining initial presentation. The description may be modified as *focal complex* if there is altered consciousness or *secondarily generalized* if there is progression to a generalized seizure after an initial focal phase.
   b. Complex partial seizures often begin with focal temporal lobe symptoms and then progress with *deja vu,* automatism, hallucinations, or mood changes.
   c. During generalized seizures, the patient is unconscious and unresponsive to stimuli from the environment, and after the event (postictal) is confused, drowsy, and disoriented.
      (1) Generalized tonic-clonic seizures: Patient exhibits synchronous tonic-clonic motor activity of all muscle groups
      (2) Absence seizures: Patient has a brief loss of consciousness, appears to stare aimlessly into space, and is unresponsive; usually affects children
      (3) Akinetic seizures: Patient loses all postural control and falls to ground unconscious

4. Evaluation
   a. Exclusion of metabolic derangements; evaluation of serum electrolytes, glucose, divalent ions, and ABG
   b. Review of medications (high-dose penicillin, imipenem, flumazenil), recent withdrawal of drugs (benzodiazepines), and history of drug abuse

    c. Brain CT scan to rule out mass lesion in trauma and postoperative patients

    d. CSF sampling to rule out infection (lumbar puncture performed after CT)

    e. EEG for localization of a focus

  5. Treatment

    a. Phenytoin (Dilantin)

      (1) Maintenance dosing 3 to 5 mg/kg/day titrated for a serum level 10 to 20 µg/ml

      (2) In status epilepticus, 50 mg/min (bolus) to achieve total loading dose of 15 to 20 mg/kg; ECG monitoring for prolonged PR interval

    b. Carbamazepine

      (1) Maintenance dosing 600 to 1200 mg/day, aiming for serum levels 4 to 8 µg/ml

      (2) No role in acute therapy of status epilepticus

    c. Diazepam

      (1) Used in short-term control of status epilepticus: 10 mg IV bolus

      (2) May repeat every 10 to 15 minutes if seizures persist, to maximum of 30 mg

      (3) May repeat course again in 2 to 4 hours as needed

    d. Prophylaxis

      (1) Prophylaxis is indicated in patients with penetrating head injury; 50% will develop seizures in the first year.

      (2) Prophylaxis is not indicated in severe nonpentrating head injury; only 5% of these patients have an acute seizure in the first year.

      (3) Phenytoin or carbamazepine may be used for prophylaxis at therapeutic serum levels.

    e. Status epilepticus

      (1) Airway secured by endotracheal intubation

      (2) IV access and blood samples

      (3) Diazepam and phenytoin as above

      (4) If seizures persist, phenobarbital 120 mg IV bolus (25 mg/min) every 15 minutes, to maximum 600 mg

      (5) If seizures persist, paraldehyde infusion 4% in NS titrated to control seizures

C. Elevated Intracranial Pressure

  1. The normal ICP is 6 to 16 mm Hg; elevated ICP is generally defined as >20 mm Hg.

2. The brain is contained within a rigid cavity (the calvarium) and any increased volume within that cavity increases pressure. The result is displacement of one of the three components of the calvaria (blood, CSF, or brain).

3. Shifts of CSF and blood serve as the normal compensatory reserve mechanisms; herniation of the brain occurs when these compensatory mechanisms are overwhelmed.

4. In addition, as ICP rises, cerebral perfusion pressure falls and cerebral perfusion is diminished.

5. Etiology of elevated ICP includes the following:
   a. Mass lesions: Hematoma (posttraumatic or postoperative), tumor, or abscess
   b. Diffuse edema: Cerebral infarct, surrounding mass lesion (tumor or infection)

6. Evaluation includes the following:
   a. Symptoms: Headache (predominant complaint), may be accompanied by nausea, vomiting, depressed/changing mental status, and focal signs of herniation
   b. Findings: Hypertension, bradycardia, irregular respiration (Cheyne-Stokes respiration); may see papilledema in longer standing increased ICP

7. Herniation syndromes of elevated ICP include the following:
   a. Uncal herniation: Medial displacement of uncus of temporal lobe over the tentorium by a lateral mass
      (1) Uncal herniation results in progressive CN III palsy and ipsilateral pupillary dilation and is followed by deteriorating mental status.
      (2) Hemiplegia in this setting indicates compression of the cerebral peduncle and may be ipsilateral or contralateral to the mass lesion.
      (3) Decerebrate rigidity and respiratory disturbance are late signs.
   b. Central herniation: Downward displacement of the brainstem secondary to a centrally placed mass lesion or diffusely increased ICP
      (1) Central herniation results in a deteriorating mental status, Cheyne-Stokes respiration, and small, reactive pupils.
      (2) Decorticate posturing is also seen relatively early.
      (3) More ominous findings include hyperventilation, decerebrate posturing, and fixed pupils; these findings signify progression.

(4) Flaccidity is a preterminal finding.

c. Upward transtentorial herniation resulting from posterior fossa mass: Results in loss of upward gaze and loss of consciousness

d. Cerebellar tonsillar herniation due to posterior fossa mass: Presents with nuchal rigidity and may result in respiratory arrest due to medullary compression

8. Considerations for monitoring ICP include the following:

a. Invasive ICP monitoring is indicated in patients with evidence of elevated intracranial pressure to allow continuous assessment of effectiveness of therapy. Two or more of the following factors are associated with a 60% incidence of elevated ICP in the severely head-injured patient:

(1) Age > 40 years

(2) SBP < 90 mm Hg

(3) Motor posturing

b. In trauma patients, elevated ICP and mortality can be predicted based on the injury pattern as seen on CT (Table 13-2).

c. All patients with these devices should be treated with prophylactic antibiotics affording gram-positive coverage (vancomycin or penicillinase-resistant penicillin).

(1) Subdural "bolt": Simple to place and has a relatively low infection rate; does not allow withdrawal of CSF

(2) Ventriculostomy: Allows therapeutic and diagnostic drainage of CSF; carries an 8% infection rate at 5 days

9. Treatment for elevated ICP includes the following:

a. Positioning: Head of bed elevated and neck extended

b. Hyperventilation to P_{CO_2} of 25 to 28 mm Hg; autoregulation reduces blood flow and thereby intracranial volume

TABLE 13-2.

Risk of Mortality after CNS Trauma

Injury	Incidence of Elevated ICP (%)	Mortality Rate (%)
"Surgical" mass lesion	70	30
Intracerebral contusion	70	6
Diffuse axonal injury	33	4

   c. Mannitol 20% solution 0.25 to 1.0 g/kg IV q3h; an osmotic diuretic that is useful in patients with an intact blood-brain barrier; serum osmolarity monitored and mannitol held if osmolarity > 305 mOsm

   d. CSF drainage through ventriculostomy catheter or lumbar drain (depending on the anatomy and source of elevated ICP)

   e. Steroids: "Stabilize" the blood brain barrier and may be helpful in cases of vasogenic edema related to tumors or postoperative edema; dexamethasone 10 to 100 mg IV, then 1 to 4 mg IV q6h, or methylprednisolone 1 gm IV followed by 40 mg IV q6h

   f. Lidocaine 100 mg IV push: May reduce ICP; mechanism unknown

   g. Barbiturate coma: Only used with ICP monitoring in place

      (1) Titrate to desired reduction of ICP or burst suppression on EEG. Systemic hypotension should be avoided.

      (2) Administer thiopental 3 to 5 mg/kg IV load followed by infusion 1 mg/kg/hr. With the exception of pupillary reflexes, all brain stem reflexes are lost.

   h. Surgical

      (1) Drainage of extraaxial blood collections

      (2) Resection of mass lesion

      (3) Resection of right anterior temporal or right frontal lobes (relatively silent areas) as a last resort to decompress when all other options have failed in the setting of herniation

D. Spinal Cord Deficits

Acute deficits in spinal cord function may present with one of several classic patterns of findings and may be caused by vascular events, cord compression by neoplastic masses, spinal stenosis, herniated disc, or trauma.

  1. Patterns

   a. Spinal shock: Bilateral loss of reflexes in all segments below the injury, spastic paralysis, loss of sympathetic tone, atonic bladder

   b. Central cord syndrome: More weakness in upper extremities than in lower extremities, variable band-like distribution of sensory deficit

   c. Brown-Sequard syndrome (cord hemisection): Ipsilateral

spastic paralysis, loss of position and vibratory sense, contralateral heat and pain insensitivity

d. Anterior cord syndrome: Complete paralysis (bilateral), loss of heat and pain sensation, position and vibration sense (dorsal columns) preserved; usually the result of vascular events such as occlusion of the anterior spinal artery, which occurs as a complication of a thoracic aneurysm repair or during descending thoracic aortic dissection

2. Evaluation
   a. History of mechanism of injury
   b. Complete neurologic examination
   c. Complete vascular examination
   d. Radiographic evaluation of entire axial skeleton to define fractures; must adequately image entire C1 to T1 region with cervical spine radiographs
   e. CT myelogram or MRI: May be indicated at a later stage

3. Treatment
   a. Airway: Use care in securing the airway to avoid exacerbation of a preexisting injury. A nasotracheal intubation or cricothyroidotomy may be indicated.
   b. Fluid resuscitation: Several liters of fluid may be necessary acutely to resuscitate the patient in spinal shock (even with no other injury) because of loss of sympathetic tone.
   c. Immobilization: The initial management of all blunt trauma patients includes the use of a cervical collar and spine board. These should be used in the field prior to patient transport and removed only when injuries have been excluded.
   d. Steroids: High-dose steroids given within the first 8 hours after injury are beneficial in blunt spinal cord injuries. They are contraindicated in injuries > 8 hours old, spinal lesions below L2, and cauda equina lesions.
      (1) Administer methylprednisolone 30 mg/kg IV load over 15 minutes.
      (2) After 45 minutes begin 5.4 mg/kg/hr infusion for the following 23 hours.
   e. Surgical decompression and stabilization: These procedures are indicated for some injuries to prevent progression of deficits

SUGGESTED READING

Bracken MB, et al: A randomized controlled trial of methylprednisolone or naloxone in the treatment of acute spinal-cord injury. Results of the second national acute spinal cord injury
study, *N Engl J Med* 322:1405, 1990.

Guthrie SK: The treatment of alcohol withdrawal, *Pharmacotherapy* 9:131-143, 1989.

Weiss GH et al: Predicting posttraumatic epilepsy in penetrating
head injury, *Arch Neurol* 43:771, 1986.

Wirth F, Ratcheson R, editors: *Neurosurgical critical care,* Baltimore, 1987, Williams and Wilkins.

PART THREE

SPECIALIZED PATIENT MANAGEMENT

TRAUMA   *14*

Mark W. Sebastian

I. **INITIAL MANAGEMENT**

Patients arriving in the SICU from the emergency department or operating room are assumed to have unrecognized problems. Late recognition of significant injuries is not uncommon in multiple-injury patients. There is significant morbidity associated with a delay in diagnosis. The initial evaluation should be identical to the initial assessment in the emergency department.

A. **Airway Management**

1. Goals of management are to secure and protect an adequate airway.

2. A cervical spine injury is assumed until radiographic clearance is confirmed. Often, semirigid collars are maintained in the SICU until all cervical views can be safely obtained.

3. As a general principle, hypothermic patients (patients with core temperatures less than 35.5° C) should remain intubated.

B. **Ventilation and Oxygenation**

1. The initial examination should include an observation of chest expansion and the confirmation of bilateral breath sounds.

2. The endotracheal tube should be examined for a properly inflated cuff, and the distance from the tip should be noted (usually 22 to 24 cm).

3. ABG analysis and CXR will provide additional data.

C. **Vascular Access**

1. IV access should be identified by location, size, and current fluid type. IV location and patency should be confirmed; this step is essential should sudden decompensation occur.

2. Arterial lines should be checked for proper placement, proper waveform, and secure position.

3. Special lines such as central venous lines and Swan-Ganz catheters should be examined.

D. Laboratory Studies

Appropriate laboratory studies should be obtained. In particular, a coagulation profile including PT, PTT, platelet count, fibrinogen level, and presence of fibrin split products facilitates rational treatment of bleeding diatheses.

E. Fluid Resuscitation

1. Upon arrival in the SICU, many patients will not be fully resuscitated.
2. Basic indices such as vital signs, assessment of peripheral perfusion via extremity temperature, capillary refill, and urine output can guide initial fluid management. Patients with multiple injuries and an unclear fluid status should undergo early invasive monitoring (Swan-Ganz catheterization). The use of Svo_2 and oximetric Swan-Ganz catheters greatly assist fluid management and the determination of need for inotropic support.

F. Physical Examination

1. A thorough head-to-toe evaluation should be performed.
2. Details of the accident should allow consideration of diagnoses associated with that mechanism of injury with attention to level of severity and possible associated injuries (Table 14-1).
3. The initial physical examination provides a baseline evaluation, enabling the detection of previously missed injuries and allowing for the monitoring of the development of complications. Special attention should be paid to the abdominal exam for presence of dullness to percussion, tympany, bowel sounds, and presence, location, and severity of tenderness, and girth.

G. Radiographs

1. An admission portable CXR allows confirmation of central line, endotracheal tube, NG tube, and chest tube placements. Careful attention should be directed to mediastinal and pulmonary structures.
2. All previous studies should be reviewed, and the final reading by the radiologists should be noted.

II. THORACIC TRAUMA

A. Pneumothorax

1. Chest pain and shortness of breath are the most common symptoms.

2. Physical findings include decreased breath sounds and decreased chest wall motion. Patients on ventilators will demonstrate significantly higher airway pressures.

3. CXR demonstrates a hyperlucent area with absent lung markings. Small pneumothoraces may only be identified on expiratory films taken with the patient upright. Other indications for a chest tube include rib fractures in a patient scheduled for the operating room, subcutaneous emphysema, and emergent decompression of a presumptive tension pneumothorax.

4. Placement of a 28F or 32F chest tube may be diagnostic and therapeutic.

   a. Incomplete reexpansion of the lung following chest tube placement results in persistent air leaks and delay in resolution. Management involves higher suction pressures or placement of an additional chest tube to accommodate higher air flow.

   b. Large air leaks should arouse suspicion of a tracheobronchial injury (Section F).

   c. Continuous air leaks that do not vary with respiration can be associated with esophageal injury (Section J).

B. Tension Pneumothorax

1. Tension pneumothorax is an immediately life-threatening problem. In the SICU, tension pneumothorax most often develops as a complication of mechanical ventilation.

2. A tension pneumothorax results from a check-valve effect, which allows accumulation of air under pressure within the pleural space but does not allow egress of air. Positive intrapleural pressures of only 10 to 15 cm H_2O significantly impede venous return to the heart.

3. The diagnosis is based on clinical findings. Respiratory compromise and hypotension associated with decreased breath sounds and hyperresonance to percussion on the affected side identify a tension pneumothorax. The trachea may shift away from the affected side. Patients requiring mechanical ventilation will demonstrate elevated airway pressures.

4. Decompression should be performed immediately, preceding radiographic confirmation. A 14-g or 16-g catheter inserted in the second or third intercostal space in the midclavicular line is effective; a rush of air confirms the diagnosis. Placement of a standard chest tube should follow the decompression.

C. **Pulmonary Contusion**
   1. Pulmonary contusion is a direct injury to the lung associated with hemorrhage and subsequent edema.
   2. Diagnosis is confirmed by radiographic findings of pulmonary infiltrates and consolidation.
   3. Mild contusions may be treated with the following:
      a. Aggressive pulmonary toilet including chest physiotherapy and endotracheal suctioning
      b. Pain control of associated rib fractures
      c. Avoidance of fluid overload
   4. Moderate to severe contusions require intubation and mechanical ventilation based on standard criteria: $Pao_2 < 60$ mm Hg, $Paco_2 > 55$ mm Hg, respiratory rate > 30.
      a. Treatment goals should be to maintain O_2 saturation > 90% while maintaining $Fio_2 < 0.5$ to prevent O_2 toxicity.
      b. PEEP is effective in increasing functional residual capacity and in improving oxygenation. Cardiac output determinations, Svo_2, and pulmonary compliance measurements allow selection of optimal PEEP settings. Optimal PEEP should be obtained through 2 to 5 minute trials with ABG sampling at graduated PEEP intervals and return to baseline PEEP while results arrive. This prevents a collapse of the alveoli, which may require 24 hours to return to ventilatory capacity.
      c. Fluid overload should be avoided. Invasive hemodynamic monitoring including PA catheterization is indicated to allow optimal fluid management.
      d. The hematocrit should be maintained at levels to optimize Do_2. Oximetric PA catheterization enables precise calculation of Do_2.
   5. Complications of pulmonary contusion include the following:
      a. Infection
         (1) The injured lung is susceptible to bacterial colonization.
         (2) Prophylactic antibiotics are not indicated.
         (3) Frequent sputum cultures should be obtained.
         (4) Antibiotic therapy is initiated for the treatment of documented pneumonia.
      b. Barotrauma: Most common manifestation is development of a pneumothorax

6. Patients with severe contusions are expected to have a gradual improvement in ABGs and clinical condition, which allows progressive ventilation weaning. Failure to demonstrate improvement should arouse suspicion of superimposed pneumonia or PE.

D. Flail Chest

1. Flail chest results when a segment of chest wall loses continuity with the remainder of the bony thorax.
2. The flail segment will demonstrate paradoxical respiratory movement; however, the primary pathophysiology results from injury to the underlying lung.
3. Therapy is directed toward the underlying lung injury.

E. Hemothorax

1. The initial treatment of hemothorax in the SICU is the placement of a 36F chest tube. Only 15% of patients require operation.
2. Indications for operation include the following:
   a. Initial output > 1000 ml
   b. Hourly output > 300 ml/hr
   c. Total output > 2000 ml
3. A hemothorax that is not evacuated by a chest tube may require a thoracotomy and evacuation of the clot.

F. Tracheobronchial Injuries

1. Only 30% of the cases are diagnosed within the first 24 hours.
2. Signs include mediastinal or subcutaneous emphysema and presence of pneumothorax. A large air leak will often be present from chest tubes. Proximity to the path of a penetrating object should arouse suspicion.
3. Diagnosis is made by bronchoscopy.
4. Treatment involves operative repair, and the incision used is determined by the site of injury.
5. The two clinical syndromes seen with delayed diagnosis are the following:
   a. In patients with incomplete injuries, the bronchus will heal with a stricture.
      (1) Atelectasis and recurrent infection will occur distally, and ultimately tissue destruction will occur.
      (2) At this point, management involves pulmonary resection.
   b. In patients with circumferential lacerations, granulation will occur at each end. The distal bronchial tree will fill

with mucus, and radiographic studies will demonstrate complete atelectasis.

G. Myocardial Contusion

1. This diagnosis should be considered in patients sustaining blunt trauma to the anterior chest and in patients demonstrating evidence of severe thoracic trauma, such as scapular fracture or high cervical rib fracture. Initial manifestations may include arrhythmias or hypotension.

2. The diagnosis is based on ECG and cardiac isoenzyme determination. ECG findings include ST segment changes, PVCs, conduction system defects, and atrial dysrhythmias.

3. Echocardiography will identify associated wall motion abnormalities in severe cases and allow identification of a pericardial effusion, if present.

4. Management of a myocardial contusion includes the following:
   a. Provide ECG monitoring for 24 hours. A lack of ECG findings rules out significant myocardial injury.
   b. Measure serial cardiac isoenzymes.
   c. Treat ventricular ectopy with lidocaine.

5. If a new postinjury murmur is found, it should be evaluated with an echocardiogram.

H. Aortic Transection

1. Injury to the intima of the aorta may occur with severe deceleration. The most common site of aortic transection is immediately distal to the left subclavian artery.

2. Diagnosis of an aortic transection involves the following:
   a. CXR: Several cardinal features are sought:
      (1) Widened mediastinum
      (2) Fractures of the first and second ribs
      (3) Scapular fractures
      (4) Deviation of the esophagus (NG tube)
      (5) Loss of definition of the aortic knob
      (6) Deviation of the trachea or depression of the left mainstream bronchus
      (7) Apical cap
      (8) Left pleural effusion
   b. Aortography: The definitive test; should maintain a low threshold for obtaining this study

3. Therapy involves left posterolateral thoracotomy with primary or graft repair.

4. Complications of an aortic transection include the following:
   a. Paraparesis or paraplegia occurs in approximately 5% of patients.
   b. Acute renal failure may occur and is usually reversible.
   c. Vigorous correction of coagulation abnormalities should be performed with correction of hypothermia. Continued bleeding after the correction of coagulation parameters suggests a mechanical source.

I. **Diaphragmatic Injury**
   1. A diaphragmatic rupture usually occurs with significant blunt trauma. The tears are usually radial and more commonly on the left side.
   2. Diagnosis can be difficult in the early postinjury period. CXR findings include irregularity or elevation of the diaphragm, a loculated hydropneumothorax, or a subpulmonary hematoma.
      a. Contrast studies are utilized to confirm the diagnosis.
      b. The presence of an NG tube or abdominal viscera in the hemithorax on plain films will establish the diagnosis.
   3. The stomach is the most frequent organ involved in herniation, and may result in gastric volvulus. Injuries to the liver and spleen are frequently associated.
   4. Diaphragmatic tears should be repaired in one or two layers with a nonabsorbable suture. For acute injuries, repairs should be performed through an abdominal approach. This facilitates reduction of herniated abdominal contents and allows for optimal examination of intraabdominal viscera and vessels for associated injury.
   5. Late repairs should be performed through a thoracotomy, since dense peritoneal adhesions are usually present.

J. **Esophageal Injuries**
   1. These injuries most commonly occur with penetrating trauma and should be suspected in all cases of penetrating chest trauma.
   2. Symptoms include dysphagia and hematemesis.
   3. Findings include subcutaneous or mediastinal emphysema, fluid levels within the mediastinum, or pleural effusion.
      a. If a chest tube has been placed, finding an air leak that does not vary with respiration suggests an esophageal leak.

b. Particulate matter in chest tube drainage also indicates an esophageal injury.

4. Gastrografin swallow is utilized in most patients who are suspected to have injury to the esophagus. Esophagoscopy can be used in patients unable to cooperate or in patients taken emergently to the operating room for associated injuries.

5. Early treatment involves debridement, primary repair, and drainage with chest tubes.

6. Complex injuries and those recognized late (>12 hours postinjury) may require diversion and drainage.

7. Adequate nutrition is an absolute priority after repair and can be delivered with TPN or with placement of an enteral tube into the jejunum.

8. Gastrografin swallow is obtained 5 to 7 days after repair. Oral feeding is resumed after documentation of no extravasation.

III. GENERAL PRINCIPLES IN ABDOMINAL TRAUMA

A. Acute Management

1. A subset of patients are managed in the SICU after sustaining abdominal trauma without having undergone abdominal exploration. A high index of suspicion for occult injuries is required, as well as repetitive and thorough physical examinations by the same examiners. Negative peritoneal lavage or CT scans do not absolutely exclude intraabdominal pathology.

2. A second group of patients will have undergone exploration. Meticulous attention must be directed toward identification of occult injuries and early recognition of complications. The SICU physician must have a thorough knowledge of the pathologic conditions identified and the therapeutic maneuvers performed during the laparotomy to assist in optimal care.

B. Occult Injuries

Significant injuries may be missed during the diagnostic workup or the laparotomy.

1. Unrecognized sources of bleeding
   a. Associated signs may include hemodynamic instability, falling hematocrit, peritoneal irritation, or increasing abdominal girth.
   b. A CT scan is a sensitive diagnostic test to evaluate the abdomen.

2. Hollow viscus perforation
   a. Signs include peritoneal irritation, continued sepsis, and clinical deterioration.
   b. Both peritoneal lavage and CT scan can miss this injury. In addition, peritoneal lavage itself may result in intestinal perforation.

C. **Late Complications**
   1. Intraabdominal abscess considerations include the following:
      a. Most patients with abscesses will have a persistent fever and an elevated WBC count with a leftward shift.
      b. Ileus and abdominal distention are frequently present. In some cases, hyperbilirubinemia or sepsis may increase in severity. MOF may follow any delay in diagnosis and treatment.
      c. A CT scan of the abdomen and pelvis is the diagnostic test of choice.
      d. Management of an abscess requires drainage.
         (1) Percutaneous catheter drainage under CT guidance
         (2) Open surgical drainage
   2. Bowel obstruction (early, postoperative) is most commonly caused by adhesions.
   3. Stress gastritis considerations include the following:
      a. Gastritis with associated upper GI bleeding is a frequent complication in the trauma patient.
      b. Prophylaxis with histamine antagonists, antacids, or sucralfate should be used.

IV. SPECIFIC ABDOMINAL INJURIES
A. **Splenic Trauma**
   1. The spleen is frequently injured in blunt trauma.
   2. Symptoms include LUQ pain and left shoulder pain (Kehr's sign).
   3. Findings may include LUQ tenderness, tachycardia, and hypotension. A falling hematocrit, in addition to radiographic findings of left lower rib fractures, an elevated left hemidiaphragm, and gastric displacement may also be found.
   4. Patients in the SICU who do not manifest an overt surgical abdomen should undergo a CT scan to establish the diagnosis in the setting of equivocal physical findings and evidence of ongoing blood loss.

5. Nonoperative management of splenic injuries has been utilized in an effort to avoid postsplenectomy sepsis in patients who have the following conditions:
   a. Documented splenic injury or CT scan which is thought to be isolated
   b. Hemodynamic stability
   c. Normal level of consciousness
   d. Absence of coagulopathy
6. Nonoperative management of splenic injuries includes the following:
   a. Bed rest
   b. Serial hematocrit determinations
   c. Serial abdominal examinations
7. Operative management of splenic injuries includes both splenic salvage and splenectomy.
   a. Splenic salvage is appropriate in patients with hemodynamic stability and no major associated injuries.
   b. Splenectomy is still commonly employed; usually for Class III or IV splenic injuries.
8. Complications of splenic injuries include the following:
   a. Hemorrhage is the most common complication after splenectomy. Coagulation abnormalities and hypothermia should be corrected. Continued evidence of blood loss mandates reexploration. Approximately 3% of patients treated with splenorrhaphy will require subsequent splenectomy secondary to postoperative bleeding.
   b. Subphrenic abscess is treated by drainage.
   c. Pancreatitis is managed with NG suction and hyperalimentation if required.
   d. Postsplenectomy sepsis is characterized by the abrupt onset of overwhelming sepsis with early death in patients with previous splenectomy.
      (1) The incidence is greatest in children.
      (2) Polyvalent pneumococcal vaccine should be given to patients prior to discharge (protective against 80% of pneumococcal strains).
      (3) Prophylactic penicillin should be given to children following splenectomy.

B. **Hepatic Injury**
   1. Recognition of liver injuries has increased in frequency since CT scanning has become used routinely in the

hemodynamically stable patient who has sustained blunt abdominal trauma.

2. Nonoperative management of hepatic injury is reserved for the hemodynamically stable patient with documented hepatic injury. Conversion to operative management is indicated with hemodynamic instability, increased intraabdominal pressure that leads to decreased urine output or an intraabdominal pressure of greater than 25 cm of H_2O (as measured by transbladder manometry), or signs of peritoneal irritation suggesting associated perforated viscus.

3. Intraoperative management of hepatic injury may include the following:
   a. Temporary control of hemorrhage
      (1) Pringle maneuver
      (2) Direct manual compression
      (3) Packing with gauze
   b. Definitive control of hemorrhage
      (1) Direct suture ligation
      (2) Debridement of nonviable tissue
      (3) Omental packing
      (4) Dexon mesh hepatorrhaphy
      (5) Hepatic artery ligation
      (6) Hepatic resection

4. Postoperative management of hepatic injury includes the following:
   a. Aggressive correction of coagulation abnormalities which can require transfusion with platelets and/or FFP
   b. Treatment of hypothermia
   c. Prevention of hypoglycemia; standard practice—administration of 10% dextrose solutions following hepatic resection

5. Subcapsular hematomas may be managed nonoperatively in stable patients with bed rest, serial physical examination, hematocrit determinations, and repeat CT scanning.
   a. One third of these patients require operation.
   b. Signs of rupture or abscess formation require immediate operative intervention.
   c. Enlargement of contained hematomas may be initially managed with arteriography and embolization but may also require operative intervention.

6. Complications of hepatic injuries include the following:
   a. Ongoing bleeding despite correction of hypothermia and

coagulation parameters should be treated with early reoperation.

b. Abscesses are common after hepatic trauma (10% to 20%), secondary to retained bile, blood, and necrotic tissue.

   (1) Clinical signs include fever, sepsis, and persistent hyperbilirubinemia.

   (2) Diagnosis is established by CT scan.

   (3) Treatment is percutaneous or open drainage.

c. Hyperbilirubinemia is a common early finding related to multiple transfusions and transient hepatic dysfunction. A persistent elevation may also indicate infection.

d. Hematobilia is a complication that has the following considerations:

   (1) Hematobilia is usually complicating subcapsular or central hematomas and may result from inadvisable closure of transcapsular lacerations.

   (2) Clinical findings include abdominal pain and GI bleeding (usually melena) with a history of abdominal trauma.

   (3) Diagnosis is established by angiography.

   (4) Embolization is usually successful. Several operative strategies have been employed including resection, ligation of hepatic artery branches, and debridement.

C. Gastric Injury

1. Gastric injuries most commonly occur with penetrating trauma. Diagnosis may be suspected if a bloody NG aspirate is present.

2. Most gastric injuries can be repaired primarily.

3. NG suction should be maintained postoperatively until peristalsis has returned.

4. Complications of gastric injury includes the following:

   a. Significant bleeding via the NG tube may originate from a suture line. Management involves reexploration for hemostasis.

   b. Subhepatic, subphrenic, or lesser sac abscesses are suspected in patients with persistent fever and elevated WBC counts. Treatment is drainage.

D. Duodenal Injury

1. Delays in the diagnosis of duodenal injuries are common.

   a. Retroperitoneal duodenal injuries may be missed at

laparotomy unless meticulous care is given to inspection of the entire duodenum.

b. Mortality rates of 25% to 40% have been reported secondary to delay in diagnosis and severity of associated injuries.

2. Clinical findings are nonspecific but include fever, tachycardia, and abdominal, back, or shoulder pain. Testicular pain is associated with retroperitoneal injuries.

3. Plain films may demonstrate free air, loss of the right psoas margin, air outlining the right kidney or right psoas muscle, or retroperitoneal gas bubbles.

4. CT scans are very helpful in evaluating pancreatic and duodenal injuries.

5. Gastrografin swallows will demonstrate duodenal leaks as well as intramural hematomas.

6. Intramural hematoma considerations include the following:

a. Intramural hematoma commonly causes partial small bowel obstruction with nausea, vomiting, and abdominal pain.

b. UGI series is diagnostic, showing a "coiled spring" appearance in the second and third portions of the duodenum.

c. Nonoperative treatment is usually successful; TPN is an essential component of nonoperative management.

7. Operative management depends on the location and severity of injury.

a. The most important procedure is to establish effective drainage.

b. Simple lacerations can be closed transversely, and repairs can be buttressed with omental or jejunal patches.

c. Resection may be required in more serious injuries.

d. Two useful techniques for severe injuries include the following:

(1) Duodenal diverticularization: Antrectomy with Billroth II gastrojejunostomy and vagotomy, closure of the duodenal stump, repair of the duodenal laceration, decompression with a tube duodenostomy, and T-tube drainage of the common duct

(2) Pyloric exclusion: Repair of the duodenal laceration followed by closure of the pylorus with absorbable suture through a gastrotomy, which is the site for a gastrojejunostomy

  e. Tube duodenostomy may be helpful in difficult injuries.
     The tube may be removed in 2 to 4 weeks.
8. Postoperative care for duodenal injuries includes the
   following:
   a. Bowel rest with NG or gastrostomy tube decompression
      should be maintained for 5 to 7 days.
   b. Water-soluble contrast studies can be obtained to evaluate the repair.
   c. Drains should be maintained until an oral diet has been
      resumed.
9. Complications include the following:
   a. Duodenal fistula
      (1) Initial management includes the following:
          (a) Maintenance of gastric decompression
          (b) Sump drainage of the fistula
          (c) TPN
      (2) Fistulas that fail to close necessitate reoperation.
   b. Intraabdominal abscess

E. Pancreatic Injury

1. Following upper abdominal trauma, patients with pancreatic
   injuries often initially display only mild symptoms. The
   development of significant pain, tenderness with loss of
   bowel sounds, and peritoneal signs may be delayed. A
   common indication for exploration in these patients is
   associated intraperitoneal injuries that require operation.
2. Serum amylase levels are not reliable indicators of pancreatic trauma; only 66% of patients with significant blunt
   pancreatic trauma have hyperamylasemia.
3. Hyperamylasemia without other signs of injury is not alone
   an indication for exploration; a CT scan should be obtained.
   Retroperitoneal injuries may be missed by peritoneal lavage.
4. Operative management is dictated by the extent of injury
   and is based on the location of the injury, involvement of the
   pancreatic duct, and associated injury to the duodenum and
   common bile duct.
   a. Isolated injuries not involving the duct should be treated
      with drainage, with or without suturing of lacerations.
   b. Body or tail injuries including the duct can be treated
      with distal pancreatectomy.
   c. Isolated head and uncinate process injuries involving the
      duct should be treated by drainage.

5. Complex injuries involving the duodenum and pancreas are associated with a high mortality rate. Surgical options include the following:
   a. Duodenal diverticularization
   b. Duodenal exclusion
   c. Whipple procedure (as a last resort); mortality rate approaches 40%, usually from hemorrhage
6. Complications of pancreatic injuries include the following:
   a. Pancreatic fistulas (occur in approximately 10% of patients)
      (1) These fistulas can usually be managed nonoperatively.
      (2) Management of high-volume fistulas should include TPN.
      (3) Octreotide may be useful in shortening the time of closure.
   b. Pancreatitis (occurs in up to 10% of patients)
      (1) Management is nonoperative and includes bowel rest. Provisions for adequate nutrition must be made.
      (2) Recurrent pancreatitis should trigger an evaluation for ductal stricture by ERCP.
   c. Pancreatic pseudocysts
      (1) Clinical findings include abdominal pain, nausea, abdominal mass, and a persistently elevated serum amylase.
      (2) Diagnostic tests include ultrasound, CT, and ERCP.
      (3) Internal drainage via cystogastrostomy or Roux-en-Y cystojejunostomy for mature pseudocysts is indicated. Clinical findings may include sepsis with associated pulmonary or renal insufficiency or progressive deterioration with fever and elevated WBC counts.
   d. Pancreatic abscess
      (1) Signs of sepsis are usually evident.
      (2) CT scanning is the diagnostic test of choice.
      (3) Management includes open drainage.
   e. Hemorrhage
      (1) Significant bleeding may occur secondary to erosion of retroperitoneal vessels.
      (2) Immediate reexploration is necessary.

F. **Small Intestine Injuries**
1. Most small bowel injuries are managed by repair or resection with reanastomosis.
2. Complications are unusual following these injuries.
   a. Intraabdominal abscess or generalized peritonitis may result from anastomotic breakdown.
      (1) Signs include fever, abdominal pain, tenderness, and leukocytosis.
      (2) Treatment is usually reexploration with resection and reanastomosis.
   b. Enterocutaneous fistulas also result from failure at a repair site or anastomosis.
      (1) Most fistulas close with nonoperative management including TPN.
      (2) High output fistulas often require resection with reanastomosis.
   c. Obstruction can also result.
      (1) Early obstruction will frequently resolve with decompression.
      (2) Criteria for operative intervention include fever, leukocytosis, tachycardia, or peritoneal signs, as well as failure of nonoperative therapy.

G. **Colon Injuries**
1. Diagnosis involves the following considerations:
   a. The majority of colon injuries are caused by penetrating trauma. Injury to the colon is identified at laparotomy.
   b. Patients with colorectal injuries secondary to blunt trauma may require further evaluation.
      (1) Both peritoneal lavage and CT may miss hollow visceral injury.
      (2) Proctoscopy is required for evaluation of concomitant rectal injury, particularly in patients with pelvic fractures.
2. Management is based on location and extent of injury as well as time to surgery.
   a. Primary repair is used in stable patients with minimal contamination and minimal delay.
   b. The repaired segment is returned to the peritoneal cavity in 10 to 14 days.
   c. Colostomy includes patients undergoing exteriorization of the injury, repair with proximal colostomy, and resection with end colostomy.

     d. Rectal injuries should be treated with proximal diversion. Drainage of the presacral space is imperative.

  3. Complications include intraabdominal abscess, which occurs in 5% to 15% of patients and can usually be managed with percutaneous drainage.

SUGGESTED READING

Hoyt DB et al: *Trauma.* In Greenfield LJ et al, editors: *Surgery: scientific principles and practice,* Philadelphia, 1993, JB Lippincott.

Jurkovich GJ, Carrico CJ: *Trauma: management of acute injuries.* In Sabiston DC, editor: *Textbook of surgery: the biological basis of modern surgical practice,* ed 14, Philadelphia, 1991, WB Saunders.

Lyerly HK, Gaynor JW, editors: *Handbook of surgical intensive care: practices of the surgical residents of the Duke University Medical Center,* ed 3, St. Louis, 1992, Mosby.

Mattox KL, Moore EE, Feliciano DV, editors: *Trauma.* Norwalk, Conn., 1988, Conn, Appleton & Lange.

Moore EE, editor: *Early care of the injured patient,* ed 4, Toronto, 1990, BC Becker.

TRANSPLANTATION *15*

Allan D. Kirk

I. THE DONOR
A. Identification of Candidates for Organ Donation

1. All deaths should initiate an inquiry for organ and tissue donation.
   a. Tissue donation
      (1) Any aged patient without viral disease
         (a) HIV infection
         (b) Rabies
         (c) Active hepatitis
         (d) Creutzfeldt-Jakob disease
      (2) No cardiovascular function necessary
      (3) Tissues for donation
         (a) Cornea
         (b) Skin
         (c) Bone and tendon
         (d) Heart valve
   b. Solid organ donation
      (1) Patient criteria
         (a) Nonseptic cadaver with beating heart
         (b) No extracranial malignancy
      (2) Other relative guidelines
         (a) All organs—no IV drug use (check for tract marks)
         (b) Renal
            (i) Absence of primary renal disease or urinary tract infection
            (ii) Stable creatinine < 1.5 or returning to normal in response to hydration
            (iii) Moderate or no pressor requirement (dopamine < 10 µg/kg/min)
            (iv) Less than 65 years of age
         (c) Pancreas

(i) Absence of diabetes mellitus (not diabetes insipidus)

(ii) No pancreatitis

(d) Hepatic

(i) Absence of primary hepatic disease, fatty infiltration, and alcoholic history

(ii) Normal hepatic enzymes

(e) Cardiac

(i) Absence of primary cardiac disease or traumatic contusion

(ii) Normal valve and wall motion on echocardiography

(iii) Normal coronary angiography (over 40 years of age)

(iv) Less than 55 years of age

(f) Pulmonary

(i) Absence of primary pulmonary disease, neurogenic pulmonary edema, chest trauma, or effusion

(ii) PEEP < 10 mm Hg, Po_2 > 300 torr on Fio_2 of 1.0, peak airway pressures < 30 mm Hg

(iii) Less than 55 years of age

2. Establish a trusting, nonconfrontational relationship with the donor's family.

a. Emphasize that the patient is dead, not being "kept alive by machines."

b. Take cultural and religious preferences into consideration.

c. Stress that donation does not cost the donor's family anything.

d. Emphasize that donation does not preclude an open-casket funeral.

B. Criteria for Brain Death Declaration

1. Definition of death as stated by the Uniform Determination of Death Act—irreversible cessation of circulatory and respiratory functions or all brain function, including brain stem

a. Declaration of death must be made in accordance with accepted medical standards.

b. Minor local variations of this act exist.

2. Conditions for the diagnosis of brain death

a. Core temperature > 32.2°C

    b. Absence of pharmacological sedation or neuromuscular blockade

    c. Absence of metabolic causes of coma

       (1) Hyperosmolar coma

       (2) Hepatic encephalopathy

       (3) Preterminal uremia

    d. Absence of shock

    e. Normal toxin screen

3. Physical exam for the diagnosis of brain death (two exams required, 6 hours apart)

    a. Absence of all cephalic reflexes

       (1) Pupillary

       (2) Corneal

       (3) Gag

       (4) Oculocephalic (doll's eyes)

       (5) Oculovestibular (tympanic membrane caloric response)

    b. Absence of decerebrate or decorticate posturing

    c. Absence of seizure activity

    d. May be presence of spinal reflexes (nonpurposeful response to pain)

4. Clinical studies for confirmation of brain death (to be performed once)

    a. Electrocerebral silence on EEG

    b. Nonresponsive apnea test

       (1) Ventilate the cadaver for 10 minutes with 100% O_2 and draw baseline ABG

       (2) Stop ventilation and begin CPAP only with 100% O_2.

       (3) Follow the O_2 saturation closely to ensure that hypoxia does not occur.

          (a) Patients in neurogenic pulmonary edema may not tolerate this maneuver.

          (b) P_{CO_2} will rise 3 torr/min in the absence of ventilation.

       (4) After approximately 10 minutes (variable depending on starting P_{CO_2}), observe the cadaver for any respiratory effort for 2 minutes.

          (a) Draw ABG to confirm a $P_{CO_2} > 60$ torr.

          (b) No respiratory effort for 2 minutes with $P_{CO_2} > 60$ torr indicates nonresponsiveness.

       (5) For cadavers with low pulmonary compliance,

hypoxia, or neurogenic pulmonary edema use the following procedures:
   (a) Ventilate with Fio_2 of 0.9 and $Fico_2$ of 0.1.
   (b) Use capnographic monitoring to establish hypercarbia.
   (c) Draw ABG to confirm a $Pco_2 > 60$ torr.
   (d) Stop ventilation for 2 minutes to observe for respiratory effort.
   c. Cerebral angiogram or nuclear medicine brain scan to demonstrate absence of cerebral blood flow (optional)
5. Logistical concerns for brain death declaration
   a. Documentation of brain death
      (1) Entered in official medical record
      (2) Carried out by two competent, independent examiners
   b. Brain death declaration
      (1) Pronounced by a brain death committee
      (2) Follows predetermined hospital approved guidelines (See Box on p. 350.)
      (3) Should exercise caution in children less than 5 years of age because of their extraordinary ability to recover function after extreme injury

C. Stabilization of Heart-Beating Cadavers
1. Ensure that all care is of therapeutic benefit to the patient until brain death is declared.
   a. Maximization of cerebral O_2 delivery, usually at the expense of O_2 delivery to visceral organs, is mandatory.
   b. At the time of brain death declaration, all care should be redirected toward preservation of O_2 delivery to the individual organs for donation.
2. Maintain core temperature at or around 37°C.
   a. Pathophysiology
      (1) Loss of cerebral thermoregulation in the hypothalamus and brainstem controlled vasomotor responses
      (2) Rapid loss of heat and eventual hypothermic-induced dysrhythmias
   b. Methods to maintain body temperature
      (1) Warm with overhead heaters and warmed blankets.
      (2) Keep the room closed and the room temperature elevated.
      (3) Warm inspired gases to 38°C.
      (4) Warm all intravenous fluids to 38°C.

Duke University Criteria for Determination of Adult Brain Death

I. CLINICAL CRITERIA

A. Known Irreversible Etiology

Exclude CNS depressants (i.e., barbiturates, benzodiazepines, etc.), hypothermia (core temperature greater than 32.2°C), and neuromuscular blockading medications within 24 hours.

B. Two Examinations*

At least 6 hours apart demonstrating the following:

1. Unresponsive coma
2. Absent brain stem function
   (a) No pupillary light response
   (b) No corneal response
   (c) No oculocephalic response
   (d) No response to caloric stimulation (50 ml cold water AU)

C. Apnea

No spontaneous respiration following appropriate testing, i.e., respiratory drive test

II. CONFIRMATORY TESTS

Confirmatory tests are recommended, especially in the setting of hypoxic-ischemic injury and in periods of observation of less than 12 hours, but remain optional at the discretion of the attending physician.

A. Isoelectric EEG

B. Arteriogram or Nuclear Medicine Study

To demonstrate absence of cerebral circulation

*The first examination may be performed by senior neurology house staff or by an attending neurologist. The second examination is performed by an attending neurologist.

3. Reduce cerebral edema by reversing hypovolemia and hyperosmolar states if present.
   a. PA catheter may be necessary to establish volume status.
   b. Transfusion to a hemoglobin > 10 mg/dl.
   c. Maintenance of a urine output of 100 ml/hr.
4. Prevent donor hypoxia.
   a. Keep Po_2 > 100 torr.
      (1) Fio_2 can be increased as needed.
      (2) Hb levels in excess of 15 mg/ml may help provide adequate O_2 delivery in hypoxic donors.
   b. Optimize pulmonary toilet and utilize bronchodilator therapy for reactive airway disease.
   c. Treat correctable injuries (chest tube insertion for pneumothorax or hemothorax).

d. Perform a CXR evaluation for pulmonary edema.
 (1) Neurogenic pulmonary edema
  (a) Low to normal filling pressures
  (b) Nonsegmental infiltrates
  (c) Treated with PEEP and O_2
 (2) Cardiogenic pulmonary edema
  (a) High filling pressures and low cardiac output
  (b) Treated with dopamine or dobutamine
 (3) Aspiration
  (a) Segmental infiltrate
  (b) Treated with pulmonary toilet
 e. Judicious use of PEEP
 (1) Hypoxia requiring PEEP usually contraindicates pulmonary donation.
 (2) Excessive PEEP may contribute to hemodynamic instability.
5. Prevent hemodynamic instability.
 a. Hypotension unresponsive to volume or low-dose inotropic support
 (1) Sign of impending complete circulatory collapse
 (2) Mandates expedient removal of viable organs
 b. Intervention
 (1) Volume expansion is the most important first step.
 (2) Administer dopamine up to 10 µg/kg/min if inotropic support is needed.
 (3) Phenylephrine < 2 µg/kg/min may improve Do_2.
  (a) SVR must be measured and followed closely.
  (b) The measurement of Svo_2 is beneficial in this setting.
  (c) Discontinue use if Do_2 does not improve.
 (4) Use of epinephrine, norepinephrine, or high-dose phenylephrine is contraindicated.
6. Treat bradycardia only if systemic perfusion is threatened.
 a. Atropine
 (1) Nonresponsiveness to atropine is the rule since cadavers have no vagal tone.
 (2) Trial dose of 1 mg may be used since postsynaptic neural tone may still be in effect.
 b. Isoproterenol 1 mg/250 ml, continuous IV infusion
 (1) Titrate to desired heart rate.
 (2) Increased splanchnic blood flow from β-adrenergic

effects may require additional volume to prevent paradoxical hypotension.

  c. Transvenous pacing occasionally required

7. Normalize ventilation and minimize ventilator induced barotrauma.

  a. Do not compromise oxygenation.

  b. Take care to protect the integrity of the alveoli for pulmonary transplantation.

  c. Sacrificing the lungs as donor organs to maintain visceral oxygenation is appropriate.

8. Correct electrolyte abnormalities.

  a. Measure serum osmolarity and serum levels of Na^+, K^+, Ca^{2+}, Mg^{2+}, and PO_4^{2-}.

  (1) Correct levels to physiologic range.

  (2) Levels may be significantly altered after premorbid aggressive diuresis.

  b. Diabetes insipidus has the following considerations:

  (1) Pathophysiology

  (a) Lack of ADH production following loss of CNS function

  (b) Subsequent massive diuresis a frequent occurrence

  (2) Treatment

  (a) Replace urine output ml-for-ml with crystalloid containing the appropriate concentration of Na^+ and K^+ as determined by urine electrolyte measurement.

  (b) Exercise caution when K^+ requirements exceed 40 mEq/hr.

  (c) Measure serum and urine electrolytes frequently.

  (d) Urine losses exceeding 500 ml/hr may require pharmacologic intervention.

  (i) Vasopressin

  aa. Initially, administer 1 to 5 U bolus IV.

  bb. Follow with infusion starting at 1 U/hr.

  cc. Titrate to keep urine output between 200 and 500 ml/hr—vasopressin is a potent renal and splanchnic vasoconstrictor. Immediately discontinue if urine output drops below 200 ml/hr.

(ii) DDAVP (alternative)

aa. Administer 2 μg as a single bolus.

bb. Repeat as needed (generally q12h).

9. Control hyperglycemia.

a. Administer insulin, 100 U in 100 ml NS by IV infusion.

b. Titrate to prevent glucosuria (usually serum glucose < 180).

10. Contact the Organ Procurement Agency.

a. Inform them of the potential donor.

b. Initiate their standard protocol for organ retrieval and tissue typing.

II. THE RECIPIENT
A. Preoperative Assessment

1. The preoperative assessment varies widely depending on institutional protocols.

2. The assessment also depends upon the specific organ(s) to be received.

3. The general guidelines for potential recipients upon arrival on the day of transplantation are the following:

a. Obtain a complete history, with emphasis on symptoms suggesting potential infection.

(1) Recent myalgia, pyrexia

(2) Oropharyngeal discomfort, dental caries

(3) Cough

(4) Dysuria

(5) Diarrhea, constipation, rectal disorders

b. Perform a complete physical exam.

c. Perform the following laboratory studies.

(1) CBC with differential

(2) Serum electrolytes, serum liver function, PT and PTT

(3) Urinalysis and urine culture (if not anuric)

(4) CMV and HSV serologies

(5) Blood type confirmation

(6) Posteroanterior and lateral CXR

(7) ECG (except for heart recipients)

d. Rule out concomitant malignancy.

(1) New, suspicious cutaneous or pulmonary lesions, adenopathy

(2) Rectal bleeding or other symptoms or signs of potential malignancy

e. Rule out presensitization.
  (1) Obtain serum for a current crossmatch between recipient serum and donor cells.
    (a) T-cell lymphocytotoxic crossmatch is standard (must be negative prior to transplant).
    (b) B-cell and monocyte crossmatching are performed at many institutions.
  (2) Rules for ABO and Rh factors in transplantation are the same as in blood transfusions.
  (3) Determine the patient's panel reactive antibody percentage.
    (a) A general measure of the humoral presensitization against all HLA
    (b) Graded from 0 (good) to 100 (bad)
    (c) If high (>30%), may warrant the use of enhanced induction therapy
f. Establish venous and/or arterial access with strict aseptic technique.
4. Organ specific evaluation procedures include the following:
  a. Renal
    (1) Perform HLA typing prior to transplantation.
    (2) Determine whether dialysis is required.
      (a) Anticipate intraoperative fluid administration.
      (b) Determine the potential delayed graft function.
      (c) Obtain the patient's "dry weight."
      (d) Document the daily urine output from native kidneys.
    (3) Culture peritoneal dialysate if applicable.
    (4) Perform a preoperative transfusion.
      (a) Utilize sparingly the day of surgery.
      (b) Use only if cardiac comorbidities mandate the need for increased O_2 carrying capacity.
  b. Pancreas
    (1) Usually transplanted with a kidney as a simultaneous kidney pancreas transplantation
    (2) Routine renal evaluation
    (3) Should stabilize glucose levels in the 150 to 200 mg/dl range
  c. Hepatic
    (1) Blood products
      (a) Estimate blood products that will be required.

     (b) Confirm availability with blood bank prior to beginning the procedure.

    (2) HLA typing: Not performed prior to transplantation

   d. Cardiac and pulmonary

    (1) HLA typing: Not performed prior to transplantation

    (2) No other special evaluations

B. Transplant Unit Logistics

 1. Assignments should be made to avoid cross-coverage with septic or infected patients.

 2. Strict hand washing by all personnel is mandatory.

 3. Private rooms are preferred.

  a. Additional isolation procedures are usually not necessary.

  b. When induction therapy is used, masks should be worn.

C. Perioperative Care

 1. Daily evaluation for signs of infection

  a. Examination of oropharyngeal region

   (1) Thrush

   (2) Herpetic or CMV lesions

  b. Otic examination for otitis; seen with the following:

   (1) Prolonged NG suction

   (2) Prolonged endotracheal intubation

  c. Skin inspection

   (1) Wounds

   (2) Skin folds and the sacral and perianal regions

  d. Body fluids

   (1) Clarity of urine and other drainage should be noted.

   (2) Prompt culture should be performed if indicated.

  e. Mental status exam (CNS infections)

 2. Laboratory studies tailored to address individual organ function

  a. CBC

   (1) Lymphopenia

    (a) May be a sign of overaggressive immunosuppression

    (b) Occurs with use of antilymphocyte preparations

    (c) CMV infection

    (d) Poor nutrition

         (2) Neutrophil proliferation
            (a) Emerging bacterial infections
            (b) Steroid induction therapy
   b. Close monitoring of serum glucose during steroid induction
   c. Routine electrolytes
   d. Serum amylase
      (1) Should be monitored periodically during induction
      (2) Used to rule out steroid-induced pancreatitis

3. Prophylactic antibiotics
   a. Same guidelines as for other surgical procedures of similar magnitude and scope
   b. Urinary prophylaxis with doxycycline 100 mg PO daily
      (1) Used for renal and simultaneous kidney pancreas recipients
      (2) Continued until the bladder anastomoses are healed (4 weeks)
   c. Pneumocystis prophylaxis
      (1) Used for pancreas, cardiac, and pulmonary grafts
      (2) Administration of trimethoprim 160 mg/sulfamethoxazole 800 mg PO 3×/wk
   d. Oral fungal prophylaxis
      (1) Nystatin oral suspension 5 ml PO swish and swallow bid, or clotrimazole lozenges, 10 mg PO qid
      (2) Appropriate for all immunosuppressed patients until the end of the induction period (usually 4 weeks)
   e. Additional organism-specific coverage if cultures from the organ transport medium or the donor return positive

4. CMV prophylaxis
   a. Indications
      (1) CMV-positive recipients
      (2) CMV-negative recipients of CMV-positive organs
      (3) All recipients undergoing treatment with an antilymphocyte antibody preparation
   b. Agents—Ganciclovir 5 mg/kg IV q12h
      (1) Should be used while IV administration is feasible
      (2) Converted to high-dose acyclovir, 400 mg PO qid, prior to discharge
      (3) CMV hyperimmune globulin (Cytogam 150 mg/kg IV qd for 14 days)

5. HSV prophylaxis
   a. Acyclovir 200 mg PO tid
   b. Should be given postoperatively to all HSV-positive patients for 4 to 12 weeks
6. Peptic ulcer prophylaxis with an H_2 antagonist
   a. Patients receiving steroids
   b. Patients that are NPO
7. Drains
   a. Should be closed-suction drains
   b. Should be removed early in perioperative course
8. Management of hypertension
   a. Appropriate adjustment of intravascular volume status
   b. Use of antihypertensives (captopril, clonidine, nifedipine, and propranolol)
      (1) Avoidance of β-blockers and thiazide diuretics in pancreas recipients
      (2) Occasional PRN use of agents to acutely lower BP
         (a) Sublingual nifedipine 10 mg
         (b) Intravenous labetalol 20 mg load, 0.5 to 2 mg/min infusion hydralazine 10 to 20 mg
         (c) Sodium nitroprusside
             (i) Avoid using this agent in recipients of hepatic allografts.
             (ii) Metabolites are hepatotoxic.
9. Maintenance of patient hygiene (oral and cutaneous)
   a. Maintenance is critical in preventing infectious complications.
   b. Patients should be bathed daily with a bacteriostatic soap.
   c. Skin desiccation can be prevented with a moisturizer such as lanolin.
10. Constipation prevention
    a. Utilize a stool softener (docusate sodium 100 mg PO tid).
    b. Above may minimize bacterial translocation during defecation and perirectal injury.
11. Enteral nutrition
    a. Reinstate as early as possible.
    b. Utilize vitamin supplementation.

D. Organ-Specific Perioperative Care
1. Renal
   a. Hourly assessment of intravascular volume status

        (1) Urine output measured hourly until stable function achieved

        (2) Physical exam

        (3) Measurement of the CVP

    b. Posttransplant diuresis

        (1) Common after short ischemic times (e.g., living related donors)

        (2) Can precipitate electrolyte abnormalities, hypovolemia, and shock

        (3) Treatment

          (a) Fluid replacement (Table 15-1)

          (b) Frequent evaluation of serum electrolytes

    c. Posttransplant oliguria

        (1) Generally secondary to ATN

        (2) Associated with long ischemic times or donor instability

        (3) Evaluation and treatment

          (a) If the patient is hypovolemic, replenish the intravascular volume.

          (b) If the patient is euvolemic, avoid fluid overload and consider dialysis.

          (c) Rule out anastomotic complications (see below).

          (d) If oliguria persists for 5 days, consider the following:

            (i) A biopsy is indicated to rule out superim-

TABLE 15-1.

Postoperative Fluid Orders After Renal Transplantation

Urine Output (ml/hr)	IV Replacement (ml/hr)*
<75	Output + 50 and reassess volume status
75-100	Output + 50
100-200	Output + 25
200-300	Output
300-400	Output − 50
400-600	Output − 100
600-800	Output − 200
>800	Output − 50 and reassess volume status†

*Use $D_{2.5}$ ½ NS. For massive output, hyperglycemia may require lower glucose concentrations.

†If severe hypovolemia ensues, additional fluid replacement may be required.

posed rejection or cyclosporine toxicity.
(ii) Consider withdrawing cyclosporine (prolonged ATN can be exacerbated by even
normal cyclosporine levels).
(iii) Consider antirejection therapy.
d. Posttransplant anuria
(1) Managed like oliguria
(2) Particular emphasis on ruling out technical complications
e. PO intake resumed on the day of surgery
f. Bladder spasm
(1) A frequent complaint in young transplant patients
(2) Treated with oxybutynin (Ditropan) 5 mg PO qid

2. Pancreas and simultaneous kidney pancreas
a. Assessment of the intravascular volume status (same as
for solitary renal allografts)
(1) Excessive hydration
(a) Increases pancreatic graft edema
(b) Increases pancreatic complications
(2) Additional caution in achieving euvolemia
b. Loss of HCO_3^- in patients with bladder drainage of
pancreatic graft
(1) May lead to chronic metabolic acidosis
(2) Fluid replacement with $D_{2.5}$ ½ NS supplemented
with 1 to 2 ampules of sodium bicarbonate/L
c. Generally normal glucose tolerance by the first postoperative
(1) An insulin drip is frequently employed to avoid
stimulating endocrine function.
(2) Hypoglycemia is treated with glucose administration.
d. Measurement of urinary amylase for patients with
bladder drainage of pancreatic graft
(1) High amylase values (10,000 to 100,000 U/L)
indicate good pancreatic function.
(2) Timed measurements to compensate for varied
urine volume should be 1000 to 8000 U/3 hr). Urinary pH should also be monitored and should be >7.
e. PO intake
(1) Can resume the day of surgery for bladder drainage
of graft

(2) Delayed for enteric drainage of graft

f. Bed rest usually extended for 72 hours
   (1) Prevents positional damage to the pancreatic graft
   (2) Should keep graft in a nondependent position

g. Venous thrombosis
   (1) Early complication
   (2) Prevention
      (a) Enteric-coated aspirin
      (b) Dipyridamole administration

3. Hepatic
   a. Veno-venous bypass
      (1) Often used during the operative procedure
      (2) Groin and axillary incision evaluations daily

   b. Management of intravascular volume—hepatic blood flow maximization
      (1) Wide portal to central venous gradient
      (2) Reduction of hepatic edema
      (3) Therapeutic intervention
         (a) Maintain a low CVP.
         (b) Utilize colloids/blood products instead of crystalloid for volume replacement.
         (c) Utilize diuretics.

   c. Coagulopathy
      (1) Common in the early postoperative period
      (2) Management
         (a) Provide a continuous infusion of FFP (50 to 100+ ml/hr)
         (b) Administer vitamin K (phytonadione 10 to 20 mg/day IV)
         (c) Provide an infusion of cryoprecipitate for fibrinogen < 100 mg/dl
         (d) Platelet consumption may require platelet transfusion.
         (e) Failure to correct suggests a primary nonfunction (see below).

   d. Electrolyte abnormalities
      (1) Frequent in those patients with massive transfusion requirements and serum electrolytes
      (2) Monitored and replace electrolytes as necessary

   e. Hypoglycemia
      (1) Results from inability to initiate gluconeogenesis in the newly transplanted liver
      (2) May require infusion of $D_{10}W$

    f. Hypoalbuminemia: Occasionally requires infusion of albumin

    g. Liver function tests

      (1) Measured daily

      (2) Should decrease rapidly in the first 2 postoperative days

        (a) Obstructive LFT elevation suggests technical biliary anastomotic problems

        (b) Hepatocellular enzyme elevation considerations follow:

          (i) Vascular complications

          (ii) Rejection

          (iii) Primary nonfunction of the graft

    h. Mental status examination daily to assess improvement in metabolic encephalopathy

    i. Bed rest extended for 48 hours

    j. Primary graft nonfunction

      (1) Occurs in approximately 5% of patients

      (2) Necessitates immediate retransplantation

4. Cardiac

    a. The transplanted heart is denervated and thus insensate.

      (1) There is no angina during ischemia.

      (2) The SA node has no direct autonomic control.

        (a) Cardiac output: Very preload dependent

        (b) Chronotropic support to maintain a rate of 100 beats/min: Direct pacing, or isoproterenol

      (3) Loss of vagal innervation increases sensitivity to catecholamines.

    b. Cardiac function should be monitored as with any postoperative cardiac procedure.

    c. Daily ECGs should be performed. (Maintain consistent lead placement.)

    d. Chest tubes and invasive monitors should be removed as early as possible.

    e. Endomyocardial biopsy should be performed.

      (1) At least weekly in the early postoperative period

      (2) Only reliable means of diagnosing rejection early

    f. Enteral nutrition and ambulation should be instituted on the second postoperative day.

5. Pulmonary

    a. Steroids may be withheld during the first postoperative week to aid in bronchial healing.

b. Transplanted lung should be kept in the nondependent position.
c. Position should be changed frequently (q1h).
d. Early extubation is critical for postoperative recovery.
e. Chest tubes and invasive monitors should be removed as early as possible.
f. Daily CXRs are performed.
   (1) Aggressively evaluate infiltrates.
   (2) Empirically treat infiltrates with antibiotics.
g. Indications for bronchoscopy include the following:
   (1) Pulmonary toilet
   (2) Diagnostic lavage and biopsy following deterioration in pulmonary function
h. Enteral nutrition and ambulation considerations include the following:
   (1) Institute on the second postoperative day.
   (2) Take special care to avoid aspiration.

III. REJECTION
A. Hyperacute Rejection
1. Caused by presensitization of the recipient to an antigen expressed by donor
2. Mediated by antibodies binding to the antigen
   a. Complement system activated
   b. Procoagulant state produced that results in graft thrombosis
3. Occurs within the first minutes to hours following graft reperfusion
4. Treatment
   a. There is no treatment.
   b. Graft loss results.
5. Prevention
   a. Preoperative verification of proper ABO matching and a negative crossmatch
   b. Prevented in 99.5% of transplants
B. Accelerated Acute Rejection
1. An anamnestic response to a donor antigen (pretransplant exposure to the antigen)
2. Occurs within the first 4 to 8 postoperative days
3. Biopsy to distinguish between two types
   a. Vascular rejection
      (1) Primarily mediated by antibody secreted by memory B cells

        (2) Not treatable
    b. Accelerated cellular rejection
        (1) Mediated by memory T cells
        (2) Sometimes responds to antilymphocyte immunosuppressants (see below)

C. Acute Cellular Rejection

1. Acute cellular rejection is caused primarily by T cells.
2. This type of rejection evolves over a period of days to weeks.
    a. Can occur at any time after the first postoperative week
    b. Most common in the first 6 months posttransplant
    c. Can be precipitated by viral or bacterial infection
3. Treatment leads to successful restoration of graft function in 90% to 95% of cases.
    a. Biopsy should precede treatment.
    b. Institute methylprednisolone bolus therapy.
        (1) Administer 250 mg-1 g IV qd for 3 to 5 days.
        (2) Follow with a taper to the patient's baseline prednisone dose.
        (3) If there is a failure to respond, consider the possibility of a steroid resistant rejection or an error in diagnosis. Use of an antilymphocyte antibody preparation may be indicated (Section E, 6, b).

D. Chronic Rejection

1. Chronic rejection occurs over a period of months to years.
2. There is no treatment.
3. Biopsy is indicated to rule out a treatable source of graft dysfunction.
4. Acute rejection can be superimposed on chronic rejection.

E. Organ-Specific Considerations

1. Acute renal graft rejection
    a. Symptoms
        (1) Graft pain and malaise
        (2) Rarely present in patients receiving cyclosporine
    b. Signs
        (1) Fever, graft tenderness (rarely present)
        (2) Rapidly rising creatinine
        (3) Mild leukocytosis
        (4) Decreased urine output
        (5) Fluid retention, edema
    c. Diagnosis
        (1) Rule out obstruction.
            (a) Flush foley with 10 to 30 ml sterile saline.

(b) Flush stent with 2 ml sterile saline.

(2) Rule out hypovolemia.

    (a) Challenge with volume if clinically indicated.

    (b) Allografted kidneys are exquisitely sensitive to hypovolemia.

(3) Rule out vascular and ureteral anastomosis problems in the first 10 postoperative days with a ^{99m}Tc DTPA renal scan.

    (a) Will determine if the graft is perfused

    (b) Will show if urine is being made but is not entering the bladder (ureteral leak)

(4) Perform a needle core biopsy under ultrasonic guidance.

    (a) Allows for histologic examination of graft

    (b) Will provide evidence either for or against rejection

(5) Currently there is no gold standard for the diagnosis of acute rejection.

    (a) Empiric therapy may be required.

    (b) If there is no evidence of rejection, reducing the cyclosporine dose may improve function.

(6) Standard treatment protocol for acute renal graft rejection is the following:

    (a) Methylprednisolone 250 to 1000 mg IV, qd for 3 days, then rapid steroid taper to maintenance doses of prednisone

    (b) Antilymphocyte antibody preparations if no improvement seen after 2 to 3 days

2. Acute pancreas rejection

  a. The most sensitive indicator of pancreatic rejection is rejection of the accompanying kidney.

  b. Isolated pancreatic rejection is more difficult to diagnose.

    (1) It is better to make the diagnosis prior to the onset of hyperglycemia.

    (2) Isolated pancreatic rejection is generally asymptomatic but may be accompanied by malaise or fever.

    (3) Decreased urinary amylase is a sign of acute pancreatic rejection.

      (a) One of the earliest signs

      (b) Occurs prior to hyperglycemia

  c. Diagnosis of acute pancreatic rejection includes the following considerations:

(1) The diagnosis is based on changing trends of the biochemical monitors of pancreas function.

(2) Graft thrombosis should be ruled out in the early postoperative period.

    (a) Clinical signs

        (i) Rapid onset hyperglycemia

        (ii) Low urine amylase

    (b) May require reexploration or arteriography

d. Empiric treatment is the standard.

  (1) Biopsy confirmation is less common.

  (2) Cystoscopic transvesical needle biopsy can be performed in bladder drainage patients.

e. Treatment for acute pancreatic rejection follows:

  (1) The treatment is the same as for renal allografts.

  (2) Treatment with methylprednisolone may precipitate hyperglycemia.

3. Acute hepatic rejection

  a. Diagnostic signs

    (1) Elevations in the serum transaminase levels

    (2) Persistent coagulopathy

    (3) Hypoglycemia

    (4) Secretion of watery bile or absence of bile flow from the T tube (if present)

  b. Evaluation

    (1) Treatment is often empiric; coagulopathy may contraindicate percutaneous biopsy.

    (2) Rule out portal or hepatic arterial thrombosis.

      (a) Perform Doppler ultrasound.

      (b) Confirm impaired blood flow by arteriogram.

    (3) Rule out hepatitis.

      (a) Serum viral antibody titers

        (i) Hepatitis A, B, and C

        (ii) Herpes, CMV

        (iii) Adenovirus

      (b) Immunosuppression reduction if positive

    (4) Rule out biliary stricture or leak.

  c. Treatment: Same as for renal allograft rejection

4. Acute cardiac rejection

  a. Cardiac rejection is asymptomatic and has no ECG changes until it reaches the later stages.

  b. The earliest ECG finding is voltage loss, especially in the limb leads.

    c. Diagnosis of acute cardiac rejection includes the following considerations:

      (1) Established by examination of routine transvenous endomyocardial biopsies

      (2) Accelerated atherosclerosis

        (a) Considered a form of chronic rejection

        (b) Confirmed by coronary angiography

    d. Treatment is generally the same as for renal allografts.

5. Acute pulmonary rejection

    a. All pulmonary recipients experience acute rejection in the first 3 postoperative months.

    b. Diagnosis of acute pulmonary rejection includes the following considerations:

      (1) Bronchoscopy and biopsy are based on reduced pulmonary function and infiltrates on CXR.

      (2) V/Q scanning is sometimes used.

      (3) Pneumonia must be ruled out.

    c. Treatment is generally the same as for renal allografts.

IV. IMMUNOSUPPRESSION
A. Induction Therapy

1. Methylprednisolone

    a. 250 to 2000 mg/day

    b. Followed with prednisone taper

      (1) Begin when oral intake resumes.

      (2) Prednisone 5 mg PO is equivalent to methylprednisolone 4 mg IV.

2. Antibody preparations directed against T cells

    a. Used in patients at high risk for rejection

      (1) All pancreas, cardiac, and lung recipients

      (2) Highly sensitized renal recipients

    b. Available preparations

      (1) OKT3 monoclonal antibody

      (2) Polyclonal antibodies (RATG)

    c. Adverse effects

      (1) Fever, rigors, and myalgias are common following the first 2 to 3 doses. Premedicate using acetaminophen 650 mg PO/PR, and diphenhydramine 50 mg IM/PO.

      (2) Pulmonary edema

        (a) Avoid fluid overload.

           (b) Institute dialysis for patients without renal function.

       (3) Development of anti-antibodies

           (a) Occurs with repeated usage of the same preparation

           (b) Inhibits effectiveness in 40% to 60% of patients

           (c) Especially common with monoclonal preparations (OKT3)

           (d) Skin testing with test doses of polyclonal preparations

       (4) Additional side effects of polyclonal preparations

           (a) Thrombocytopenia, neutropenia

           (b) Serum sickness

       (5) OKT3: Associated with a reversible encephalopathy

    d. Dosage

       (1) The dosage is variable for polyclonal preparations.

       (2) OKT3 is given 5 mg/day.

       (3) Treatment lasts for 10 to 14 days.

B. Maintenance Therapy

  1. Glucocorticosteroids

    a. Primarily methylprednisolone or prednisone

    b. Side effects of steroid use

       (1) Glucose intolerance

       (2) Peptic ulceration

       (3) Delayed wound healing, skin friability

       (4) Psychosis

       (5) Fluid retention

       (6) Adrenal suppression

       (7) Osteoporosis with avascular necrosis

       (8) Increased susceptibility to bacterial, fungal, and viral infections

    c. Dosage

       (1) Use high doses (1.25 mg/kg/day of prednisone) for induction.

       (2) Taper to moderate doses (0.5 mg/kg/day) in early perioperative period.

  2. Azathioprine

    a. Side effects

       (1) Leukopenia

       (2) Hepatotoxicity

       (3) GI intolerance

   b. Dosage
      (1) Begin at 2 mg/kg/day rounded to the nearest 50 mg.
      (2) Reduce dose by half if patient is dialysis dependent.
   c. Required monitoring of the total leukocyte count
      (1) Reduce dose if this parameter < 7000/mm^3.
      (2) Withhold dose if this parameter < 3500/mm^3.
3. Cyclosporine
   a. Side effects
      (1) Nephrotoxicity
         (a) Nephrotoxicity can occur regardless of the serum drug level.
         (b) Biopsy may aid in diagnosis.
      (2) Other side effects
         (a) Hypertension
         (b) Hirsutism
         (c) Hypercholesterolemia
         (d) Hyperkalemia
         (e) B cell lymphoma
         (f) Acne vulgaris
   b. Dosage
      (1) Begin at 1 to 4 mg/kg IV given over 6 to 12 hours.
      (2) Convert to 8 to 15 mg/kg PO when oral intake is feasible (oral dose = 3 × IV dose).
      (3) Taper dose over the first several weeks to approximately 1 to 3 mg/kg daily.
   c. Monitoring of serum drug levels.
      (1) Desired levels
         (a) Levels are kept between 100 and 250 ng/ml if measured by HPLC.
         (b) Levels are kept in the 500 to 700 ng/ml range if measured by RIA.
      (2) Drugs that lower serum levels
         (a) Rifampin, trimethoprim IV, isoniazid
         (b) Carbamazepine
         (c) Phenobarbital
         (d) Phenytoin
      (3) Drugs that raise serum levels
         (a) Anabolic steroids
         (b) High-dose methylprednisolone
         (c) Ketoconazole
         (d) Calcium channel blockers

4. Other agents
   a. FK506
      (1) The function and toxicity profiles are similar to that of cyclosporine.
      (2) FK506 may allow for lower steroid dosage.
   b. Mycophenolate mofetil (RS61443) may have a wider therapeutic window than azathioprine.

V. COMPLICATIONS
A. Technical Complications

1. Renal
   a. Vascular compromise
      (1) Arterial stenosis and venous outflow obstruction may be related to the following:
         (a) Anastomosis
         (b) Position of transplanted kidney
      (2) Evaluate perfusion with a ^{99m}Tc DTPA renal scan.
      (3) Postoperative bleeding may require evacuation of hematoma to prevent vascular compromise.
   b. Ureteral compromise
      (1) Ensure Foley catheter patent by flushing with 30 ml sterile saline q4h.
      (2) Ensure stents are patent by irrigating 2 ml of sterile saline q4h.
      (3) Ultrasound examination of the kidney can reveal perigraft collections suggestive of urinoma.
      (4) Evaluate excretion with a ^{99m}Tc DTPA renal scan.
      (5) Evaluate anatomy with a stentogram if a stent is in place.

2. Pancreas
   a. Vascular compromise—presentation
      (1) Rapid rise in serum amylase
      (2) Drop in urine amylase (bladder drainage only)
      (3) Hyperglycemia
   b. Exocrine drainage breakdown
      (1) Bladder leak and/or leak of enteric contents
      (2) Mandates immediate reoperation
   c. Graft pancreatitis

3. Hepatic
   a. Vascular compromise

(1) Vascular compromise presents as a rapid deterioration in graft function.

(2) Venous thrombosis leads to rapid accumulation of ascites.

(3) Aterial thrombosis leads to graft dysfunction or leak from an ischemic bile duct.

(4) Doppler ultrasound is the diagnostic test of choice.

b. Management

(1) Thrombosis usually requires emergent retransplantation.

(2) Biliary leaks are treated with drainage or reoperation.

(3) Strictures can usually be stented nonoperatively.

4. Cardiac transplant complications related to CPB (See Chapter 16.)

5. Pulmonary—early technical problems

a. Most often related to bronchial anastomosis

b. Require reoperation

B. Infectious Complications

Infectious complications are common and diverse.

1. Infections in the early perioperative period

a. Preexisting infections in the recipient

(1) Urinary tract infections

(2) Pneumonia

(3) Contaminated vascular access

(4) Reactivated hepatitis B or herpes simplex

(5) Infection with *Strongyloides stercoralis*, an intestinal nematode

(a) Can present as overwhelming gram-negative sepsis related to *Escherichia coli*

(b) Treatment: Oral thiabendazole and IV antibiotics for the gram-negative sepsis

(c) 50% mortality rate

b. Infections arising from the donor

(1) Check cultures from the transport media.

(a) Institute appropriate prophylaxis if *Pseudomonas* or *Candida* organisms cultured

(b) Treat other organisms based on clinical indications

(2) Treat the CMV seropositive donor with ganciclovir 5 mg/kg IV q12h.

        (3) Other blood borne diseases can be transmitted via the graft.

   c. Wound infections (usually related to technical problems)

   d. Intraabdominal infection

      (1) All transplant patients with unexplained fever should be evaluated by abdominal CT.

      (2) Symptoms will be muted or absent as a result of immunosuppression.

      (3) Differential diagnosis include the following:

         (a) Diverticulitis

         (b) Cholecystitis

         (c) Peptic perforation

         (d) Appendicitis

   e. Pneumonia (common)

2. Infections beyond the first month

   a. Bacterial superinfection

      (1) Prolonged intubation

      (2) Drains in place for long periods of time

   b. Viral infections

      (1) CMV infection considerations include the following:

         (a) Presentation

            (i) Pneumonia

            (ii) Esophagitis, colitis, gastritis

            (iii) Retinitis

            (iv) Hepatitis

            (v) Unexplained fever

            (vi) Falling leukocyte count

         (b) Immunosuppressive effects of CMV can lead to opportunistic infection.

         (c) Treat with ganciclovir as above.

      (2) EBV, HSV, VZV, and adenoviral infection

      (3) Late presentation of hepatitis C

   c. Fungal infections

      (1) Primarily pneumonia or nasopharyngeal infection

      (2) Superinfection of transcutaneous catheters

      (3) Metastatic infection (common)

         (a) Cutaneous infections should be excised.

         (b) CT scan of the chest and brain to evaluate metastatic spread.

      (4) Treatment with amphotericin or fluconazole (required)

    (5) Fungal CNS infections
        (a) Alterations in neurologic examination
        (b) Lumbar puncture and CT investigations
    (6) Specific fungal pathogens
        (a) *Pneumocystis carinii*
            (i) Presents as life-threatening pneumonia
            (ii) Prophylaxis with trimethoprim sulfameth-
                oxazole for most patients
            (iii) Pentamidine therapy added if infection
                develops
        (b) *Listeria monocytogenes*
            (i) CNS infection is empirically assumed if
                bacteremia is present.
            (ii) Treat with ampicillin and gentamicin.
        (c) Mycobacterial infection
            (i) Presentation same as in nonimmunosup-
                pressed patients
            (ii) Standard treatment regimen

SUGGESTED READING

Bollinger RR et al: *Immunosuppressive pharmacology.* In Lumb PD, Shoemaker WC, editors: *Critical care medicine: state of the art,* vol 12, Fullerton, Calif., 1991, The Society of Critical Care.

Burdick JF: An anatomy of rejection, *Transplant Rev* 5:81, 1991.

Flye MW, editor: *Principles of organ transplantation,* Philadelphia, 1989, WB Saunders.

Rubin RH, Young LS, editors: *Clinical approach to infection in the compromised host,* ed 2, New York, 1988, Plenum Medical Book.

Starzl TE, Demetris AJ, editors: *Liver transplantation,* Chicago, 1990, Mosby-Year Book.

Sutherland DER et al: A 10-year experience with 290 pancreas transplants at a single institution, *Ann Surg* 210:274 1989.

CARDIAC SURGERY

16

Cemil M. Purut

I. INITIAL POSTOPERATIVE ASSESSMENT

A. Physical Examination

1. Significant cardiopulmonary destabilization may occur during transport from the operating room to the ICU. Thus upon arrival to the ICU, the physician should briefly note the operation performed, then proceed directly to the physical examination in a manner patterned after the advanced trauma life support protocol.

   a. Airway

     (1) Check the endotracheal tube position and cuff pressure.

     (2) Listen for air leaks around the cuff.

     (3) Check the integrity of the ventilator tubing.

   b. Breathing

     (1) Auscultate to ensure bilateral breath sounds and absence of wheezing.

     (2) Examine the chest for symmetric respiratory motion.

     (3) Initial ventilator settings should be TV 12 to 15 ml/kg, Fio_2 100%, PEEP 5 cm H_2O, and IMV 8 to 12 breaths/min.

   c. Circulation

     (1) Palpate bilateral femoral and pedal pulses (especially in the presence of the IABP)

     (2) Assess capillary refill time in the feet.

     (3) Auscultate the heart for murmurs, rubs, or arrhythmias. Rubs are often present when mediastinal chest tubes are used and are of no significance.

   d. Neurologic condition

     (1) Upon arrival in the ICU, patients are usually under the influence of intraoperative anesthetics and para-

lytics, so the initial assessment may be limited to pupillary responses.

(2) Response to commands and movement of all extremities should be ascertained before the patient is given additional sedatives and pain medications.

2. An abbreviated physical examination should be performed in a timely fashion after the initial assessment.

a. Note vital signs, including HR, BP, PA pressure, PCWP, temperature, and respiratory rate.

b. Note dosages of inotropic, antiarrhythmic and vasoactive drugs.

c. If used, check the IABP for proper timing and function. Also note BP with the IABP turned off temporarily.

3. Chest suction devices and pacemakers are examined for proper function at this time.

a. A complete understanding of the principles of three-bottle suction is mandatory for the physician, even if all-in-one proprietary commercial devices are utilized.

(1) Note the number and location of each chest tube. Normally one or two tubes are placed in the mediastinum and exit just below the xyphoid. Left and right pleural tubes exit more laterally.

(2) Insure that suction tubing is attached and that bubbling is present in the proper chambers.

(3) Note amount of collected blood at the time of arrival in the ICU.

(4) Check for the presence of air leaks. These may be a result of intraoperative injury to the lung or more commonly, to leaking of air around the chest tube insertion site or around a tubing connector. Determination of the magnitude of air leak should be made early in the patient's ICU stay.

b. External pacemakers

(1) External pacemakers are typically DVI devices (**D**ual chamber pace, **V**entricular sense, **I**nhibit pacing in response to native beat).

(2) By convention, ventricular pacing wires exit the left chest, while atrial wires exit the right chest.

(3) Ventricular and atrial pacing capture thresholds should be determined by initiating pacing at a rate higher than the heart's intrinsic rate, then gradually reducing the output current until loss of pacing

occurs. These numbers should be recorded for both atrial and ventricular pacing in the patient's ICU record. Ideally, the threshold current is 4 to 6 mA. If more than 15 mA are required, a high current output pacemaker should be made readily available.

(4) If external pacing is required, the output current of the pacemaker should be set to twice the threshold level.

(5) If pacing is not required, the pacemaker should be set to the demand mode at a "backup" rate of 60 beats/min.

4. Blood should be sent for ACT (to assess reversal of heparin), CBC with differential, serum electrolytes, glucose, BUN, creatinine, ABG, DIC screen (PT, PTT, fibrinogen, and fibrin split products), ionized calcium, and magnesium. A urinalysis should also be sent.

5. Obtain a stat CXR and ECG.

B. Review of Patient History

1. Cardiac
   a. Previous MI, ongoing preoperative angina (graded to the NYHA scale), congenital cardiac anomalies
   b. Results of invasive and noninvasive tests (cardiac catheterization, MUGA cardiac ultrasound)
   c. Previous cardiac therapies such as CABG, PTCA, thrombolytic therapy

2. Pulmonary: Tobacco use, asthma, COPD, previous pulmonary surgery, recent URI, pneumonia

3. Neurologic: Previous CVA, symptoms of ongoing TIA

4. Hematologic: History of bleeding disorders, history of anticoagulant and antiplatelet drug use, history of heparin-induced thrombocytopenia

5. Peripheral vascular disease
   a. History of claudication, previous vascular procedures (especially with respect to the femoral arteries, since these may be required for CPB or IABP access)
   b. History of previous DVT or vein stripping (especially important for CABG procedures)

6. Renal
   a. History of renal insufficiency
   b. Symptoms of ongoing urinary tract infection
   c. Symptoms of bladder outlet obstruction, especially in men

7. Gastrointestinal
   a. Dental caries, especially in patients undergoing valvular procedures
   b. History of peptic ulcer disease, cirrhosis, or hepatitis
   c. Previous abdominal surgery
8. Endocrine: Presence of diabetes mellitus, thyroid, or adrenal dysfunction.

II. POSTOPERATIVE COURSE
A. Standard Postoperative Orders
1. Vital signs: Usually q15min for 1 hour, then q30min for 4 hours, then qh thereafter
2. Activity: Bedrest $\times$ 24 hours, then up to chair after extubation and removal of PA catheter
3. Chest tubes to 20 cm H_2O suction
4. NPO; NG to continuous low wall suction until extubation
5. Foley catheter to straight drain
6. Ventilator settings
7. Pacemaker settings
8. Medications
   a. Antibiotics
   b. Analgesics and sedatives: Morphine 1 to 4 mg IV q30min for pain, midazolam 2.5 to 5.0 mg q1-2h for agitation
   c. Inotropic, antiarrhythmic, and vasoactive drugs: May give wide latitude to experienced nurses to adjust vasodilators as needed to maintain a stable BP during patient rewarming
   d. Ulcer prophylaxis: Ranitidine 50 mg IV q8h or cimetidine 300 mg IV q6h. Oral antacids may be given NG to keep gastric pH > 6
   e. Acetaminophen: 650 to 1300 mg suppository q2h PRN temperature > 38.2°C
   f. Diabetic management: May require continuous insulin infusion with hourly blood glucose measurements for refractory hyperglycemia

B. Immediate Postoperative Course
First 15 minutes after arrival
1. The initial assessment should be performed as described previously, and is done while the nursing staff transfers IV lines, attaches suction to the chest tube bottles, and connects monitoring equipment.
2. Hypothermia is the hallmark of the immediate postoperative

patient, even if patient reached normal core body temperature prior to discontinuing CPB.

    a. Vasoconstriction

    b. Depressed myocardial contractility

    c. Impaired blood coagulability

3. Abrupt changes in BP may occur immediately upon arrival in the ICU, often as a result of the short-lived pressors administered by the transporting physician en route from the operating room.

C. Early Postoperative Course

First several hours after arrival

1. Hemodynamics

    a. Hypothermia-induced vasoconstriction characterizes this period. The resultant hypertension is typically treated using an easily titratable, short, half-life IV vasodilator, such as sodium nitroprusside. Mean BP should be maintained in the range of 80 to 100 mm Hg. Sudden episodes of hypotension may be encountered resulting from rewarming vasodilatation and instability of vascular tone. For this reason, hypothermic patients who require inotropic support should receive an agent which does not itself induce vasodilatation.

    b. The cardiac index should be maintained above 2 L/min/m^2. A cardiac index below this is associated with a greater postoperative mortality rate. The treatment algorithm for low cardiac output is given in Section III.

    c. Weaning of inotropes is typically delayed until after several hours of stability have been achieved.

    d. In rare cases patients manifest a hyperdynamic state postoperatively, characterized by tachycardia, hypertension, and elevated cardiac index. These patients may be treated judiciously with labetolol 2.5 mg IV bolus. Repeated administration q10min at twice the preceding dose may be performed until the desired effect is achieved.

    e. Shivering is commonly seen and may not be related to hypothermia. Mild shivering requires no treatment. Excessive shivering causes increased Vo_2 and may be treated with meperidine 50 to 100 mg IV.

2. Respiratory

    a. Typically, weaning from the ventilator is delayed for several hours after arrival to ensure hemodynamic stability. Note that narcotics or sedatives given as patients emerge from anesthesia may compromise spontaneous breathing.

b. In cooperative patients who undergo relatively short procedures, rapid extubation may be accomplished after an IMV wean over 4 to 6 hours.

c. Generally accepted parameters for extubation in a cooperative patient are the following: TV > 10 to 15 ml/kg, respiratory rate 8 to 12 breaths/min, negative inspiratory force < −25 cm H_2O, and Sao_2 > 90%, with the Fio_2 = 40%.

3. Renal

a. Urine output should be maintained above 0.5 ml/kg in all patients. Depending on the length of the procedure and the skill of the CPB perfusionist, the patient may arrive in the ICU several kg over preoperative weight due to intraoperative fluid administration. Furosemide 10 to 20 mg IV is usually effective in inducing diuresis in patients with adequate cardiac output. Ethacrynic acid 25 to 50 mg IV may be effective in patients who are unresponsive to furosemide.

b. Upon arrival in the ICU serum creatinine may be *lower* than baseline as a result of CPB-induced hemodilution, even in patients with renal insufficiency. Serum creatinine may be expected to rise to baseline over a period of hours and often exceeds baseline by a small degree. This is a result of mild renal injury from CPB and should not be interpreted as ongoing renal ischemia.

c. Patients who have baseline renal insufficiency, who suffer intraoperative renal injury, and whose serum creatinine continues to rise postoperatively may be treated with dopamine 2.5 to 3.0 µg/kg/min to increase renal blood flow.

4. Wound/chest tubes

a. Pleural drainage may be >200 ml/hr for the first 1 to 6 hours. Ideally, drainage should taper off gradually to 20 to 30 ml/hr. Abrupt decrease in output should alert the physician to the possibility of obstructing thrombus within the chest tube.

b. Obstructing thrombus may be removed by gently milking or "stripping" the chest tube using devices designed for this purpose or with lubricated fingers. Fogarty thrombectomy of occluded chest tubes requires sterile technique and extreme care, since disastrous consequences accompany inadvertent dislodgment of newly placed arterial grafts.

c. Nonobstructing thrombus within the chest tube should be mobilized by a gentle squeezing action. If stripping of chest tubes is too vigorous, it may exacerbate bleeding.

D. Intermediate Postoperative Course

6 to 12 hours after arrival

1. Hemodynamics

    a. Hypothermia-induced vasoconstriction should be resolved, and most patients will require no continuation of vasodilator drugs. Persistently hypothermic patients should be treated with external warming devices until normothermia is achieved. Patients who require continued vasodilation despite normothermia may be treated with prazosin 1 to 2 mg via NG. Absence of bowel sounds is not a contraindication to the enteral administration of prazosin.

    b. Cardiac output should continue to improve and inotropic drugs should be slowly weaned with the goal of discontinuance 12 to 18 hours postoperatively.

2. Respiratory

    a. Progress should be made toward extubation in terms of an IMV and Fio_2 wean. Many centers avoid extubation in the late evening and early morning hours for safety considerations.

    b. If extubation is to be delayed until morning, ventilation settings should be chosen in order to reduce the work of breathing overnight. Fio_2 may be weaned as appropriate.

3. Renal

    a. Urine output may diminish despite adequate cardiac output and BP. Furosemide should be given for urine output < 0.5 ml/kg/hr after assuring an adequate cardiac output.

    b. Significant kaliureses is common, especially when diuretics are employed, and necessitates frequent (q4-6h) measurements of serum potassium with IV supplementation as needed.

4. Wound/chest tubes

    a. Chest tube output should be no more than 30 to 50 ml/hr. For excessive chest tube output, see below.

b. Sternal wound should be stable with minimal spotting on the dressing.

E. **Late Postoperative Course**

12 to 24 hours after arrival

1. Hemodynamics
   a. Inotropes should no longer be required to maintain cardiac index > 2 L/min/m^2.
   b. In stable patients not needing inotropes, PA catheters are pulled after extubation.
   c. Oral β-blockers (atenolol 25 mg bid or propranolol 10 mg qid) may be administered to patients with preoperative ejection fraction of > 35% as prophylaxis against atrial arrhythmias.

2. Respiratory
   a. >90% of patients should be extubated by 24 hours postoperatively.
   b. Supplemental oxygen (2 to 4 L/min by nasal prongs) is often needed for 48 to 72 hours postoperatively until patients achieve their preoperative weight.

3. Renal
   a. Continued diuresis with furosemide is maintained until patients achieve their preoperative weight.
   b. Hypokalemia (serum K < 4.5 mEq/L) is treated with oral potassium supplementation.

4. Wound/chest tubes
   a. Chest tubes may be pulled when output is less than 20 ml/hr for 3 to 4 hours, no air leak is present, and the CXR demonstrates no undrained fluid.
   b. Chest tubes should always be pulled *after* extubation.

III. POSTOPERATIVE COMPLICATIONS

A. Low Cardiac Output

In the postoperative setting, low cardiac output is usually a result of impaired pump performance, excessive afterload, insufficient preload or a combination of these factors. An algorithm for the treatment of low cardiac output is given in the Table 16-1.

1. Possible causes of impaired pump performance:
   a. Bradycardia
      (1) Cardiac output increases with increasing HR. However increased HR also increases myocardial oxygen demand.

TABLE 16-1.

Treatment Guidelines for Postoperative Cardiac Dysfunction

Mean Left Atrial Pressure (mm Hg)	Mean Systemic Pressure (mm Hg)	Cardiac Index (L/min/m^2)		
		<2	2-3	>3
≤7	Any	VE*	VE	NT
8-14	<100	VE	VE	NT
	>100	VE and SNP	VE and SNP	NT
15-19	<80	VE; and D, Do, or E	VE; and D, Do, or E	NT
	>80	D, Do, or E; and SNP or NG	NT	NT
>20	<80	D, Do, or E	D, Do, or E	NT
	>80	D, Do, or E; and SNP or NG	SNP, NG, or NT	SNP, NG, or NT

*VE = volume expansion; NT = no treatment if urine output is adequate;
SNP = sodium nitroprusside; D = dopamine; Do = dobutamine; E = epinephrine;
NG = nitroglycerin.

    (2) In general, a HR < 60 beats/min should be treated by atrial pacing to a rate of 100 to 110 using temporary epicardial wires. Increasing HR above 110 seldom provides further increases in cardiac output and may be detrimental in terms of increased myocardial oxygen demand.

    (3) Atrial pacing is preferred, but AV pacing may be used in patients with complete AV block. Ventricular pacing alone may be associated with a 10% to 20% decrement in cardiac output.

    (4) Patients with no epicardial pacing wires may be paced using a PA catheter equipped with pacing electrodes.

  b. Myocardial dysfunction

    (1) Mild diastolic dysfunction (decreased ventricular compliance) is universal after hypothermic cardiac arrest. Therefore it is imperative that preload be maximized before attributing poor cardiac output to lack of myocardial contractility.

    (2) Systolic dysfunction may be a result of inadequate revascularization, acute graft occlusion, myocardial

"stunning," or insufficient cardiac reserve to meet postoperative demands.

(3) Systolic function may be enhanced with inotropic drugs. It is important that a drug's inotropic, chronotropic, and vasoactive properties be considered when choosing an appropriate agent.

(4) Inotropic drugs should be started at low doses, then titrated to desired effect. Similarly, once started these drugs should be weaned gradually (as tolerated). Abrupt cessation may result in fatal hemodynamic decompensation.

c. Tamponade

(1) Pericardial fluid can develop in >80% of postoperative patients, but only 1% develop clinically significant tamponade.

(2) Beck's triad (associated with elevated CVP, hypotension, and muffled heart tones) is tamponade in the postoperative setting. Additional signs are low cardiac output, CVP which exceeds mean PA pressure, progressive widening of the mediastinal shadow on the CXR, and tachycardia, often occurring after abrupt cessation of mediastinal chest tube output.

(3) The diagnosis is usually made on clinical indexes, but it may be confirmed by bedside cardiac ultrasound showing poor RV filling due to free wall compression.

(4) The treatment is vigorous volume expansion and immediate decompression of the pericardium. Vigorous stripping of mediastinal chest tubes may be effective, but patients are usually returned to the operating room for direct evacuation of pericardial clot. Acute, life-threatening tamponade demands immediate opening of the sternotomy with evacuation of clot in the ICU. Reclosure of the sternum is performed in the operating room.

2. Excessive afterload

a. The normal systemic afterload is 900 to 1400 dyne/sec/cm^{-5}.

b. Sodium nitroprusside 1 to 10 µg/kg/min is the vasodilator of choice because of its short half-life and relative specificity as an arterial vasodilator. Doses > 2 µg/kg/

min should not be used for prolonged periods (>24 hours). Toxicity occurs as a result formation of cyanide and is manifested as an elevation of mixed venous O_2, metabolic acidosis, convulsions, disorientation, muscle spasms, and anorexia. Treatment for cyanide intoxication is IV infusion of 25% sodium thiosulfate 150 μg/kg over 15 minutes.

c. Nitroglycerin is primarily a venous vasodilator but does have limited arterial vasoactivity as well. It also has the added benefit of being a coronary arterial vasodilator. Dosage is 0.5 to 3.0 μg/kg/min. Nitroglycerin is absorbed by polyvinyl chloride IV tubing, thus the actual administered dosage is less than the calculated dosage until the tubing is saturated (unless special IV tubing is employed).

3. Insufficient preload
   a. All patients manifest decreased ventricular compliance resulting from myocardial edema after cardioplegia-induced cardiac arrest. Thus postoperative filling pressures often exceed preoperative values to obtain the same degree of ventricular filling.
   b. LV preload is generally limited by the development of pulmonary edema at filling pressures greater than about 20 mm Hg (although this is somewhat patient-specific).
   c. No significant difference in outcome exists between the various choices of fluids given to increase preload. In practical terms, blood should be transfused when the postoperative hematocrit < 25%. Otherwise, the choice of fluid is based on individual preference, with the recognition that crystalloid solutions are generally needed in greater volume than colloid or starch solutions but are also slightly easier to eliminate after the immediate postoperative period.

B. Arrhythmias

1. Atrial fibrillation
   a. Atrial fibrillation occurs in up to one third of patients and usually occurs in the first three postoperative days.
   b. Prevention of atrial arrhythmias is preferable and is achieved by prompt treatment of hypokalemia and hypomagnesemia, maintenance of Sao_2 > 90%, and prevention of serum acidosis.
   c. Ventricular response rates of 100 to 130 that do not cause hemodynamic instability may be slowed with digoxin

0.5 mg, 0.25 mg, and 0.25 mg IV 2 hours apart (1 mg total loading dose) while a cause for the arrhythmia is sought by measuring serum electrolytes (including calcium and magnesium), ABG, and pH.

d. Rapid ventricular response to atrial fibrillation demands prompt treatment. After loading with digoxin 0.5 mg IV, verapamil 10 mg IV bolus may slow the ventricular rate enough to restore hemodynamic stability.

e. Acutely unstable patients should undergo electrical cardioversion with a synchronizing defibrillator at 50 to 150 joules.

f. Procainamide 13 to 17 mg/kg bolus followed by 1 to 3 mg/kg/hr IV infusion should be reserved for patients who develop atrial fibrillation despite normal electrolytes and ABG and are poorly tolerant of their arrhythmia.

g. As a last recourse in patients who persist in hemodynamically significant atrial fibrillation despite correction of electrolytes and ABG, administration of digoxin and procainamide, and attempts at electrical cardioversion, lidocaine 100 mg IV may be effective in maintaining sinus rhythm.

2. Atrial flutter

a. Diagnosis is facilitated by the finding of a regular atrial rate of 250 to 350 beats/min (typically 300 beats/min) on an atrial ECG obtained using the external atrial pacing wires.

b. In patients with external atrial pacing wires, rapid atrial pacing may restore sinus rhythm. The two following techniques are possible:

(1) Ramp technique: Begin atrial pacing with 10 to 20 mA current at 10 beats/min > the flutter rate, then gradually increase the rate. When the atrial complex in lead II becomes positive, either abruptly discontinue pacing or gradually slow the pacing to the desired rate.

(2) Constant rate technique: Atrially pace at 10 beats/min faster than the flutter rate for 30 seconds, then abruptly stop pacing. If this is ineffective, repeat up to 6 times.

3. Ventricular arrhythmias

a. PVCs are common postoperatively. Unifocal PVCs raise the possibility of endocardial stimulation by a misplaced PA catheter tip. Treatment is relocation of the catheter;

lidocaine is ineffective in suppressing mechanically induced PVCs. Multifocal PVCs are more likely a result of global metabolic insult and should prompt a thorough search for electrolyte imbalances, hypoxia, or myocardial ischemia. PVCs which occur > 10 to 12/min may be treated with a test dose of lidocaine 100 mg IV. Successful suppression of PVCs with the test dose may be followed by lidocaine 1 to 2 mg/kg IV continuous infusion.

   b. Ventricular tachycardia/fibrillation is treated with immediate cardioversion and lidocaine 100 mg IV followed by lidocaine 1 to 2 mg/kg IV infusion.

C. Hemorrhage

1. Excessive postoperative bleeding is either a result of a coagulopathy or intraoperative technical error. Excessive bleeding cannot be ascribed to mechanical causes until an underlying coagulopathy is corrected.

2. Consideration of return to the operating room should be made if chest tube output is > 500 ml/hr for 4 or more hours. Hemorrhage which results in hemodynamic instability demands immediate operative intervention.

3. The order of treatment of coagulopathy is (1) reversal of heparin, (2) correction of hypocalcemia and hypothermia, (3) replacement of clotting factors, and (4) correction of thrombocytopenia.

   a. Heparin reversal is guided by the ACT. Prolonged ACT is treated by repeated administration of protamine and measurement of ACT until a normal value is achieved. Heparin "wash-out" may cause delayed prolongation of the ACT after initially normal values and is treated with protamine as above. Fear of protamine-induced coagulopathy (the existence of which is controversial) should not be allowed to interfere with adequate reversal of heparin.

   b. Administration of clotting factors in the form of FFP and cryoprecipitate is guided by the DIC panel (PT, APTT, fibrinogen, and fibrin split products). Prolongation of the PT/APTT indicates the need for FFP; hypofibrinogenemia requires cryoprecipitate.

   c. Thrombocytopenia (platelet count < 50,000/mm^3) is treated with pooled platelets. Patients who receive aspirin preoperatively and bleed postoperatively should receive one pooled unit of platelets regardless of absolute platelet count. Acetaminophen 650 mg PR and diphenhydramine 25 mg IV may ameliorate transfusion-related fever.

4. Adjunctive techniques to control bleeding include the following:

   a. Elevating the head of the bed 45° is helpful in decreasing venous pressure in the thorax and controlling persistent venous oozing.

   b. PEEP 10 cm H_2O will increase intrathoracic pressure and help tamponade diffuse bleeding.

   c. Aminocaproic acid 5 g IV bolus followed by 1g IV q1h bolus $\times$ 5 hours inhibits clot lysis and is sometimes helpful. Careful use is advisable since it is associated with obstructive clotting of blood in the chest tubes and tamponade.

D. Renal Failure

1. Mild elevation of the serum creatinine is not an uncommon occurrence 24 to 48 hours postoperatively and is thought to be caused by mild ischemic injury from CPB; it requires no treatment.

2. Hemodilution while on CPB may lower the serum creatine below the preoperative value. A return to the preoperative value is expected with postoperative diuresis, and this should not be interpreted as a sign of renal dysfunction.

3. Although commonly used, low-dose dopamine (2.5 to 3.5 µg/kg/min) administered postoperatively has not been shown to ameliorate the renal dysfunction caused by intraoperative ischemia. However, in some patients with postoperative oliguria (despite adequate cardiac output), low-dose dopamine may potentiate the effect of diuretic drugs.

4. Oliguria (<30 ml/hr) is treated with diuretics only after assuring adequate cardiac output. The first drug of choice is usually furosemide 20 mg IV. Increasing doses up to 200 mg IV may be used q2h until the desired rate of urine output is achieved. If furosemide is ineffective, try ethacrynic acid 50 mg initially, followed by increasing doses to 200 mg. Finally, refractory oliguria may respond to metolazone 2.5 to 20 mg via NG.

5. In patients requiring dialysis, peritoneal dialysis is preferred because of its minimal effect on hemodynamics. It is

appropriate to insert the peritoneal dialysis catheter in the ICU.

E. Gastrointestinal Complications

1. Cholecystitis after cardiac surgery may be acalculous. Diagnosis is made by ultrasonography of the gallbladder with the finding of pericholecystic fluid, gallbladder wall thickening, and often sludge in the gallbladder. Treatment is percutaneous drainage via tube cholecystostomy, followed by cholecystectomy at a later date. Patients who fail to respond to percutaneous drainage should undergo immediate open cholecystectomy. The risk of pneumothorax and pneumomediastinum with laparoscopic cholecystectomy in the immediate poststernotomy period has not been established but may be significant.

2. Perforation most commonly occurs as a result of a duodenal ulcer and is manifested as free air on the lateral abdominal X-ray in association with abdominal pain with peritoneal signs. Duodenal perforation is rare in patients receiving adequate prophylaxis with H_2 blockers and/or buffering agents.

3. Ischemia may occur intraoperatively because of insufficient flow during CPB or postoperatively because of low cardiac output or embolus. Intraoperative ischemia may not manifest symptoms for the first 2 to 3 postoperative days, even with frank bowel necrosis. The cecum is the most commonly involved bowel segment.

4. For unclear reasons, pancreatitis occurs in relation to CPB and rarely results from obstruction of the pancreatic duct.

F. Infections

1. Infections are rarely apparent before the patient leaves the ICU.

2. Mediastinitis is suspected in all patients with an unstable sternum. Sternal stability is assessed by gently rocking the sternum with hands placed to either side of the sternotomy. An alternative method is to placing a hand on the upper third of the sternal incision and asking the patient to cough. In either case, a "clicking" sensation is indicative of an unstable sternum.

3. Sternal instability in association with an unexplained fever and leukocytosis is sufficient for the diagnosis of mediastinitis, even in the absence of purulent drainage.

4. Preferred treatment of mediastinitis is immediate reopening of the sternal wound, thorough irrigation of the mediastinum, IV antibiotics, and q12h dressing changes. Delayed closure with appropriate muscle or omental flaps is accomplished in 4 to 5 days.

IV. FEATURES OF SPECIFIC CARDIAC OPERATIONS

A. Coronary Artery Bypass Grafting

1. Graft occlusion: Sudden graft occlusion within 24 hours of surgery is rare. Signs of graft occlusion include sudden hypotension, abrupt loss of contractility (not explainable by other mechanisms), and typical ECG changes (ST segment elevation). Therapy consists of immediate reoperation to replace the occluded graft.

2. Mammary artery spasm: This phenomenon is poorly understood, but its effects are equivalent to those of a graft occlusion. Initial therapy should consist of nifedipine 10 mg SL followed by SNP and NTG infusions in an attempt to abort the spasm. Refractory spasm which results in hemodynamic instability is treated with reoperation and replacement of the mammary artery with a vein graft.

B. Valvular Operations

1. Anticoagulation: Therapeutic anticoagulation should be delayed for at least 48 hours postoperatively to ensure hemostasis.

2. Arrhythmias: Operations on both the mitral and aortic valves may result in injury to the cardiac conduction system and result in AV conduction delays or complete AV dissociation. The injury may be apparent immediately postoperatively or 24 to 48 hours later as a result of progressive inflammation and/or myocardial edema. Prophylactic digoxin is avoided in these patients.

3. Excessive preload: Patients undergoing mitral valve replacement for mitral stenosis require special attention with respect to blood volume expansion, since these patients exhibit a pronounced descending limb of the Starling curve. Acute fluid overload may initiate a downward spiral of reduced myocardial contractility resulting in remarkably rapid death.

4. Elevated systemic BP: Close vigilance is required to maintain a mean BP near 100 mm Hg, since even transient

hypertensive episodes may disrupt an aortotomy incision or dislodge a newly placed prosthetic aortic or mitral valve.

C. Ventricular Aneurysmectomy

1. Resection of a ventricular aneurysm results in an increase in ventricular ejection fraction which should not be interpreted as improvement in myocardial contractility.

2. Excessive resection of aneurysmal tissue may result in a small ventricular chamber and poor diastolic performance. Cardiac output in these patients is especially dependent upon heart rate.

SUGGESTED READINGS

Cohn LH: The role of mechanical devices, *J Card Surg* 5(suppl 3)278-81, 1990.

DiSesa VJ: Pharmacologic support for postoperative low cardiac output, *Semin Thorac Cardiovasc Surg* 3(1):13-23, 1991.

Hendren WG, Higgins TL: Immediate postoperative care of the cardiac surgical patient, *Semin Thorac Cardiovasc Surg* 3(1):3-12, 1991.

Inada E: Blood coagulation and autologous blood transfusion in cardiac surgery, *J Clin Anesth* 2(6):393-406, 1990.

Kirklin JW, Barratt-Boyes BG: *Postoperative care in cardiac surgery,* ed 2, New York, 1993, Churchill Livingstone.

Mangano DT: Myocardial ischemia following surgery: preliminary findings. Study of perioperative ischemia research group, *J Card Surg* 5(suppl 3):288-93, 1990.

Scott WJ, Kessler R, Wernly JA: Blood conservation in cardiac surgery, *Ann Thor Surg* 50(5):843-51, 1990.

PEDIATRIC SURGERY

17

Andrew M. Davidoff

I. GENERAL PERIOPERATIVE MANAGEMENT

A. Neonatal Transitional Physiology

1. Respiratory
   a. Fetal respiratory gas exchange occurs across the placenta.
      (1) O_2 uptake is enhanced by left-shifted dissociation curve of fetal Hb.
      (2) Carrying capacity is improved by high Hb concentration (14 to 20 g/dl).
   b. Bronchial tree differentiation occurs between 24 and 28 weeks of gestation.
      (1) Cells lining the bronchial tree differentiate into type I lining cells or type II pneumocytes.
      (2) There is subsequent development of alveoli through 36 weeks of gestation.
   c. Pulmonary surfactant is a combination of surface-active phospholipids and proteins.
      (1) Produced by type II pneumocytes
      (2) Lines terminal lung air spaces
      (3) Essential for maintaining alveolar stability
         (a) A change in pattern of amniotic fluid phospholipids (ratio of lecithin to sphingomyelin) reflects lung maturity (L/S > 2).
         (b) Inadequate surfactant may result in hyaline membrane disease.
         (c) Surfactant replacement therapy may be efficacious in preterm infants.
   d. Chest wall compliance decreases with increasing gestation.
      (1) Premature infants with pliable, compliant chest walls

may be inefficient in generating effective negative intrathoracic pressure for inspiration.

(2) The work of breathing is great for newborns with lung disease and high chest wall compliance.

(3) Fetal fluid disappearance from the airways and alveoli occurs in conjunction with increased lung lymphatic flow after birth to permit gas exchange.

2. Cardiovascular
   a. Anatomic differences in fetal/postnatal circulation
   b. Fetal circulation
      (1) High fetal pulmonary vascular resistance
      (2) Low systemic resistance associated with placental circulation
      (3) Results in right-to-left flow across the ductus arteriosus
   c. Changes at birth
      (1) Lung expansion with increased alveolar P_{O_2}
      (2) Resultant PA vasodilation and decreased pulmonary vascular resistance
      (3) Increased arterial and mixed venous O_2 tension which mediates umbilical artery and ductus arteriosus constriction
         (a) Ductus arteriosus and PA smooth muscle remain sensitive to changes in O_2 tension postnatally.
         (b) Hypoxemia from lung disease may lead to PA vasoconstriction.
            (i) Ductus dilation with worsening shunt
            (ii) Hypoxemia
      (4) Increased pulmonary venous return and systemic venous resistance
         (a) Increase in LAP to level above that of RA
         (b) Functional closure of right-to-left shunt through the foramen ovale

3. Nutritional
   a. All fetal nutrients are supplied by mother.
   b. Glucose is most important energy substrate for the fetus.
      (1) Diffusion across the placenta maintains a fetal blood glucose at 75% of the maternal level.
      (2) Fetal gluconeogenesis and glycogen stores are low.
         (a) Low glucagon levels
         (b) High insulin levels

    (3) Maintenance of postnatal glucose levels includes the following:
        (a) Oral intake
        (b) Increased glucagon levels
        (c) Decreased insulin levels
    (4) Newborns have limited ability to utilize fat or protein to synthesize glucose.
    (5) Hypoglycemia (<30 mg/dl) considerations include the following:
        (a) Manifestations
            (i) Apathy, weak cry
            (ii) Cyanosis
            (iii) Seizures
            (iv) Asymptomatic
        (b) Risk inversely related to gestational age
    (6) Hyperglycemia considerations include the following:
        (a) Result of reduced insulin response
        (b) Most frequently seen in immature infants receiving parenteral nutrition
        (c) May result in intraventricular hemorrhage and fluid/electrolyte derangements
c. Calcium is also important in fetal development.
    (1) Necessary for normal fetal bone mineralization
    (2) Delivered to fetus by active transport across the placenta (especially third trimester)
    (3) Resolution of transient hypocalcemia by second day of life
        (a) Loss of maternal source
        (b) Renal immaturity
        (c) Parathyroid suppression from high fetal calcium
    (4) Persistent hypocalcemia
        (a) Infants at risk
            (i) Preterm or surgical infants
            (ii) Infants requiring transfusions
            (iii) Infants of diabetic mothers
        (b) Symptoms
            (i) Jitteriness
            (ii) Seizures
            (iii) Increased muscle tone

        (c) Treatment
           (i) 10% calcium gluconate 1 ml/kg IV over 10 minutes
           (ii) Continuous ECG monitoring
    (5) Hypomagnesemia
        (a) May accompany hypocalcemia
        (b) Treated with 50% magnesium sulfate 0.2 mg/kg IM

4. Thermoregulatory
  a. Thermal protection from intrauterine environment
  b. Heat production in the newborn
    (1) Newborns cannot shiver.
    (2) Heat produced through reflexive increases in non-shivering thermogenesis with a capacity proportional to body weight.
  c. Heat loss in the newborn
    (1) Loss of amniotic fluid insulation at birth can result in significant heat loss.
    (2) Heat loss is proportional to body surface area.
        (a) Newborns are at a disadvantage since their body surface area is quite large in proportion to their body weight.
        (b) The rate of heat loss may quickly overwhelm the heat-producing capacity in a newborn.
    (3) Heat loss may necessitate use of a thermally controlled environment.

B. Fluids and Electrolytes
1. Renal function
  a. GFR in a newborn is 25% that of an adult.
    (1) GFR reaches adult levels by 18 to 24 months.
    (2) GFR in a preterm infant is slightly lower than in a full term infant.
  b. Concentrating ability in infants is lower than in adults.
    (1) Preterm infant—400 mOsm/kg
    (2) Full term infant—600 mOsm/kg
    (3) Adults—1200 mOsm/kg
  c. Premature neonates must diurese significant extracellular and postnatal total body water in a short period after birth.
    (1) Total body water
        (a) 80% of body weight at 32 weeks gestation

       (b) Falls to 75% by the end of the first post-
          natal week

       (c) Adult levels (60%) by 18 months

    (2) Extracellular fluid volume

       (a) 45% body weight at birth

       (b) Decreases to 20% by 24 months

2. Fluid and electrolyte requirements include the following:

  a. Insensible water loss

    (1) Loss from the respiratory tract

       (a) Respiratory loss is about one third of the total
          loss.

       (b) Loss is 12 ml/kg/day for full term infants in a
          thermoneutral environment and 50% humidity.

       (c) Loss increases (up to 10×) with increasing
          prematurity.

    (2) Loss from skin

       (a) Stratum corneum

          (i) Major barrier component of the skin

          (ii) Less well developed in premature infants

       (b) Warmers, phototherapy

          (i) May increase skin loss by up to 50% in full
             term infants

          (ii) May increase skin loss by up to 100% in
             premature infants

       (c) Perspiration

          (i) Full term infants sweat if body temper-
             ature > 37.5°C.

          (ii) Premature infants do not sweat at birth.

  b. Renal water requirements

    (1) Requirements depend on solute load and concentrat-
       ing ability of the kidneys

    (2) The concentrating ability of kidneys depends on
       gestational age

    (3) Solute loads are the following:

       (a) The solute load at birth is 15 mOsm/kg/day.

       (b) The solute load after the second week of life is
          30 mOsm/kg/day.

       (c) Increased solute load results from oral diet,
          catabolic state, and postsurgery/trauma.

  c. Gastrointestinal water loss

    (1) Normal stool water loss is relatively inconse-
       quential.

(2) Vomiting, diarrhea, and fistula output should be measured and replaced.

d. Sodium
  (1) 2 mEq/kg/day for full term newborns
  (2) 4 to 5 mEq/kg/day for critically ill premature infants
  (3) Newborns able to retain sodium but cannot excrete excess well

e. Potassium
  (1) Two mEq/kg/day, required
  (2) Significant catabolic state with protein and potassium loss may require more

f. Bicarbonate
  (1) Metabolic acidosis from underperfusion
    (a) Treat underlying cause.
    (b) Manage temporarily with dilute bicarbonate solutions (1 mEq/kg).
  (2) Metabolic alkalosis accompanying vomiting or orogastric suctioning
    (a) Result of dehydration and loss of gastric HCl
    (b) Correction with appropriate fluid/electrolyte replacement

3. Monitoring of fluids and electrolytes includes the following:
  a. Body weight
    (1) Acute changes result from changes in total body water.
    (2) Newborns have significant diuresis on the first day of life.
      (a) 10% loss of body weight in the first week
      (b) Normal
  b. Urine output
    (1) Urine output monitoring is a sensitive, noninvasive method to assess the adequacy of fluid resuscitation.
    (2) Normal output is 1 to 2 ml/kg/hr.
    (3) Urine specific gravity may also be helpful.
  c. Laboratory evaluation
    (1) Serum values
      (a) Sodium
      (b) Urea nitrogen
      (c) Creatinine

                    (d) Hematocrit
                    (e) Osmolarity
                (2) Fractional excretion of sodium (See Chapter 8.)
C. Nutrition (See Chapter 22.)
    1. Assessment
        a. Physical variables (weight, length, head circumference, triceps skin fold)
        b. Laboratory assessment
            (1) Serum albumin
                (a) 2.8 to 3.5 g/dl suggests moderate malnutrition.
                (b) <2.8 g/dl indicates severe malnutrition.
                (c) Normal newborns may have low levels.
            (2) Serum transferrin
                (a) More sensitive than albumin
                (b) Shorter half-life (9 vs. 20 days) than albumin
            (3) Lymphocyte count
    2. Fluid/electrolyte requirements
        a. The volume requirement calculation is based on the infant's weight.
            (1) First 10 kg—100 ml/kg/day (4 ml/kg/hr)
            (2) Next 10 kg—50 ml/kg/day (+100 ml/day for first 10 kg)
            (3) Every kilogram thereafter—20 ml/kg/day (+1500 ml/day for first 20 kg)
        b. The volume requirement may increase because of increased insensible losses.
    3. Caloric/protein requirement
        a. Typical age-dependent requirements are listed in Table 17-1.
        b. Ideal diet (percent in calories)
            (1) 50% carbohydrate

TABLE 17-1.

Age-Dependent Calorie and Protein Requirements

Age (years)	Kilocalories (kcal/kg)	Protein (kg)
0-1	90-120	2-3.5
1-7	75-90	2-2.5
7-12	60-75	2
12-18	30-60	1.5
18	25-30	1

   (2) 35% fat

   (3) 15% protein (230 nonprotein kcal/g nitrogen)

  c. Requirements increased during certain periods

   (1) Fever increases caloric requirements 12%/°C greater than 37°C.

   (2) Major surgery increases caloric requirements 20% to 30%.

   (3) Severe sepsis increases caloric requirements 40% to 50%.

   (4) Long-term growth failure increases caloric requirements up to 100%.

  d. The metabolic rate can be calculated from oxygen consumption (See Chapter 1.)

  e. A positive nitrogen balance is achieved in an anabolic state.

 4. Enteral nutrition

  a. Always preferable to use GI tract for feedings

   (1) Breast milk is the preferred source of nutrition for infants.

   (2) Commonly used formulas are listed in Table 17-2.

   (3) Enteral nutrition may be most efficient if it is delivered through a feeding tube.

  b. Typical protocol for enteral feeding of neonates

   (1) Begin with 15 ml Pedialyte every 3 hours.

   (2) Increase volume 5 ml with each feed for a day.

   (3) Advance to half-strength formula for a day.

   (4) Advance to full-strength formula.

  c. Special considerations

TABLE 17-2.

Commonly Used Infant Formulas

Formula	Calories (kcal/ml)	Na (mEq/L)	K (mEq/L)	Ca (mEq/L)	P (mEq/L)	Fe (mEq/L)	Osmolarity (mOsm/L)
Breast milk	0.67	7	14	340	162	1.5	100
Cow's milk	0.67	25	35	1240	950	1	270
Enfamil	0.67	11	19	546	462	<1	285
Nutramigen	0.67	14	17	630	473	13	450
Portagen	0.67	14	21	630	473	13	210
Pregestimil	0.67	14	17	630	473	13	311
ProSobee	0.67	18	19	788	525	13	250
Similac	0.67	11	19	580	430	<1	285

(1) Hyperosmolar feeds may produce diarrhea.

(2) Nonlactose-containing formulas (e.g., Isomil, Pro-Sobee) may be better tolerated in the early postoperative period.

(3) Predigested formulas may be better tolerated in patients with short gut syndrome.

(4) Increases in volume are usually better tolerated than increases in osmolarity.

5. Parenteral nutrition
   a. Route of delivery
      (1) Central venous catheterization
         (a) Permits administration of hypertonic solutions
         (b) Carries the risks of central line placement
      (2) Peripheral route
         (a) Short-term parental alimentation
         (b) Partial nutritional support
   b. Indications
      (1) Newborns expected to be without enteral nutrition for more than 5 days
      (2) Gastrointestinal disease
         (a) Short bowel syndrome
         (b) Necrotizing enterocolitis
         (c) Inflammatory bowel disease
         (d) Gastroschisis
         (e) Omphalocele
         (f) Intestinal atresia
   c. Initiation
      (1) Protein
         (a) Begin at 1 g/kg/day.
         (b) Increase to 2 to 3 g/kg/day.
      (2) Glucose
         (a) Begin at 7 g/kg/day
         (b) Increase to about 20 g/kg/day
      (3) Fat (lipid): 1 to 4 g/kg/day as a 10% to 20% emulsion
   d. Monitoring
      (1) Daily weight
      (2) Serum electrolytes twice per week
      (3) Serum triglycerides, albumin, liver enzymes, calcium, phosphorous, and magnesium each week
      (4) Vitamins A, D, B_{12}, folate, and zinc each month
      (5) More frequent laboratory assessment at initiation of TPN

e. Complications
  (1) Electrolyte abnormalities, hyperlipidemia, trace element deficiencies
  (2) Fluid overload
  (3) Catheter sepsis
  (4) Hepatic dysfunction, cholestatic jaundice, hyperammonemia

D. Ventilatory Support

1. Monitoring
  a. Variance of normal respiratory rate with age (Table 17-3)
  b. Apnea monitor
    (1) The tendency for apnea is greater with premature infants.
    (2) Many other pathologic conditions increase the frequency and severity of apneic events.
  c. Pulse oximetry
    (1) Measures Sao_2 by absorption spectrophotometry
    (2) Benefits
      (a) Rapid response time
      (b) Continuous monitoring
      (c) No calibration required
    (3) Limited usefulness
      (a) Patients with poor arterial pulsations
      (b) Anemia
      (c) Jaundice, dark skin
  d. End-tidal carbon dioxide
    (1) Noninvasive, continuous monitor of alveolar, and therefore arteriolar, CO_2
    (2) Based on absorption of infrared light by carbon dioxide gas
  e. ABG

TABLE 17-3.

Normal Vital Signs of Children

Age (years)	HR (beats/min)	BP (mm Hg)	Respiratory Rate (breaths/min)
0-1	120	80/40	40
1-5	100	100/60	30
5-10	80	120/80	20

(1) May use umbilical artery in newborn

(2) Useful for monitoring adequacy of oxygenation, ventilation, and perfusion

2. Mechanical ventilation

  a. Indications

   (1) Severe respiratory acidosis (pH < 7.2)

   (2) Severe hypoxemia (Pao_2 < 60 mm Hg, Fio_2 > 70%)

   (3) Neonatal apnea

   (4) Pulmonary toilet

   (5) Airway obstruction

  b. Endotracheal tubes

   (1) Size

    (a) Premature infants: 3 mm

    (b) Full term newborns through 6 months: 3.5 mm

    (c) Age greater than 6 months: 4+ (age in years/4) mm

   (2) Uncuffed tube for infants and young children

   (3) May remain in place for weeks before tracheostomy needs to be considered

  c. Ventilatory mode

   (1) Older children can be managed with volume-cycled ventilators.

   (2) Infants are best managed with pressure-cycled ventilators.

    (a) PIP

     (i) Increasing PIP increases tidal volume, improves CO_2 elimination

     (ii) 12 to 18 cm H_2O (normal lungs), 20 to 25 cm H_2O (respiratory distress syndrome)

    (b) PEEP

     (i) Prevents alveolar collapse

     (ii) Increasing PEEP

      aa. May increase oxygenation because of alveolar recruitment

      bb. Decreases ventilation

    (c) I:E ratio

     (i) Normally 1:3

     (ii) Reversal of I:E ratio

      aa. May improve oxygenation

      bb. Will increase mean airway pressure and barotrauma

    (d) Increasing Fio_2

     (i) May improve oxygenation temporarily

(ii) Complications

aa. Atelectasis

bb. Bronchopulmonary dysplasia

(3) High-frequency ventilation

(a) Theoretically improves oxygenation at lower peak airway pressures

(b) Results in less barotrauma

(4) ECMO: For patients with reversible cardiopulmonary disease who fail conventional ventilatory methods (See Chapter 20.)

E. Hemodynamic Support

1. Monitoring

a. HR and rhythm

(1) Monitor with continuous ECG.

(2) Normal values vary with age (Table 17-3).

(3) Increase in cardiac output is achieved by increase in HR.

(4) Bradycardia frequently results from hypoxia and may be seen in patients in shock

b. BP

(1) Normal values vary with age. (See Table 17-3.)

(2) Doppler ultrasound is the most accurate noninvasive method.

(3) Intraarterial monitoring can be used for critically ill patients.

(a) Radial, dorsalis pedis, and temporal arteries are common sites.

(b) The umbilical artery may be used in newborns.

(4) Hypotension usually occurs very late in profound shock.

c. Central venous catheters

(1) CVP reflects volume status in the absence of cardiopulmonary disease.

(a) Catheter tip should be in the superior vena cava or RA.

(b) Conditions which will elevate CVP include the following:

(i) Positive-pressure ventilation

(ii) Pneumothorax

(iii) Pericardial tamponade

(iv) Abdominal distension

(c) The CVP trend is more useful than absolute numbers.

(2) Preferred sites for placement include the following:
  (a) Older infants and children—subclavian vein
  (b) Younger infants—facial vein
  (c) External or internal jugular or basilic veins acceptable
  (d) Femoral catheter placement less preferable because of contamination from groin

d. PA catheters
  (1) Allow measurement of PA and pulmonary artery wedge pressures.
  (2) Allow calculation of cardiac index (normal: 3.5 to 4.5 $L/min/m^2$) and Vo_2.

2. Shock
  a. Sepsis
    (1) Most common cause of shock in infants and children
    (2) Insufficient Do_2
      (a) Severe decrease in SVR with maldistribution of blood flow
      (b) Cardiac output generally elevated, but can be depressed
    (3) Usually caused by gram-negative bacteria
    (4) Associated conditions
      (a) Intestinal perforation
      (b) Urinary tract infection
      (c) Respiratory tract infection
      (d) Contaminated IV catheters
    (5) Neonates—particularly susceptible because of immature host defenses
      (a) Decreased storage pool of poorly functioning neutrophils
      (b) Reduced immunoglobulin levels
    (6) Treatment
      (a) Fluid resuscitation
      (b) Broad-spectrum antibiotic administration
      (c) Vasoactive support
      (d) Correctable surgical conditions ruled out
      (e) Experimental treatments
        (i) Granulocyte transfusions
        (ii) Granulocyte colony-stimulating factors
        (iii) Intravenous immunoglobulin
        (iv) Antibodies to endotoxin or TNF
  b. Hypovolemic shock

    (1) Dehydration
        (a) Causes
            (i) Sensible losses (e.g., vomiting, diarrhea)
            (ii) Insensible losses (e.g., evaporative, third-spacing)
        (b) Fluid lost usually hypotonic
            (i) More water lost than electrolytes
            (ii) Results in a hypertonic dehydration
        (c) Emergency treatment with hypotonic solutions of NaCl
    (2) Hemorrhage
        (a) May be due to trauma, coagulation abnormality
        (b) Resuscitation with blood/blood products
        (c) Must control hemorrhage
            (i) Operative control if indicated
            (ii) Coagulation factors replaced
  c. Diagnosis
    (1) Clinical evidence of impaired tissue perfusion
        (a) Slow capillary refill (>3 seconds), weak pulses, cool extremities
        (b) Tachypnea, tachycardia, hypoxemia, acidosis
        (c) Oliguria
        (d) Altered mental status
        (e) Thrombocytopenia
    (2) Data from invasive monitoring
3. Resuscitation
  a. Fluids
    (1) Lactated Ringer's 20 ml/kg, by rapid IV infusion
        (a) Some prefer colloid (e.g., 5% albumin solution).
        (b) Blood may be used if the hemorrhage is the etiology for shock.
        (c) If there is no response, administer second bolus.
    (2) Acidosis should be treated with $NaHCO_3$
    (3) Consider placing a central venous catheter.
    (4) Search for sites of ongoing fluid loss.
  b. Pharmacologic support
    (1) May be necessary to optimize cardiac output and Do_2
    (2) Discussion in Chapter 2
  c. Progress closely monitored
  d. Underlying cause of hemodynamic instability treated

II. GASTROINTESTINAL EMERGENCIES IN THE NEONATE

A. General Strategy for Evaluation
1. Rule out mechanical obstruction (congenital atresias).
2. Evaluate other causes.

B. Initial Assessment
1. History
   a. Maternal hydramnios
      (1) Normal amniotic fluid dynamics
         (a) Swallowed by the fetus
         (b) Resorbed by the intestine
         (c) Excreted by the kidney
      (2) Fetal GI obstruction
         (a) Fetal GI obstruction interrupts the amniotic fluid cycle, causing hydramnios (>21 amniotic fluid).
         (b) 15% to 20% of these newborns will have GI obstruction.
      (3) Decreased amniotic fluid (oligohydramnios) associated with renal disorders
   b. Bilious emesis
      (1) Suggests obstruction distal to the ampulla of Vater
         (a) This is a surgical emergency.
         (b) Consider mechanical obstruction, specifically malrotation with midgut volvulus.
      (2) Non–bile-stained vomitus
         (a) Possible prepyloric obstruction (pyloric atresia/stenosis)
         (b) May be due to nonsurgical, nonobstructing conditions (e.g., GE reflux)
   c. Delay of postnatal events
      (1) Normal bowel gas pattern
         (a) Air to the cecum by sixth hour of life
         (b) May take another 20 hours for air to reach rectum
      (2) Failure to pass meconium within 24 hours suggests obstruction
2. Physical examination
   a. Abdomen
      (1) Scaphoid: Suggests proximal GI obstruction
      (2) Distended
         (a) Suggests distal GI obstruction

(b) Rapid distension: Possible esophageal atresia with distal TE fistula
  b. Obvious anomalies
    (1) Incarcerated hernia
    (2) Gastroschisis
    (3) Omphalocele
    (4) Imperforate anus
3. Evaluation
  a. Place orogastric tube.
    (1) Aspirate contents; obstruction is suggested if aspirate > 10 ml or fluid is bile-stained.
    (2) Insufflate 25 ml air and clamp tube.
  b. Obtain chest/abdominal radiograph.
    (1) Tube coiled in the neck—esophageal atresia (with distal TE fistula if air present in GI tract)
    (2) Free air seen under diaphragm on upright radiograph—hollow viscus perforation
    (3) Intraabdominal calcifications associated with prenatal perforation
    (4) Failure of air to pass through to the distal bowel
      (a) Suggests intestinal obstruction
      (b) May be difficult to distinguish small from large bowel in a neonate
  c. Obtain contrast study to further evaluate possible intestinal obstruction.
    (1) Proximal bowel obstruction
      (a) Cecum is in the right upper quadrant by barium enema in malrotation.
      (b) Follow a normal barium enema by an upper GI series.
        (i) A barium enema may only be suggestive of malrotation.
        (ii) A barium enema will not demonstrate other causes of proximal obstruction.
      (c) Proceed directly to upper GI series without barium enema.
        (i) If KUB suggests obstruction
        (ii) If suspicion for malrotation is high
      (d) Performing upper GI first may preclude immediate subsequent barium enema because of the residual contrast.
    (2) Distal obstruction

  (a) Contrast enema performed with a high-osmolar, water-soluble agent

  (b) May be therapeutic as well as diagnostic

C. Specific Conditions

  1. Esophageal atresia (with TE fistula)

   a. Presenting symptoms/radiograph dependent on anatomic configuration

    (1) Pure atresia (5%), or atresia with a proximal fistula (<1%)

     (a) Inability to swallow, excess secretions, tachypnea with aspiration of saliva

     (b) Orogastric tube coiled in mediastinum, no GI air

    (2) Atresia with distal fistula (85%)

     (a) Respiratory distress as a result of reflux of gastric contents in the lungs

     (b) Orogastric tube coiled in mediastinum, normal GI gas pattern

    (3) Fistula alone (5%)

     (a) More subtle symptoms

      (i) Intermittent choking

      (ii) Cyanosis with feeding

      (iii) Recurrent pneumonia

     (b) Plain film usually normal

   b. Preoperative management

    (1) Patient should be upright, in the prone position with a suction catheter in the proximal esophageal pouch.

    (2) Assess for associated anomalies (occur in 30% to 40% of cases).

    (3) Preoperative bronchoscopy may be helpful in defining fistula(s).

    (4) Gastrostomy may be placed as a temporizing measure in patients not ready for operative repair.

    (5) "Wide-gap" atresia may benefit from gradual stretching with metal sounds.

   c. Postoperative considerations

    (1) Maintain an upright position with neck flexed and orogastric tube securely in place.

    (2) Use nebulized air and intermittent endotracheal suctioning.

    (3) Obtain an esophagram on the fifth postoperative day.

(a) Remove orogastric tube and initiate feeds if no leak present.

(b) Remove extrapleural chest tube once feeds have been tolerated for 24 hours.

2. Malrotation

a. Anatomy

(1) Small bowel primarily on the right side of abdomen

(2) Colon on the left

(3) Partial distal duodenal obstruction and failure of the duodenal C loop to cross back to the left upper quadrant

b. Clinical presentation

(1) Acute midgut volvulus

(a) Sudden onset of bilious vomiting

(b) With or without abdominal distention and pain

(c) Results from ischemia due to occlusion of the superior mesenteric artery by twisted mesentery

(2) Duodenal obstruction

(a) May have acute or chronic symptoms

(b) Results from complete/partial obstruction by peritoneal bands and/or midgut volvulus

c. Management

(1) Vigorous fluid resuscitation

(2) Broad-spectrum antibiotics

(3) Radiographic evaluation

(4) Emergent operative intervention

(a) Neonates with bilious emesis in whom malrotation cannot definitively be excluded

(b) Immediate exploration since acute midgut volvulus is a potentially catastrophic event

3. Abdominal wall defects

a. Gastroschisis

(1) Intestinal herniation through a perforation in the umbilical ring

(a) Probably result of atrophy of the right (usually) embryonic umbilical vein

(b) Not associated with other anatomic anomalies

(2) Pathophysiologic consequences

(a) No peritoneal covering over eviscerated bowel

(b) Inflammation of this bowel a result of irritating effect of amniotic fluid in utero

(c) Significant fluid loss from the exposed inflamed bowel after birth

(3) Immediate therapy

    (a) Vigorous fluid resuscitation

    (b) Bowel supported and wrapped in moistened gauze

    (c) Neonate placed in a plastic bag with only head outside

    (d) Operative repair

b. Omphalocele

(1) Arrest in development of the anterior abdominal wall

(2) Associated anomalies in 35% of patients

(3) Immediate treatment

    (a) Fluid losses not excessive if peritoneal lining or sac is intact

    (b) Peritoneal sac protected from rupture preoperatively with petroleum gauze

    (c) Operative repair

c. Perioperative considerations

(1) Prolonged ventilatory support and TPN are likely to be required.

(2) Use of a Silastic silo may be necessary.

    (a) Required if the bowel cannot be safely returned to the abdominal cavity because of respiratory compromise

    (b) Permits gradual return of intestines into abdomen over one week

4. Necrotizing enterocolitis

a. Most common acquired GI emergency in neonates

b. 50% overall mortality rate

c. Pathophysiology

(1) Acute inflammatory process involving the intestine

    (a) Gut ischemia/hypoxia

    (b) Bacterial overgrowth or abnormal flora in the presence of enteral feeding

(2) Associated conditions

    (a) Prematurity

        (i) Average birthweight is 1.5 kg.

        (ii) Average gestational age is 31 weeks.

    (b) Hypoxia, shock

    (c) Cytopenia

    (d) Umbilical artery catheterization

d. Presentation
   (1) Symptoms
       (a) Lethargy
       (b) Abdominal distension with edema/erythema of the abdominal wall
       (c) Bloody diarrhea, bilious emesis
       (d) Usually seen within the first two weeks of life
       (e) May progress to MOF
   (2) Radiographic findings
       (a) Dilated loops of the intestine may be the only abnormality.
       (b) Characteristic pneumatosis intestinalis may be present.
       (c) Portal venous gas suggests advanced disease.
       (d) Contrast enema is contraindicated.
e. Management
   (1) Nonoperative interventions
       (a) Fluid resuscitation and cardiopulmonary support
       (b) Bowel rest/decompression and parenteral nutrition
       (c) Broad-spectrum antibiotics
       (d) Frequent examinations of the abdomen with serial abdominal radiographs
   (2) Indications for surgical intervention
       (a) Intestinal perforation and pneumoperitoneum
       (b) Evidence of intestinal necrosis
           (i) Erythema/edema of the abdominal wall
           (ii) Fixed/tender abdominal mass
           (iii) Fixed loop on radiograph
           (iv) Clinical deterioration

III. RESPIRATORY DISTRESS IN INFANTS AND CHILDREN

A. Presentation

1. Assessment
   a. Early signs of respiratory distress
      (1) Restlessness, feeding difficulties
      (2) Tachypnea, retractions and stridor
   b. Later signs
      (1) Bradycardia, cyanosis
      (2) Unresponsiveness and cardiopulmonary arrest
2. Initial management

    a. Chest radiograph
- (1) Chest radiographs should be performed for all patients with signs of respiratory distress.
- (2) Chest radiographs helps differentiate surgical from nonsurgical conditions.
- (3) Place radio-opaque orogastric tube for assessment of TE anomalies in newborns.
- (4) Lateral soft-tissue films of neck are useful in children with upper airway obstruction.
- (5) Inspiratory/expiratory x-rays or fluoroscopy may demonstrate air-trapping resulting from bronchial obstruction with a radiolucent object.

    b. Monitoring
- (1) Observation in an intensive care setting
- (2) Continuous pulse-oximetry
- (3) Serial ABG determinations to assess adequacy of oxygenation, ventilation

    c. Maintenance of patent airway
- (1) Endotracheal intubation, tracheostomy if indicated
- (2) Removal of oral, pharyngeal, tracheal secretions with suctioning
- (3) Use of humidified supplemental O_2

B. Specific Conditions
1. Congenital diaphragmatic (Bochdaleck's) hernia
   a. Failure of closure of the posterior pleuroperitoneal canal
   b. Permits herniation of abdominal contents into the chest
   c. Pathophysiologic consequences
   - (1) Inhibition of ipsilateral lung growth
   - (2) May also be retard contralateral lung growth with mediastinal shift
   - (3) Pulmonary vascular immaturity
   - (4) May develop pulmonary hypertension and persistent fetal circulation

   d. Presentation
   - (1) May be diagnosed in utero (maternal referral to tertiary care center indicated)
   - (2) May be asymptomatic or have cardiopulmonary collapse
   - (3) Physical examination
     - (a) Respiratory distress
     - (b) Decreased breath sounds in one chest, usually the left (90%)

        (c) Cyanosis

        (d) Scaphoid abdomen

    (4) Bowel gas and nasogastric tube in the chest shown by CXR

    (5) Differential diagnosis

        (a) Diaphragmatic eventration

        (b) Congenital cystic adenomatoid malformation

  e. Management

    (1) Orogastric tube for GI decompression

    (2) Endotracheal intubation and mechanical ventilation

        (a) Low P_{CO_2}, high pH maintained

        (b) Tube thoracostomy as needed

    (3) Additional therapies

        (a) ECMO considered for patients not adequately oxygenated with conventional or high-frequency jet ventilation

        (b) Pulmonary vasodilators

    (4) Operative repair of diaphragmatic defect once patient stabilized

2. Congenital cystic adenomatoid malformation

  a. Multicystic mass of pulmonary tissue with a proliferation of bronchial structures

  b. May be symptomatic in the early neonatal period

  c. Treatment

    (1) Surgical excision, usually lobectomy

    (2) Indicated even if the patient is asymptomatic

3. Congenital lobar emphysema

  a. Hyperinflated, poorly ventilated lobe (usually upper)

  b. Pathophysiology

    (1) A cartilaginous deficiency is in the tracheobronchial tree.

    (2) Bronchial obstruction develops.

    (3) Progressive distress results from compression of surrounding normal parenchyma.

  c. High incidence of associated cardiac anomalies

  d. Diagnosis

    (1) A CXR does not always demonstrate hyperaeration.

    (2) A diagnosis can be made by V/Q or CT scan.

  e. Lobectomy—curative; may require emergent surgery

4. Pneumothorax

  a. Frequent complication of mechanical ventilation, especially in premature infants

b. Treatment
   (1) May resolve spontaneously in otherwise healthy infants (may hasten resolution by high, inspired Fio_2 improving the gradient for poorly diffusing nitrogen)
   (2) Indications for tube thoracostomy (See Chapter 5.)
       (a) Symptomatic pneumothoraxes
       (b) Pneumothoraxes in patients requiring positive-pressure ventilation
   (3) Should perform needle aspiration of chest for immediate decompression of suspected tension pneumothorax
5. Airway obstruction
   a. Potentially fatal necessitating thorough, early, rapid evaluation
   b. Relationship of stridor to site of obstruction
       (1) Inspiratory—vocal cord, cervical trachea
       (2) Expiratory—intrathoracic trachea
       (3) Biphasic—subglottic
   c. Evaluation
       (1) Awake laryngoscopy in the stable patient can identify the following:
           (a) Palatal defects
           (b) Hypopharyngeal tumors, subglottic masses
           (c) Laryngomalacia
       (2) Lateral airway film may demonstrate the following:
           (a) Epiglottitis
           (b) Supraglottic obstruction
       (3) Unstable patients should be taken to the operating room.
           (a) Intubation or tracheostomy
           (b) Bronchoscopy for complete evaluation from oropharynx to proximal tracheobronchial tree
   d. Causes of airway obstruction (See box on following page.)

IV. PEDIATRIC TRAUMA
A. General Principles
1. Leading cause of death in children (ages 1 to 15)
   a. Over 10,000 deaths annually
   b. More than 100,000 cases of permanent disability per year
2. Differences from the management of adult trauma

Causes of Airway Obstruction in Children

Congenital
Choanal atresia
Macroglosia/mandibular hypoplasia
Laryngomalacia
Laryngeal web, cyst
Hemangioma
Acquired
Adenoid hypertrophy
Vocal cord paralysis
Subglottic stenosis
Inflammatory
Epiglottitis
Croup
Bacterial tracheitis
Tonsillar hypertrophy
Peritonsilar/retropharyngeal abscess
Foreign body
Tumor

    a. Accident patterns
      (1) Most accidents result from blunt trauma (80%).
      (2) Head trauma is very common.
        (a) Results in most morbidity and mortality
        (b) Orthopedic injuries responsible for almost all remaining morbidity
    b. Physiologic
      (1) Small amounts of blood loss represent a significant percentage of total body blood volume.
      (2) Water and heat loss can be much greater than in adult trauma.
      (3) Gastric dilatation is common in children.
        (a) Vomiting
        (b) Aspiration
      (4) Basal metabolic rate/nutritional requirements are higher
    c. Psychological
      (1) Patients may have difficulty in expressing complaints and assessing pain.
      (2) Fear and stress may result in misleading signs and physical findings.
  3. Trauma score (Table 17-4)

TABLE 17-4.

Pediatric Trauma Score

Criteria	Score
Size (kg)	
>20	+2
10-20	+1
<10	−1
Airway	
Normal	+2
Maintainable	+1
Not maintainable	−1
Systolic BP	
>90 mm Hg (palpable wrist pulse)	+2
50-90 mm Hg (palpable groin pulse only)	+1
<50 mm Hg (pulse not palpable)	−1
CNS status	
Awake	+2
Partially conscious or unconscious	+1
Comatose or decerebrate	−1
Open wounds	
None	+2
Minor	+1
Major	−1
Skeletal injury	
None	+2
Closed fracture	+1
Open/multiple fractures	−1

a. Reflects severity of injury
b. Patient transferred to pediatric trauma center if score < 9

B. Emergency Management
1. Standard ABCs of CPR
2. Vascular access
    a. Place a large-bore peripheral intravenous line.
        (1) If not possible, use the following:
            (a) Subclavian line in larger patients
            (b) Distal saphenous vein cutdown in smaller patients
        (2) Groin lines are less favored.
    b. Intraosseous catheters may be placed in neonates and infants.

3. Shock
    a. Almost always due to hemorrhage
    b. Treated with vigorous fluid resuscitation
C. **Abdominopelvic Trauma**
    1. Penetrating trauma (20%) is managed in a similar manner as adults.
    2. Abdominal trauma in children is usually blunt.
    3. Evaluation includes the following:
        a. Abdomen assessed through serial examinations
        b. Serial laboratory studies (hematocrit, urinalysis, amylase, liver enzymes)
        c. CT scanning
            (1) Indications
                (a) Stable patients with history or exam suggestive of intraabdominal injury
                (b) Multiple system injury, especially head trauma
                (c) Significant volume requirement without obvious source of fluid loss
            (2) Can be useful for subsequent follow-up
        d. Management
            (1) Nonoperative
                (a) Nonoperative management is safe for patients with stable liver or spleen injuries.
                (b) Splenic preservation avoids potential complication of postsplenectomy sepsis.
            (2) Indications for laparotomy
                (a) Ongoing hemorrhage and instability
                (b) Acute deterioration
                (c) GI perforation
                (d) Transfusion requirement of >50% blood volume in 24 hours
D. **Burns (See Chapter 19.)**
E. **Child Abuse**
    1. Incidence is probably over 50,000 cases per year
        a. Demographics
            (1) Children are usually younger (<2 years old)
            (2) Low socioeconomic background
            (3) Young parents
            (4) Average age for sexual abuse is older (10 years of age)
        b. Includes physical injury, emotional abuse, neglect, and sexual abuse

TABLE 17-5.

Pediatric Emergency Drugs and Doses

	Dose
Epinephrine (1:10,000)	0.01 mg/kg (0.1 ml/kg)
Atropine (0.1 mg/ml)	0.01 mg/kg (0.1 ml/kg)
Lidocaine 1% (10 mg/ml)	1 mg/kg 0.1 ml/kg)
Sodium bicarbonate (1 mEq/ml)	1 mEq/kg (1 ml/kg)
Calcium chloride 10% (100 mg/ml)	30 mg/kg (0.3 ml/kg)
Dextrose 50%	0.5 gm/kg (1 ml/kg)
Naloxone (0.4 mg/ml)	0.01 mg/kg (0.025 ml/kg)
Dilantin	10 mg/kg
Phenobarbital	10 mg/kg
Ativan	0.05 mg/kg
Valium	0.05 mg/kg
Defibrillation	2 J/kg
Transfusion (ml PRBC)	(blood volume) (desired Hb−present Hb)/23

2. Clues to the possibility of child abuse
    a. Parents with flat affect or depressed mood, poor hygiene
    b. Delay in seeking medical attention by parents for child
    c. Inconsistent physical history, one that does not fit with physical findings in case of injury
    d. Injuries often burns, fractures, soft-tissue injuries, or head trauma
    e. Radiographic clues
        (1) Multiple healing fractures of different ages
        (2) Liver, splenic, or pancreatic fractures or duodenal hematoma
3. Required to report suspected child abuse by state law
F. Birth Trauma
    Incidence is about 0.5% of all births
    1. Larger infants and those with significant congenital anomalies are at greater risk.
    2. Typical injuries include the following:
        a. Fractures (e.g., clavicle—in cases of shoulder dystocia)
        b. Nerve injuries (especially the brachial plexus)
        c. Visceral injuries
    3. Treatment usually conservative, since most resolve with time
    4. Hemoperitoneum

a. May result from compression and fracture of liver, spleen, or adrenals
b. May necessitate blood transfusion

V. PEDIATRIC EMERGENCY DRUGS AND DOSAGES (TABLE 7-5)

SUGGESTED READING

Coran AG: Perioperative care of the pediatric surgical patient. In Wilmore DW et al, editors: *Care of the surgical patient,* New York, 1988, Scientific American.

Filston HC, Izant RJ Jr: *The surgical neonate: evaluation and care,* Norwalk, Conn., 1985, Appleton-Century-Crofts.

Smith SD, Rowe MI: Physiology of the patient. In Ashcraft KW, Holder TM, editors: *Pediatric surgery,* Philadelphia, 1993, WB Saunders.

BURNS

18

Scott K. Pruitt

I. **INITIAL MANAGEMENT**
A. **Stopping the Burning Process**
   1. Extinguish flames and remove all involved clothing.
   2. Flush chemical burns with copious amounts of water.
B. **Standard ABCs of CPR**
C. **Establishment of Venous Access**
   1. Insert a 14 or 16 gauge IV catheter; place through unburned skin, if possible.
   2. Peripheral veins are almost always adequate.
D. **History**
E. **Physical Examination**
   1. Examine for associated injuries.
      a. Examine for evidence of inhalation injury.
      b. Examine for evidence of musculoskeletal and thoracoabdominal trauma.
   2. Monitor vital signs hourly.
   3. Obtain baseline body weight.
F. **Laboratory Evaluation**
   1. ABG with carboxyhemoglobin level
   2. CBC
      a. RBC loss proportional to extent of full thickness burn injury
      b. Normal hematocrit within 48 to 72 hours postburn
   3. Electrolytes, BUN, and creatinine
   4. Urinalysis
   5. Type and crossmatch
G. **Tetanus Prophylaxis**
   1. 0.5 ml tetanus toxoid IM
   2. Unknown history of tetanus immunization
      a. 250 to 500 U of tetanus-immune globulin IM
      b. Active immunization with tetanus toxoid

H. **Estimate Extent of Burn**
1. Use the Rule of 9's for approximation of BSA burned (Fig. 18-1).
2. The patient's palm is approximately 1% BSA.
3. Children have an increased percentage of BSA in the head and neck as compared with an adult.

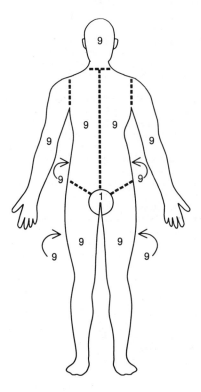

FIG 18-1.
"The rule of nines." Each of the above regions represent approximately 9% of BSA.

I.   **Estimation of Burn Depth**
    1. Partial thickness burn
        a. Pink or mottled red color
        b. Wet appearance
        c. Covered with vesicles or bullae
        d. Often severely painful
    2. Full thickness burns—all epithelial elements destroyed
        a. Charred—may appear translucent
        b. Dry appearance
        c. May have thrombosed superficial veins
        d. Insensate—nerve endings destroyed
        e. Often requires excision
        f. Always requires cutaneous autografting for wound closure

J.   **Indications for ICU or Burn Center Admission**
    1. Adults with ≥ 25% BSA burn
    2. Children with ≥ 20% BSA burn
    3. Full thickness burns ≥ 10% of BSA
    4. Burns of face, hands, feet, eyes, ears, or perineum
    5. High voltage electric injury
    6. Inhalation injury or associated trauma
    7. Other medical conditions which increase medical risk

II.   **FLUID RESUSCITATION**
A.   **Mandatory IV Hydration for all Burns ≥15% BSA**
B.   **Physiologic Considerations**
    1. Blood volume decreases and edema forms most rapidly during the first 8 hours postburn; these processes decrease over the first postburn day.
    2. Capillary permeability begins to return to normal on the postburn day 2; edema resorption also begins.
    3. Pulmonary edema
        a. Uncommon during initial resuscitation
        b. Most often occurs during the resorptive phase (commonly 3 to 6 days postburn)

C.   **IV Fluid Therapy**
    1. Duke method of initial resuscitation
        a. Isotonic fluid (150 to 160 mEq Na/L) for resuscitation during first 48 hours post*burn*
            (1) Add 1/2 ampule of $NaHCO_3$ to each L of lactated Ringer's.

        (2) Infuse 3 ml/kg/% BSA burn.

           (a) Administer half of the calculated volume over the first 8 hours postburn.

           (b) Administer the remaining half of the calculated volume over the next 16 hours.

        (3) Reduce the rate of fluid administration.

           (a) Attempt to decrease infusion rate during the second 24 postburn hours after the patient is stable.

           (b) Reduce the infusion rate by 25% every 3 hours, as tolerated.

   b. Colloid infusion

        (1) reserved until capillary permeability returns to normal (second postburn day)

        (2) Infusion of salt-poor albumin if serum albumin level < 2.5 g/dl

2. Modified Brooke formula for initial resuscitation

   a. Lactated Ringer's for fluid resuscitation during the first 24 hours

        (1) Infuse 2 ml/kg/% BSA burn in adults (3 ml/kg/% BSA burn in children).

        (2) Administer half of the calculated volume over the first 8 hours post*burn*.

        (3) Administer the remaining half of the calculated volume over the next 16 hours.

   b. Colloid-containing fluid for fluid resuscitation during the second 24 postburn hours

        (1) Add 25 g albumin (1 ampule) to 500 ml NS to yield a concentration of 5 g/dl.

        (2) Estimate the plasma volume deficit (based on BSA burn) and replace it with colloid-containing fluid over 24 hours.

           (a) 30% to 50% BSA burn, infusion of 0.3 ml/kg/% BSA burn

           (b) 50% to 70% BSA burn, infusion of 0.4 ml/kg/% BSA burn

           (c) >70% BSA burn, infusion of 0.5 ml/kg/% BSA burn

        (3) Utilize an electrolyte-free water infusion to maintain adequate urine output.

           (a) IV D_5W in the adult

   (b) Children
     (i) Children tend to develop hyponatremia with D_5W infusion.
     (ii) Infuse D_5 ¼ NS or D_5 ½ NS.

 3. Estimation of insensible fluid losses (important after initial resuscitation)
  a. Insensible water loss (ml/hr) = (25 + % BSA burn) × total BSA (m^2).
  b. Replace insensible losses with D_5W.
  c. Inadequate free water replacement may lead to hypernatremia.
  d. Anticipate a decreased evaporative loss when open wounds are grafted or covered with biologic dressings.

 4. Transfusion of PRBC to maintain hematocrit between 30% and 35%

 5. In children, may require maintenance fluid in addition to calculated resuscitation volume

D. Evaluation of the Adequacy of Fluid Resuscitation

 1. Monitor hourly urine output.
  a. Most readily available index of adequate volume resuscitation
  b. Insertion of Foley catheter and hourly urine output measurements
  c. Adequate urine output—30 to 50 ml/hr in an adult; 1 ml/kg/hr in children <30 kg
   (1) Low urine output
    (a) Usually prerenal oliguria
    (b) Acute renal failure extremely uncommon in burn patients
    (c) Administration of additional IV fluid as a fluid challenge
    (d) Maintenance adjustments and fluid infusion replacement based on urine response
   (2) High urine output—>75 ml/hr in adult; >2 ml/kg/hr in children
    (a) Indicates overhydration, unless secondary to glucosuria
    (b) Decrease in fluid administration

 2. PA catheterization indications include the following:
  a. Poor response to adequate volume resuscitation
  b. Underlying cardiac disease
  c. Age extremes

3. Body weight should be measured upon admission and every day after.
   a. First 48 hours postburn—weight gain of 10% to 20% with adequate resuscitation
   b. After 48 hours—1% to 2% weight loss occurs every day
   c. 7 to 10 days postburn—return to preburn weight
4. Hematocrit is not an accurate indicator of the adequacy of volume resuscitation.

III. VASCULAR CONSIDERATIONS
A. Vascular Compromise
1. May occur in full thickness encircling burns of the extremities because seared tissue will not expand as edema develops
2. Signs and symptoms
   a. Progressive paresthesia and deep tissue pain
   b. Cyanosis
   c. Impaired capillary refill
3. Doppler ultrasonic flow meter
   a. Useful in evaluation because tissue edema may make palpation of pulses difficult
   b. Examination of palmar arch pulses in the upper extremity
4. Prevention
   a. Elevation of the circumferentially burned limb above heart level
   b. Active exercise and muscular contraction
      (1) Periods of 2 to 3 minutes q2h during first 24 to 48 hours postburn
      (2) May enhance venous return and reduce edema
5. Indications for escharotomy to release compressing eschar
   a. Absence of pulsatile arterial flow
   b. Progressive decrease in pulse on serial examination
6. Escharotomy technique
   a. Sterile bedside procedure
   b. No anesthesia necessary (no sensation in areas of full thickness burn)
   c. Scalpel or electrocautery
   d. Midmedial and/or midlateral incision through nonviable eschar
      (1) Make incisions only through full thickness burns.

  (2) Proceed from proximal to distal and always incise eschar across involved joints.

  (3) Stay anterior to the medial epicondyle of the upper extremity to avoid the ulnar nerve.

  (4) Incise through the superficial fascia.

   (a) Incise down to, but not through, underlying subcutaneous tissue.

   (b) Cut eschar edges should separate.

 e. Return of distal pulses within a few minutes

  (1) Facilitate venous return by extremity elevation and exercise.

  (2) Failure of pulses to return may have several etiologies, including the following:

   (a) Hypovolemia

   (b) Subfascial edema secondary to electrical or deep thermal burn, prolonged ischemia, or trauma; may need fasciotomy

 f. Topical antimicrobial agent applied to all escharotomy (and fasciotomy) incisions until fully healed (Section V, B)

B.   **Fasciotomy (Section VIII, A, 7)**

IV.   **PULMONARY CONSIDERATIONS**
A.   **Carbon Monoxide Intoxication**
 1. Signs and symptoms
  a. Palpitations
  b. Mild muscular weakness
  c. Mild headache
  d. Dizziness
  e. Confusion
 2. Carboxyhemoglobin level
  a. The carboxyhemoglobin level is determined with ABG.
  b. Hb with bound carbon monoxide cannot transport O_2, so tissue hypoxia may occur.
  c. If the carbon monoxide level > 40%, the patient may experience progressive collapse, coma, or death.
 3. Treatment
  a. 100% O_2
  b. May be beneficial to use hyperbaric O_2
B.   **Inhalation Injury**
 1. Rarely a cause of immediate hypoxia (onset often delayed > 24 hours postburn)

2. Risk factors
   a. Impaired mental status (ethanol or other drug intoxication, neurologic disease)
   b. Head trauma
   c. Burns from petroleum products
   d. Burns sustained in a closed space
3. Signs and symptoms of inhalation injury
   a. Inflammation of oropharyngeal mucosa
   b. Facial burns and singed nasal hair
   c. Hoarseness, stridor, wheezing, and rales
   d. Unexplained hypoxemia
   e. Carbonaceous sputum production (most specific sign)
4. Evaluation of possible inhalation injury
   a. CXR—notoriously insensitive
   b. Flexible fiberoptic bronchoscopy
      (1) Perform this procedure when the patient is hemodynamically stable.
      (2) Anesthetize the nasal mucosa with topical agents.
      (3) Administer 100% O_2 to patient for 3 minutes prior to examination.
      (4) Place an appropriately sized endotracheal tube over the scope prior to examination.
      (5) If intubation is necessary, the tube can easily be passed into the trachea over the scope.
      (6) Signs of inhalation injury include the following:
         (a) Mucosal erythema, edema, blisters, ulcers, or hemorrhage
         (b) Carbon particles in major airways
   c. Xenon-133 perfusion lung scan—significant inhalation injury suggested by a delay of more than 90 seconds in xenon clearance
   d. ABG—for evidence of hypoxia and carboxyhemoglobinemia
5. Treatment of inhalation injury
   a. Administer warm, humidified O_2
   b. Pulmonary toilet—postural drainage, chest percussion, incentive spirometry, IPPB
   c. Bronchospasm treatment
   d. Therapeutic bronchoscopy to clear debris
   e. Intubation indications
      (1) Progressive hypoxia

(2) Vocal cord edema threatening airway occlusion (on bronchoscopic examination)

  f. Prophylactic steroids

    (1) *Not* beneficial

    (2) May increase the risk of infection

  g. Prophylactic antibiotics

    (1) *Not* beneficial

    (2) May lead to the emergence of resistant strains of bacteria

  h. High-frequency positive-pressure ventilation

C. Circumferential Burns of the Thorax

  1. May mechanically impair ventilation

  2. Signs and symptoms

    a. Progressive use of accessory muscles of respiration

    b. Increase in inspiratory pressures in mechanically ventilated patients (most common indication for thoracic escharotomy)

    c. Tachypnea

  3. Thoracic escharotomy

    a. Use the technique described in Section III, A, 6.

    b. Incisions are made bilaterally in anterior axillary lines.

    c. Extend incisions from the clavicle to the costal margin.

    d. Connect these escharotomies with a costal margin escharotomy if the full thickness burn involves the anterior abdominal wall.

D. Unexpected Respiratory Depression in a Patient Accepted in Transfer from Another Hospital

  1. The patient may have been given IM or subcutaneous narcotics.

  2. These drugs will be systemically absorbed as resuscitation increases tissue perfusion.

  3. Treat with IV naloxone (Narcan).

V. WOUND CARE

A. General Care

  1. Daily examination of wound until totally healed

  2. Daily gentle cleansing with a non–alcohol-containing surgical detergent

  3. Gentle debridement of nonviable tissue after cleansing

    a. Continue debridement to the point of pain or bleeding.

      b. Administer IV analgesia as needed.

      c. Wash in a shower or Hubbard tank, but do not immerse.

   4. Wound and adjacent margin shaved of approximately 1 inch (do *not* shave eyebrows)

   5. Wound allowed to air dry

B. Topical Antimicrobial Agent Application (q12h)

   1. Sulfamylon (11.1% mafenide acetate)

      a. Wound left open (no dressing)

      b. Removed with shower for daily debridement

      c. Advantages

         (1) Broadest spectrum of activity, especially against *Pseudomonas* organisms.

         (2) Penetrates eschar well

      d. Disadvantages and side effects

         (1) Causes pain in areas of partial thickness burn

         (2) Hyperchloremic metabolic acidosis from carbonic anhydrase inhibition

   2. Silvadene (1% silver sulfadiazine)

      a. Wound left open (no dressing)

      b. Advantages

         (1) Nontoxic

         (2) Not painful

      c. Disadvantages

         (1) Less effective penetration of eschar

         (2) Narrower spectrum of antimicrobial activity compared to sulfamylon

         (3) Neutropenia (resolves with cessation of application)

   3. Silver nitrate solution (0.5%)

      a. Applied with multilayered dressings

      b. Reserved for those patients allergic to sulfonamides

      c. Disadvantages

         (1) Joint motion limited by dressings

         (2) Leaching of electrolytes—supplemental sodium, potassium, and calcium may be needed

         (3) Poor eschar penetration

         (4) Stains environment

C. Burn Wound Excision

   1. Performed only after resuscitation is complete

   2. Indications

    a. Full thickness burns
    b. Patients requiring debridement of high voltage electric injury
  3. Contraindications
    a. Hemodynamic instability
      (1) Burn excision is accompanied by large volume blood loss.
      (2) Limit excision to 20% BSA or 2 hours operative time.
    b. Pulmonary complications
    c. Superficial partial thickness injury
  4. Technique
    a. Should be adequate levels of systemic antibiotics present before excision
    b. Method of excision
      (1) Tangential "shaving" method
      (2) Excision to fascia
    c. Control of hemorrhage
      (1) Thrombin and/or epinephrine moistened gauze dressings
      (2) Tourniquet for excision on extremity
      (3) IV or subeschar infiltration with vasopressin
    d. May graft immediately or delay

D. Biologic Dressings
  1. Indications and uses
    a. Coverage of freshly excised wounds
    b. Decreases bacterial proliferation and promotes granulation tissue formation
    c. May be used to determine readiness of a site for grafting
    d. Decreases the pain of partial thickness burns and maintains joint mobility
    e. Decreases evaporative water loss
  2. Types of biologic dressings
    a. Human cutaneous allografts
      (1) Dressing of choice
      (2) Donor must be minimal risk, documented HIV seronegative
    b. Porcine xenografts
      (1) Readily available
      (2) Less effective than allografts in decreasing bacterial proliferation

      c. Bilaminate synthetic dressing

        (1) Only when allografts or xenografts are not available

        (2) Ineffective in decreasing bacterial proliferation

  3. Technique

      a. Reapply new dressings every 3 to 5 days.

      b. Remove and replace dressings more frequently if suppuration occurs between the wound and dressing.

E. Burn Wound Infection

  1. Signs of burn wound infection

      a. Intraeschar hemorrhage (black or dark hemorrhagic discoloration)

        (1) Most common sign

        (2) May be secondary to minor trauma

      b. Conversion of a partial thickness burn to full thickness injury—pathognomonic of burn wound infection

      c. Erythema and edema at wound edges

      d. Degeneration of granulation tissue

      e. Marked subeschar suppuration

      f. Premature or unexpected eschar separation

      g. Hemorrhagic fat necrosis

      h. Metastatic abscesses in unburned skin (ecthyma gangrenosum)

      i. Vesicular lesions on healing partial thickness burns—suggest viral infection

  2. Diagnosis of burn wound infection

      a. A surface culture is unreliable.

      b. Wound biopsy is the method of choice.

        (1) Should be performed if any signs of infection are present

        (2) Biopsy viable tissue subjacent or adjacent to the burn wound

        (3) Excision of a 500 mg lenticular portion of tissue—tissue sample divided in half

          (a) Send one half of the sample for culture and sensitivity.

            (i) Greater than or equal to 10^5 organisms/g of tissue suggestive but not diagnostic of infection

            (ii) May be due to surface colonization

          (b) Send one half of the sample for histological examination.

(i) Place the sample in 10% formalin for rapid processing or examine by frozen section.

(ii) Invasive infection is present if bacteria are detected in unburned tissue that is adjacent to the wound.

3. Treatment of documented bacterial wound infection
   a. Change topical antimicrobial agent to sulfamylon.
   b. Administer systemic antibiotics based on the sensitivities of the offending organisms.
   c. Use a subeschar injection of antibiotics into the infected burn wound.
      (1) Especially useful in treatment of focal pseudomonal infections
      (2) Prior to excision of infected wound to reduce bacteremia
      (3) Technique
         (a) One-half daily dose of semisynthetic penicillin (Piperacillin) in 150 to 1000 ml NS q12h
         (b) Injected beneath eschar using a #20 spinal needle to minimize the number of injection sites
   d. Excise all infected tissue.
      (1) Adequate blood levels of antibiotics should be present prior to excision.
      (2) Debride any infected tissue (may be necessary to amputate)
      (3) Cover immediately with a biologic dressing.
4. Nonbacterial burn wound infection
   a. *Candida* organisms
      (1) Frequently colonize but rarely cause invasive infection
      (2) Systemic therapy if fungemia occurs
         (a) Amphotericin-B
         (b) With or without 5-fluorocytosine
   b. HSV: Systemic AraA, or acyclovir

VI. COMPLICATIONS
A. GI Complications
1. Curling's ulcer
   a. Acute ulceration of the upper GI tract

b. May progress to hemorrhage or perforation and can be life-threatening

c. Preventive therapy—gastric pH > 5 maintained

(1) H_2 blockers

(2) Early feeding and antacids (30 ml q1-2h PRN pH < 5)

2. Ileus

a. Almost always present in burns ≥ 20% BSA

b. Usually resolves spontaneously 2 to 3 days postinjury

c. Treat with NG suction, IV fluids

3. Acalculous cholecystitis

a. Usually causes right upper quadrant pain and jaundice

b. Diagnosis confirmed using abdominal ultrasound

c. Cholecystectomy if distended gallbladder is detected by ultrasonography

B. **Respiratory Complications**

Pneumonia is the most common infectious complication in burn patients.

1. Most commonly resulting from *Staphylococcus aureus* and gram-negative bacteria

2. Can result from hematogenous spread

a. Can occur with wound infection (usually late in the hospital course)

b. Other sources—infected veins, soft tissue abscesses, and perforated viscus

C. **Suppurative Thrombophlebitis**

1. Local signs in less than half of the patients

a. Maintain a high index of suspicion in a septic patient with no identifiable source of infection.

b. Every previously cannulated vein is a potential site for infection.

2. Exploration of vein

a. Recovery of normal-appearing blood from the vein is a negative result.

b. Intraluminal pus confirms the diagnosis.

c. Excise veins which contain intraluminal clots.

(1) Send one segment for histologic examination.

(2) Send another segment for culture and sensitivity.

3. Treatment

a. IV antibiotics

b. Complete surgical removal of infected vein

    4. Prevention—all IV catheters, including central lines, changed at least every 72 hours

D. Acute Bacterial Endocarditis
1. Right heart involvement is the most common.
2. All valves can potentially be affected.

VII. NUTRITION

An enteric tube feeding is usually necessary initially. Avoid TPN if possible (high risk of catheter-related sepsis).

A. Control of Diarrhea
1. Reduced caloric density of feedings
2. Paragoric

B. Caloric and Protein Requirements
1. Based on percent BSA burn and preburn weight
2. Requirements for patients with > 40% total BSA burn
    a. 2000 to 2200 calories/total BSA(m^2)/day
    b. 12 to 18 g nitrogen/total BSA(m^2)/day

VIII. SPECIAL CONSIDERATIONS

A. Electrical Injury
1. Arrhythmias are common, especially asystole and ventricular fibrillation.
    a. ACLS as needed
    b. Indications for continuous cardiac monitoring (for a minimum of 48 hours)
        (1) Loss of consciousness
        (2) Abnormal ECG
2. Associated skeletal fractures are common.
    a. Falls often associated with the electrical injury (falls from high-voltage towers)
    b. Current-induced muscle contractions
        (1) May cause vertebral fractures
        (2) Must exclude cervical spine injury with appropriate radiographs
3. Vascular damage must be excluded.
    a. The electrical current may damage the intima, producing thrombosis and/or hemorrhage
    b. Arteriography may be useful.
        (1) Identification of extent of tissue damage
        (2) Determination of level for amputation
4. There may be renal damage secondary to hemochromogens (hemoglobin and myoglobin).

a. Common after electric injury
b. May also occur with burn-associated crush injuries
c. Prevention
   (1) Increase infusion of IV fluids.
      (a) Maintain a urine output of 1 ml/kg/hr.
      (b) Continue until no hemochromogens are present in the urine.
   (2) If excretion of hemochromogens continues or there is a risk of hypervolemia consider the following:
      (a) Mannitol 25 g IV bolus
         (i) Administer up to 300 g every 24 hours.
         (ii) Mannitol prevents tubular deposition of pigment.
      (b) IV sodium bicarbonate
         (i) Keep the urine pH > 6.
         (ii) Alkalinization of urine facilitates hemochromogen excretion.

5. Neurologic damage includes spinal cord deficits.
   a. Deficits which appear early may be transient.
   b. Deficits which appear late are generally permanent.
6. Cataract formation occurs days to months after head or neck electric injury.
7. Wound care includes the following:
   a. Fasciotomy
      (1) Indications
         (a) Cyanosis and impaired distal capillary refill
         (b) Hard, stony muscle by palpation
         (c) Progressively diminishing or absent pulses by Doppler ultrasound examination
         (d) Compartment pressure by wick catheter > 30 mm Hg
      (2) Technique
         (a) Perform in the operating room.
         (b) Incise the fascia of each involved muscle compartment.
         (c) If distal pulses do not return after compartment release, amputation may be indicated.
   b. Operative debridement
      (1) Delay until resuscitation is complete.
      (2) Debride all necrotic tissue; amputate if necessary.
      (3) Pack the wound open.

        (4) Reexplore the wound 24 to 72 hours later.
           (a) Carry out further debridement if necessary.
           (b) If all necrotic tissue has been removed, close the wound by skin approximation or grafting.
    c. Daily wound inspection with further debridement as necessary

B. Chemical Burns

1. Initial treatment
    a. Remove all involved clothing.
    b. Flush with large amounts of water.
        (1) Do not waste time searching for specific neutralizing agents.
        (2) Chemicals burn continuously until washed off.
    c. Utilize IV fluid resuscitation as with other burns.

2. Agents for which specific therapy is indicated
    a. Hydrofluoric acid
        (1) Prolonged irrigation with benzalkonium chloride
        (2) Topical application of calcium gluconate gel
        (3) Local injection of 10% calcium gluconate into damaged tissue for treatment of severe pain
        (4) Treatment of hypocalcemia as necessary
    b. Phenol
        (1) Initial water lavage
        (2) Lipophilic solvent wash (polyethylene glycol, propylene glycol, or glycerol) to remove residual phenol
    c. White phosphorus
        (1) Irrigate wound with saline.
        (2) Cover with moist gauze dressing to prevent ignition.
        (3) 0.5% to 1% copper sulfate wash followed by copious irrigation will turn retained particles blue-gray.
           (a) Facilitates identification of particles
           (b) Impedes ignition
    d. Tar and bitumen burns
        (1) Hot material cooled with cold water
        (2) Wound care
           (a) Do *not* remove material with a petroleum-based solvent.
           (b) Cover with a petroleum-based ointment and dress daily.

3. Treatment of chemical eye injury
   a. Continuous irrigation with water for at least 30 minutes
   b. Topical antimicrobial agent
   c. Cycloplegic eye drops to decrease synechia formation
   d. Lubricant ointments without eye patches
   e. Daily monitoring of intraocular pressure
   f. Early consultation with an ophthalmologist

SUGGESTED READING

McManus WF, Pruitt BA Jr: *Thermal injuries.* In Mattox KL, Moore EV, Feliciano DV, editors: *Trauma,* Norwalk, Conn, 1988, Appleton & Lange.

Moylan JA: *Burn injury.* In Moylan JA, editor: *Trauma surgery,* ed 2, Philadelphia, 1991, JB Lippincott.

Pruitt BA Jr: The burn patient. I. Initial care. II. Later care and complications of thermal injury, *Curr Prob Surg* 16(4 and 5), 1979.

Pruitt BA Jr, Goodwin CW Jr, Pruitt SK: *Burns: including cold, chemical and electrical injuries.* In Sabiston DC Jr, editor: *Textbook of surgery,* ed 14, Philadelphia, 1991, WB Saunders.

Pruitt BA Jr, Goodwin CW Jr: *Thermal injuries.* In Davis JH, editor: *Clinical surgery,* vol 1 & 2, St. Louis, 1987, Mosby.

Waymack J, Pruitt BA Jr: Burn wound care, *Adv Surg* 23: 261, 1990.

EXTRACORPOREAL *19* MEMBRANE OXYGENATION

James R. Mault

I. INTRODUCTION

ECMO is an extrathoracic CPB technique applied for extended periods in patients with severe but potentially reversible pulmonary and/or cardiac disease. ECMO sustains the patient's oxygenation and hemodynamic requirements while allowing the basic disease to resolve under optimal conditions. It is most commonly applied to neonates with acute respiratory failure but has also been used in children and adults.

II. INDICATIONS AND PATIENT SELECTION

ECMO is indicated for newborns and children with acute respiratory failure that is refractory to conventional management. An objective evaluation of the mortality risk of respiratory failure is the oxygenation index (OI) which is calculated as follows:

$$OI = \left\{ \frac{\text{Mean Airway Pressure} \times \text{Fio}_2}{\text{Pao}_2} \right\} \times 100$$

When treated by conventional management alone, patients with an OI of 25 have a predicted mortality rate of greater than 50%; an OI of 40 defines a mortality rate of 80%. Currently, patients are considered candidates for ECMO after demonstrating three of five OIs greater than 40 on maximal conventional therapy within a 4 hour period. Cerebral and cardiac anomalies must be excluded by cranial ultrasonography and echocardiography prior to consideration for ECMO. Newborns under 34 weeks gestation or less than 2 kg are usually excluded from ECMO. Mechanical ventilation with high Fio_2 for longer than 5 days is a relative contraindication; longer than 10 days is an absolute contraindication to ECMO because of the likelihood of irreversible lung damage. The most common diagnoses of neonates placed on ECMO are as follows:

A. **Meconium Aspiration Syndrome (MAS)**

During delivery, meconium-stained amniotic fluid indicates fetal distress and results from sustained hypoxemia that causes hyperperistalsis and sphincter relaxation. At birth, the neonate may aspirate meconium into the distal airways, causing airway obstruction, inflammation, and chemical pneumonitis. Infants who aspirate meconium may have mild, moderate, or severe respiratory distress at birth. Patients with MAS and severe respiratory distress refractory to conventional therapy are candidates for ECMO.

B. **Persistent Pulmonary Hypertension of the Newborn (PPHN)**

In the newborn lung, severe pulmonary vasoconstriction often occurs in response to factors such as hypoxia, hypercarbia, acidosis, and sepsis. The resultant elevation in pulmonary vascular resistance can cause right-to-left shunting of blood flow away from the lungs and through the ductus arteriosus and foramen ovale. As this negative cycle perpetuates, the neonate becomes severely hypoxemic and acidotic. Standard therapy for PPHN consists of mechanical ventilation, induced respiratory alkalosis, and use of various pharmacologic agents. However, approximately 2% to 5% of neonates fail to respond to this therapy and are considered for ECMO.

C. **Congenital Diaphragmatic Hernia (CDH)**

During the embryonic formation of the diaphragm, a defect may result from incomplete closure of the posterolateral communication between the abdominal and thoracic cavities. With incomplete development of the posterior diaphragm, abdominal contents herniate into the chest cavity and interfere with lung development and prevent inflation after delivery. Severe respiratory distress presents as PPHN and surgical repair is required. Postoperatively, neonates experience a "honeymoon period" of improved pulmonary function, often followed by intractable respiratory failure. ECMO is indicated in patients failing conventional treatment after a honeymoon period. The absence of this honeymoon period is considered evidence of pulmonary hypoplasia and is therefore a contraindication to ECMO.

D. Following Cardiac Surgery

Venoarterial ECMO can also serve as a form of mechanical assist in patients with severe cardiac failure. This may be applied preoperatively and or postoperatively in patients with correctable cardiac anomalies that experience reversible mechanical failure resulting from severe pulmonary hypertension or depressed myocardial function.

III. ECMO PROTOCOL

After obtaining informed consent to administer ECMO support to a patient, the ECMO team is mobilized. This team usually consists of a select group of respiratory therapists, perfusionists, nurses, and physicians who have combined to establish a safe and reliable protocol for initiating, maintaining, and concluding extracorporeal life support.

A. Techniques of Extracorporeal Support

ECMO is performed by draining venous (deoxygenated) blood, pumping it through an artificial lung where carbon dioxide is removed and oxygen is added, and returning the blood to the circulation via an artery (venoarterial ECMO) or a vein (venovenous ECMO). The features of venoarterial and venovenous ECMO are listed in Table 19-1.

  1. The ECMO circuit
     a. The components of a standard ECMO circuit are illustrated in Fig. 19-1.
     b. Deoxygenated blood drains passively into a distensible

TABLE 19–1.

Comparison of Venoarterial and Venovenous ECMO

Parameter	VA ECMO	V V ECMO
Organ support	Gas exchange and cardiac output	Gas exchange only
Pulse contour	Reduced pulsatility	Normal pulsatility
CVP	Unreliable	Reliable
PA pressure	Unreliable	Reliable
Circuit Svo$_2$	Reliable	Unreliable
Circuit recirculation	None	15%-50%
Arterial O$_2$ saturation	≥95%	80%-95%
Ventilator settings	Minimal	Moderate

silicone bladder which operates as the control point of a servo-regulated roller pump that draws blood from the bladder. If the pump flow exceeds the passive venous return, the bladder will collapse and the roller pump will automatically slow down or shut off until it reexpands. Blood is then pumped through a silicone rubber membrane lung which is designed for extended periods of ECMO. After passing through a counter-current heat exchanger, the warmed, oxygenated blood is then returned to the patient via the arterial or venous infusion cannula. A tubing bridge is created between the drainage and perfusion catheters to allow recirculation of the ECMO circuit during priming and weaning. Heparin and fluids are infused into the circuit immediately proximal to the bladder.

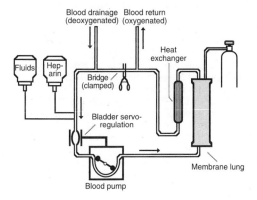

FIG 19-1.
ECMO circuit schematic. Deoxygenated blood drains passively to a sealed bladder. If negative pressure occurs within the bladder, the roller pump is automatically shut off. After passing through the membrane lung, oxygenated blood is circulated through a countercurrent heat exchanger and back to the patient. Heparin and other infusions are delivered into the circuit immediately before the bladder.

2. Cannulation
   a. Venoarterial (VA) ECMO: The functions of both the heart and the lungs are partially or totally replaced. Deoxygenated blood is drained from the RA via a cannula inserted into the right internal jugular or femoral vein while oxygenated blood is pumped through a cannula placed into the right common carotid artery. VA ECMO is the standard configuration for neonatal ECMO.
   b. Venovenous (VV) ECMO: This type provides gas exchange but no cardiac support. Venous drainage and infusion cannulae are placed into the RA or vena cavae via the right internal jugular or femoral veins. Alternatively, a double-lumen catheter may be positioned in the RA through the right internal jugular vein for both drainage and infusion. In either case, blood is drained from and returned to the venous circulation at the same rate. Therefore, ECMO candidates who are hemodynamically unstable and require cardiovascular support should be placed on VA ECMO. In addition, a portion of newly-oxygenated blood is removed by the drainage catheter in VV ECMO, and this recirculation fraction increases with the circuit blood flow.

B. Initiation and Management of ECMO

Cannulation is performed by cut-down and ligation of vessels with strict sterile technique at the ICU bedside, with an operating room team and a complete set of instruments. In the neonate, a 12F or 14F venous cannula and 10F or 12F arterial cannula (for VA ECMO) are inserted into the right internal jugular vein and right common carotid artery, respectively, after receiving a heparin loading dose of 100 U/kg. Since circuit blood flow is limited by the available venous drainage, the venous drainage cannula should be as large as possible.

C. Circuit Management

1. Blood flow: The blood flow setting of the ECMO circuit is determined by the Do_2 requirements of the patient. Typical blood flow rates are 100 to 150 ml/kg/min in neonates and 80 to 120 ml/kg/min in children.
   a. VA ECMO: Blood flow during VA ECMO is usually 80% of the total cardiac output, resulting in a diminished but observable pulse pressure. The exact flow rate is best

managed by continuous, in-line monitoring of the Svo_2. An Svo_2 of 75% or greater indicates adequate Do_2. Inadequate Do_2, indicated by a falling Svo_2, is treated by increasing the circuit blood flow.

b. VV ECMO: Blood is drained and returned to the venous circulation at the same rate and thus has no influence on cardiac output or hemodynamics. As a result of recirculation of oxygenated blood, the circuit flow for total respiratory support with VV ECMO is 20% to 50% higher than VA ECMO for the same patient. In addition, the Svo_2 will be falsely elevated and a less reliable source for assessing the adequacy of Do_2. Continuous pulse oximetry provides better information for monitoring Do_2 during VV ECMO.

2. Oxygenation: Oxygenation is controlled by the Fio_2 of the gas connected to the membrane lung. In both VA ECMO and VV ECMO, a postoxygenator Po_2 of 200 to 300 mm Hg is maintained.

   a. VA ECMO: The systemic Po_2 during VA ECMO results from the combined bypass and nonbypass Do_2. In most conditions (80% bypass and poor native lung function) the patient's ABG will be fully saturated with a Po_2 of 150 to 250 mm Hg.

   b. VV ECMO: Because of the recirculation of VV ECMO, the patient's Sao_2 will have a range of 85% to 95%, with a Po_2 of 60 to 80 mm Hg. Patients undergoing VV ECMO may appear slightly cyanotic, although Do_2 is usually adequate if the cardiac output and Hb are maintained in their normal ranges. If Do_2 is inadequate during maximal settings on VV ECMO, extracorporeal support should be converted to the VA mode.

3. Carbon dioxide removal: Pco_2 is maintained at a value of 35 to 50 mm Hg by adjusting the "sweep" flow of gas. Frequently, however, 5% CO_2 is added to the lung gas flow because of the high efficiency of CO_2 removal by membrane lungs.

4. Anticoagulation: Continuous heparin infusion is required throughout the ECMO course. To monitor heparinization, the ACT is measured hourly. The ACT, which is a measure of whole blood clotting ability, is normally 100 seconds. During ECMO, the heparin infusion is titrated to maintain an ACT of 150 to 200 seconds.

D. Patient Care During ECMO

Upon initiation of ECMO support, there is usually immediate improvement of the patient's condition and several aspects of care are modified.

1. Pulmonary care
   a. During ECMO support, ventilator management should be adjusted to minimal settings to provide lung rest and optimum conditions for pulmonary recovery.
   b. With VA ECMO, ventilator settings should be reduced to an Fio_2 of .21, peak airway pressure of 20 cm H_2O, and a respiratory rate of 5 to 10 breaths/min.
   c. With VV ECMO, the ventilator is usually maintained at moderate settings with an Fio_2 of 40%, peak airway pressure of 30 cm H_2O, and a respiratory rate of 10 to 20 breaths/min. A PEEP of at least 8 cm H_2O should be maintained to prevent profound atelectasis. When based on compliance measurements, higher levels of PEEP have also resulted in earlier recovery of pulmonary function.
   d. Aggressive pulmonary toilet should be performed several times per day and a chest film should be ordered daily.
2. Medications and fluids
   a. An accurate record of fluid balance and daily weights is essential.
   b. Blood is transfused to maintain a hematocrit between 40% and 45%.
   c. Platelets are routinely administered at the initiation of ECMO and daily thereafter to maintain a count greater than 150,000/mm^3.
   d. Prophylactic antibiotics are usually given daily while on bypass.
   e. Full nutrition should be administered throughout the duration of ECMO support.
   f. Patients requiring ECMO are usually hypervolemic upon initiation of support. In these cases, pharmacologic diuresis is instituted to remove excess fluid and return patients to their dry weights. If diuretics are insufficient, a small, hollow-fiber hemofilter may be placed into the ECMO circuit to supplement urine output and provide hemoconcentration.
   g. Minimal pharmacologic sedation should be applied during ECMO. Seizure activity must be treated promptly.

3. Laboratory studies
   a. Prior to initiation of ECMO, baseline determinations of CBC, electrolytes, liver function tests, and coagulation parameters must be obtained.
   b. During ECMO, the CBC, electrolytes, and coagulation parameters are measured every 8 hours.
   c. ABG is obtained every 8 to 12 hours, and continuous pulse oximeter monitoring is used. Head ultrasound is performed daily on neonates to rule out intracranial hemorrhage.

E. **Weaning and Decannulation from ECMO**
   ECMO support is usually maintained for 4 to 5 days. Indications of lung recovery include an increasing Svo_2 and systemic Po_2, or decreasing Pco_2 while ECMO flow and ventilator settings are constant. Other signs of improvement are noted by increased pulmonary compliance and a normalizing CXR. Cardiac recovery is noted by increased pulse pressure, cardiac output, and Svo_2, in addition to improved contractility as monitored by serial echocardiography.
   1. Weaning from VA ECMO
      a. When significant improvement is documented in native lung or cardiac function, VA ECMO blood flow is gradually reduced over a period of hours. When the native lung and heart can provide adequate Do_2 and gas exchange at 20% of the baseline VA ECMO flow, a brief trial off bypass (cannulae clamped, bridge open) is attempted on moderate ventilator settings.
      b. If this is successful, VA ECMO is started again and the patient is prepared for the sterile decannulation procedure. Anticoagulation of the circuit should be maintained until decannulation is initiated.
   2. Weaning from VV ECMO
      a. A trial wean from VV ECMO consists of decreasing and capping the gas flow to the membrane lung while continuing extracorporeal flow.
      b. If the native lungs provide adequate gas exchange, ECMO can be discontinued and the cannulae removed. Anticoagulation of the circuit should be maintained until decannulation is initiated.

F. **Emergencies During ECMO**
   Infrequently, an emergency situation such as circuit disruption or air embolism may occur and require immediate exclusion

from the ECMO circuit. If this situation develops, the following steps must be followed sequentially:

1. Clamp the venous drainage line.
2. Open the tubing bridge.
3. Clamp the infusion line.
4. Increase patient ventilator settings to full support.
5. Disconnect the gas line to the membrane lung.
6. Repair or replace the source of emergency.
7. Evaluate the need for starting ECMO again.

G. Complications

1. Mechanical complications occur in approximately one-tenth of ECMO applications. These range from frequent minor events, such as cracks in connectors and kinking of tubing, to rare major problems, such as oxygenator failure and raceway rupture. While the direct effects of these technical problems on ECMO survival has been about 3%, physiologic instability may be significant until the source has been corrected.

2. Medical complications include the following:

   a. Bleeding is the most common complication during ECMO. Intracranial hemorrhage is the most significant bleeding complication and occurs in 10% to 15% of ECMO cases. Other locations of bleeding include the GI tract and the vascular access sites. Bleeding complications are best managed by titrating heparin to a lower ACT target of 150 seconds and aggressively maintaining a platelet count greater than 150,000/mm^3. ECMO is usually discontinued in response to confirmed intracranial hemorrhage or uncontrollable bleeding.

   b. Neurologic: During cannulation for VA ECMO, the right common carotid artery is ligated, with only rare attempts to repair it after ECMO. As a result of collateral blood flow to the brain, acute neurologic sequelae directly related to this ligation are rare, although seizures have been reported at 5% of patients while on ECMO.

   c. Other complications encountered during ECMO include hemolysis, hyperbilirubinemia, renal insufficiency, cardiac arrhythmias, pulmonary hypertension, and sepsis.

IV. OUTCOME

As part of its charter, the Extracorporeal Life Support Organization (ELSO) maintains an international registry of all patients treated with ECMO. As of April 1994, the registry for neonatal ECMO has recorded 8913 cases performed at 78 medical centers. The overall hospital survival of this population was 7213 neonates (81%). By diagnosis, babies suffering MAS or PPHN had survival rates of 93% and 83%, respectively, while the survival rate of patients with CDH or postcardiac surgery averaged 60%. Several reports of long-term follow-up including prospective, randomized trials using neurodevelopmental testing describe approximately 75% of ECMO survivors as normal children.

V. FUTURE DIRECTIONS

The near future of ECMO consists of several technical innovations as well as new patient applications. Extracorporeal circuits with special, nonthrombogenic surfaces have demonstrated early clinical success and will ultimately allow ECMO to be performed with little or no systemic anticoagulation. Automation and miniaturization of various pumps and in-line blood gas analyzers are also in various stages of clinical development and will lead to compact, bedside ECMO conducted with increased safety and reduced cost. Widening patient applications include pediatric as well as adult ECMO for severe, acute respiratory failure secondary to viral pneumonia, pulmonary contusion, or bridge to transplantation have shown promise in early clinical results.

SUGGESTED READING

Anderson HL, et al: Multicenter comparison of conventional venoarterial access versus venovenous double-lumen catheter access in newborn infants undergoing extracorporeal membrane oxygenation, *J Pediatr Surg* 28:530, 1993.

Bartlett RH: Extracorporeal life support for cardiopulmonary failure, *Curr Prob Surg* 27:623, 1990.

Schumacher RE, et al: Extracorporeal membrane oxygenation in term newborns: a prospective cost-benefit analysis, *ASAIO J* 39:873, 1993.

Wildin SR, Landry SH, Zwischenberger JB: Prospective controlled study of developmental outcome in survivors of extracorporeal membrane oxygenation, *Pediatrics* 93:404, 1994.

PART FOUR

SELECTED PROBLEMS IN PATIENT MANAGEMENT

INFECTION AND SEPSIS   *20*

Mark W. Sebastian

I. **FEVER AND DISORDERS OF TEMPERATURE HOMEOSTASIS**
A. **Normal Temperature Homeostasis**
   1. Normal range for core temperature
      a. 36.7° C to 37.6° C
      b. Superimposed normal diurnal variation, usually peaking in the evening
   2. Normal homeostatic mechanisms
      a. Thermal control originates from the preoptic nucleus of the anterior hypothalamus, which directs the autonomic nervous system to regulate cutaneous vasomotor tone, perspiration, cutaneous muscular tone, and endocrinologic effectors of metabolic activity.
      b. Nonshivering thermogenesis, the exaggerated metabolic activity of brown fat (significant in neonates only), and skeletal muscle (adults and neonates) can increase heat production 40% to 100%.
   3. Measurement
      a. Accurate measurement of core temperature in the SICU is via a thermal sensor-equipped PA catheter, although this is rarely an indication for PA catheter insertion.
      b. Esophageal probes are suited only for unconscious patients.
      c. Rectal temperature is the best noninvasive method.
      d. Oral measurement is suitable for patients able to maintain an oral seal.
      e. Use automated devices for tympanic membrane (external canal) monitoring.
B. **Fever**
   1. Pathophysiology: In response to noxious stimuli (such as endotoxin, complement activation, immune complexes,

tissue injury), activated macrophages or lymphocytes release cytokines (primarily IL-1, IL-2, IL-6, TNF, and interferons), which ultimately raise the hypothalamic thermal set point.

2. Treatment of fever: Fever should be treated to reduce the discomfort of associated myalgias or to ameliorate increased metabolic activity that stresses a compromised cardiovascular system.

   a. Drugs affecting prostaglandin synthesis (acetaminophen, NSAID) should be used.

   b. Topical cooling does not reduce fever and actually increases metabolic demand unless the hypothalamic driven effectors of temperature regulation are blocked; this can be accomplished in extreme instances by sedation and pharmacologic paralysis.

   c. Specific treatment should be directed to the underlying infection or damaged tissue.

3. Complications of fever: Major complications related to fever are the result of the causative agent or illness, not the elevated temperature.

   a. Febrile seizures rarely occur after the age of 6 years and are usually benign.

   b. Patients with marginal cardiovascular reserve can suffer serious consequences (stroke, MI, dysrhythmia, CHF) if unable to meet the increased Vo_2 (7% increase in Vo_2 for each 1° C fever) or decreased SVR of pyrexia; aggressive treatment is indicated in these instances.

C. **Hyperthermia**

   1. Examples include malignant hyperthermia, thyroid storm, dehydration, heat stroke, and hypothalamic injury (trauma, tumor, infarction).

   2. Hyperthermia cannot be distinguished from fever based on the magnitude of pyrexia; certain clinical situations produce a readily apparent diagnosis, but endocrinologic and hypothalamic disorders require extensive testing.

   3. Treatment includes the following:

      a. Therapy is directed to the underlying disorder.

      b. Offending drugs are withdrawn.

      c. Hydration is maintained.

      d. Specific pharmacotherapy (dantrolene, propylthiouracil) is employed when indicated.

e. Topical cooling should be used for temperatures >40° C.

D. Hypothermia

1. The most common causes of hypothermia (core body temperature <35° C) in the SICU are prolonged abdominal surgery, cooling during CPB, sepsis, and environmental exposure following burns or trauma.

2. Metabolic causes include hypoglycemia, hypopituitarism, hypothyroidism, and hypothalamic dysfunction.

3. The most important problems stem from dysfunction of excitable tissues.
   a. Ventricular fibrillation, which occurs at 30° C to 32° C, is the most common cause of death.
   b. Depressed mentation progresses to a flat EEG around 20° C.
   c. Coagulation factors work poorly at less than 35° C, substantially complicating trauma resuscitation and recovery from CPB.
   d. A leftward shift in the O_2 dissociation curve prevents adequate unloading of O_2 to the tissues.

4. Passive rewarming is used if temperature > 30° C and the patient's homeostatic regulatory mechanisms (shivering) are intact.
   a. Monitor ECG and core temperature.
   b. Administer 100% O_2.
   c. Warm the room.
   d. Utilize heat lamps or body warmers.
   e. Warm all IV fluids and inspired gases to 39° C.

5. Active rewarming is used for temperatures < 30° C or when normal regulatory mechanisms are impaired.
   a. Continue passive rewarming.
   b. Consider gastric, colonic, or peritoneal lavage with 39° C lactated Ringer's solution.
   c. Consider warming via CPB or hemodialysis.

II. SURGICAL INFECTIONS

A. Signs and Symptoms

1. Signs and symptoms include fever, leukocytosis, and local signs of infection, such as inflammation, wound drainage, or foul sputum.

2. The classic signs of infection are usually (but not always) present, especially in immunocompromised patients.

    a. Tachycardia
    b. Tachypnea
    c. Hypoxemia
    d. Ileus
    e. Hyperglycemia (insulin resistance)
    f. Altered mental status
    g. Hypotension
    h. Hypovolemia
    i. DIC
    j. Hypothermia

3. Risk factors which increase the likelihood and severity of infections include advanced age, diabetes, malnutrition, immunocompromise (steroids, burns, AIDS), and multiple organ dysfunction syndrome.

B. Systemic Manifestations

1. Bacteremia: The presence of viable bacteria in the blood
2. Sepsis: Infection plus signs of systemic response; tachypnea, tachycardia, hyperthermia, or hypothermia
3. Sepsis syndrome: Sepsis plus evidence of altered organ perfusion
   a. $Pao_2/Fio_2 < 280$ mm Hg
   b. Elevated lactate
   c. Oliguria
   d. Altered mental status
4. Septic shock: Clinical diagnosis of the sepsis syndrome plus hypotension refractory to fluid administration or pharmacologic intervention
5. Systemic inflammatory response syndrome (SIRS): Systemic response characterized by uncontrolled inflammatory response due to multiple mediators, leading to endothelial cell damage with organ damage or death
6. Multiple organ dysfunction syndrome: The presence of altered organ function in an acutely ill patient such that homeostasis cannot be maintained without intervention
7. Risk factors for SIRS
   a. Use of indwelling catheters
   b. Implantation of prosthetic devices
   c. Immunodeficient patients (HIV, transplant, compromised nutrition, cancer, elderly)
   d. Immunosuppressive drug administration: Corticosteroids, chemotherapy
   e. Broad-spectrum antibiotic use

      f. Long-term antibiotic use

      g. Other risk factors: Multiple trauma, burns, pancreatitis, hemodynamic instability, complex elective operations, major postoperative complications, and overwhelming infections, especially intraabdominal.

      h. Most commonly associated with gram-negative sepsis

         (1) Endotoxin: Lipopolysaccharide moiety of bacterial wall; active component is termed lipid A

         (2) Antibody against lipid A effective in treatment of gram-negative septicemia and sepsis syndrome

C. Mediators in Sepsis

  1. TNF-α

      a. TNF-α is produced by macrophages and endothelial cells.

      b. TNF-α is seen early in systemic inflammatory response syndrome.

      c. TNF-α levels are elevated in a variety of septic states.

      d. Endotoxin and enterotoxin induce macrophage release of TNF-α.

      e. Injection of a lethal dose of endotoxin causes a rise in TNF-α levels.

      f. Injection of TNF-α causes similar signs and symptoms to septic shock (neutropenia, hypotension, vascular permeability).

      g. Administration of antibody to TNF-α abrogates lethal effects of a subsequent endotoxin challenge in animal models.

      h. TNF-α acts as paracrine (local) rather than endocrine (systemic) type mediator.

      i. TNF-α acts to decrease levels of thrombomodulin; a promoter of anticoagulation when bound to thrombin.

  2. IL-1

  3. IL-4

  4. IL-6

  5. IL-8

  6. Arachidonic acid breakdown products: Leukotrienes, prostaglandins, thromboxane-A_2, prostacyclin

III. EVALUATION AND MANAGEMENT OF FEVER

A. Evaluation of Fever

  1. Within 48 hours after surgery or trauma, the most common causes of fever are atelectasis, clostridial or streptococcal wound infections, infections related to anastomotic leak,

and generalized immune activation following major trauma.

a. Fever in the first 48 hours postoperatively is usually caused by atelectasis; measures to prevent this include providing adequate analgesia, encouraging deep breathing, incentive spirometry, and early ambulation.

b. Early cellulitis is due to either streptococcal or clostridial infection; the wound should be examined to exclude this cause of early fever.

c. An anastomotic leak or perforation may cause fever in the early postoperative period; usually these patients are hypovolemic and may appear systematically ill.

d. The presence of a preoperative infection may be the cause of early postoperative fever.

2. Beyond 48 hours, more extensive evaluation is required.

a. Wounds should be examined, including all sites of transcutaneous catheters.

b. A thorough HEENT examination for signs of otitis, sinusitis, or meningitis is especially important in patients with an intubated nasopharynx or oropharynx.

c. Thoracic examination should detect areas of pulmonary consolidation, effusions, or bronchospasm.

d. Abdominal examination is used to evaluate cholecystitis, pancreatitis, intraabdominal abscess, or intestinal obstruction.

e. Prostatitis and perirectal abscess is evaluated by rectal examination.

f. Look for signs of thrombophlebitis.

g. Laboratory studies include CBC with differential, urinalysis, and two sets of blood cultures drawn during the febrile episode from separate sites.

h. CXR should be obtained.

i. More extensive testing (e.g., abdominal CT scan, ventilation-perfusion scan, lumbar puncture, sinus films, echocardiogram) are performed as indicated.

B. **Management of the Febrile Patient**

1. In the hemodynamically stable patient:

a. Diagnostic evaluation prior to initiating therapy

(1) History and physical examination

(2) Laboratory and radiographic studies

(3) Blood cultures, Gram's stain, and appropriate fluid cultures prior to beginning antibiotics

    b. Identified infectious source
       (1) Initiate treatment appropriate for diagnosis.
       (2) The clinical response is the standard by which therapy is assessed.
       (3) Antibiotics are altered as culture and sensitivity results become available.
    c. Unidentified infectious source
       (1) Empiric therapy is based on the most likely diagnosis.
       (2) Alternatively, therapy may be withheld pending culture results or repeat examination.
2. In the hemodynamically unstable patient:
    a. Patients with surgical infections may present in septic shock.
       (1) Sepsis is usually presents in adults as fever, tachycardia, tachypnea, and at least one manifestation of organ dysfunction.
       (2) A patient with multiple risk factors for infection is more likely to present with respiratory or cardiovascular instability.
    b. Resuscitation is the first line of therapy of the patient in shock.
       (1) Intubation may be required in patients with respiratory insufficiency.
       (2) Hypotension should be treated with volume resuscitation and cardiovascular agents as appropriate.
       (3) A PA catheter may be helpful in guiding resuscitation.
       (4) Do_2 and consumption relationships should be assessed to ensure optimal physiology exists.
    c. After resuscitation and stabilization, begin a diagnostic evaluation for infection.
    d. When the source of infection is known, a specific treatment based on the most likely pathogens can begin; however, the source of infection is often not obvious and empiric therapy should be instituted in the unstable patient.
    e. Broad-spectrum antibiotics should be started when all cultures have been obtained.
       (1) Ampicillin, gentamicin, and metronidazole are often started as empiric therapy.

    (2) The empiric use of aminoglycosides in the patient at risk for renal failure as a result of sepsis syndrome is cautioned; alternatively, gram-negative coverage can be effectively instituted with aztreonam.

    (3) Third-generation cephalosporins and imipenem may be used as broad-spectrum therapy, especially if renal insufficiency is present.

    (4) Fungal sepsis must be considered in patients who manifest septic physiology while on antibiotics.

  f. Specific surgical therapy is instituted as indicated; it is rarely necessary to perform an exploratory laparotomy in a patient without a specific diagnosis.

IV. SPECIFIC PATHOGENS
A. Bacterial Pathogens
  1. Gram-positive cocci

    a. *Staphylococcus aureus* is often a cause of wound- and catheter-related infections. Treat preferentially with nafcillin or oxacillin.

    b. Methicillin-resistant *S. aureus* (MRSA) has same virulence as *S. aureus* but requires treatment with vancomycin.

    c. *S. epidermidis* is often associated with infections of prosthetic materials; since the organism is part of normal skin flora it may appear as a contaminant in blood cultures. Treat with vancomycin.

    d. Streptococci are often a cause of cellulitis and endocarditis; Group A are causative in scarlet fever, erysipelas, and rheumatic fever. Treat with penicillin G.

    e. Enterococci are often associated with infections involving IV devices and biliary sepsis. Treat with ampicillin and gentamicin.

  2. Gram-positive rods

    a. *Clostridium* organisms

      (1) *Clostridium tetani* and *C. perfringens* are anaerobic bacteria which cause tetanus and gas gangrene, respectively. Treatment requires debridement and high-dose penicillin G.

      (2) *C. difficile* is the major cause of pseudomembranous colitis and is treated with vancomycin (oral) or metronidazole (oral or IV).

b. *Corynebacterium diphtheriae* is the causative organism in diphtheria. Prevention is by immunization with diphtheria toxoid which is usually given with tetanus toxoid. Treat with diphtheria antitoxin and penicillin G.

3. Gram-negative cocci
   a. *Neisseria gonorrhoeae* causes gonorrhea. Treat with penicillin.
   b. *N. meningitidis* causes meningitis and septic shock. Treat with penicillin.

4. Gram-negative rods
   a. *Bacteroides* organisms are anaerobic bacteria of the GI tract, often involved in intraabdominal abscesses; *B. fragilis* is the most eminent. Treat with metronidazole or clindamycin.
   b. The *Enterobacteriaceae* family includes *Escherichia coli* and *Klebsiella, Enterobacter, Serratia,* and *Proteus* organisms; they are involved in biliary, urinary, and GI-related infections. Treat with aminoglycosides; alternatively, a second- or third-generation cephalosporin may be used.
   c. *Haemophilus influenzae* may cause meningitis, epiglottitis, or pneumonia. Treatment is with aztreonam, imipenem, β-lactam agents combined with a β-lactamase inhibitor, or third-generation cephalosporin (ampicillin-resistant strains now common).
   d. *Pseudomonas aeruginosa* is common in nosocomial infections; wound infections typically have greenish exudate with fruity odor. Treat with two synergistic drugs to avoid resistance (usually mezlocillin, aztreonam, or ceftazidime combined with an aminoglycoside).

B. Fungal Pathogens
1. Candidal infections are the most common.
   a. Predisposing factors
      (1) Immunosuppression, including patients on steroids or those with T-cell dysfunction
      (2) Long-term illness
      (3) Long-term antibiotic use, especially broad-spectrum antibiotics
   b. *Candida* endophthalmitis: Indication for systemic therapy
   c. *Candida* organisms: Isolated from more than three separate sites with negative blood cultures; usually

necessitate empiric amphotericin B therapy for presumed disseminated candidiasis

d. Symptomatic urinary tract infection with candidal cultures: Treatment may consist of amphotericin bladder irrigation or oral fluconazole for more severe infections

e. Oral or esophageal candidiasis
   (1) Prophylaxis against oral candidiasis is best accomplished with oral nystatin.
   (2) Candidiasis may be treated with either oral nystatin or fluconazole.

2. Other fungal pathogens include *Cryptococcus histoplasma, Mucor* organisms, and *Aspergillus* organisms.

3. The decision to treat a presumed fungal infection is based upon the clinical setting in conjunction with culture results.
   a. When a positive blood culture is drawn through an indwelling catheter, the catheter should be changed and catheter tip sent for culture.
   b. Persistent positive blood cultures after catheters have been changed or removed usually necessitates parenteral amphotericin B or fluconazole.

C.   Viral Pathogens

1. Hepatitis B
   a. Hepatitis B is transmitted by blood, blood products, or sexual contact and can result in chronic active hepatitis and cirrhosis.
   b. Needle sticks from carriers can be treated by hepatitis B immune globulin and vaccination.
   c. Prevention is best managed by immunization with hepatitis vaccine.

2. HIV
   a. Needle sticks from seropositive patients carry 1 in 250 to 1 in 300 risk of infection.
   b. Exposure to blood of seropositive patients should be managed by serotesting the exposed health care worker and repeated testing 6 weeks, 3 months, 6 months, and 12 months after exposure.
   c. Protocols exist for use of AZT in exposed health care workers (AZT 250 mg PO q4h × 6 to 7 weeks).

3. Herpes viruses
   a. CMV infection is usually seen in immunocompromised

patients, especially in bone marrow and organ transplant patients.

   b. Attempts to limit transmission have included organ depletion of leukocytes which harbor the virus and screening donors for CMV serologic markers.

   c. Diagnosis is by viral titer, inclusion bodies seen on biopsy, viral culture, or polymerase chain reaction.

   d. Severe infections are treated with ganciclovir.

   e. HSV causes oral and genital skin eruptions, pneumonitis, and encephalitis. Treat with acyclovir.

   f. VZV is the causative agent in both chickenpox (primary) and zoster (reactivation). Treat with acyclovir.

V.   PREVENTION OF SURGICAL WOUND INFECTIONS

A.   Bacterial Contamination

1. The presence of infection prior to surgery increases the risk of wound infection; elective surgery should be postponed until the infection has been treated.

2. Antiseptic showers prior to surgery decrease wound infection rate; skin is prepared with chlorhexidine or povidone-iodine.

3. Prophylactic antibiotics are chosen according to the pathogen likely to be present in the operative field.

4. Wound infection rates are the following:

   a. Clean case—no gross contamination (hernia, thyroidectomy); wound infection rate < 1%

   b. Clean-contaminated case—minor contamination (biliary surgery); wound infection rate 2% to 5%

   c. Contaminated case—major contamination (gross spillage from unprepared bowel); wound infection rate 5% to 30%

   d. Dirty case—contamination from infected source (drainage of appendiceal abscess); wound infection rate > 30%

B.   Patient Risk Factors

1. Hyperglycemia interferes with WBC function.

2. Steroids are immunosuppressive; their use is associated with increased wound infection rates and poor healing.

3. Advanced age is associated with poor wound healing.

4. Malnutrition is associated with poor wound healing.

5. Renal failure is associated with poor wound healing.
6. Obese patients have higher wound infection rates, which may be related to poorly vascularized fat.
7. Radiation and chemotherapy interfere with normal wound healing processes.
8. Neutropenia results in increased risk of wound infection.

VI. TREATMENT OF INFECTION AND SEPSIS IN THE ICU

A. Respiratory Tract (See Chapter 7.)

1. Respiratory infections are common in postoperative patients; prolonged intubation and underlying lung disease are associated with an increased risk of pneumonia.
2. Sputum production, pleuritic chest pain, and auscultatory findings of consolidation are usually present.
3. Gram's stain of sputum reveals leukocytes; the predominant organism identified is used to guide antibiotic therapy.
4. CXR may reveal a pulmonary infiltrate.
5. Treatment involves aggressive pulmonary toilet and appropriate antibiotics; the choice of antibiotics is guided by the clinical situation and the Gram's stain results.

B. Urinary Tract

1. Urinary tract infections may occur any time during hospitalization; urinary retention and instrumentation predispose to urinary infections.
2. Dysuria, frequency, hesitancy, and inability to void are frequent symptoms of cystitis; flank pain, fever, and ileus may be due to pyelonephritis.
3. Urinalysis and urine culture should be performed.
   a. The presence of pyuria, leukocyte esterase, nitrite, and bacteriuria should be noted.
   b. A positive culture is reported as >100,000 colonies/ml of urine of a specific organism.
4. Treatment includes adequate urinary drainage and appropriate antibiotics; usual organisms are gram-negative rods (*E. coli* and *Klebsiella, Proteus,* and *Pseudomonas* organisms).

C. Wound Infections

1. Wound infections are usually evident by physical examination—erythema, drainage, and the presence of crepitus.

2. Cellulitis is manifested by a tender, warm, erythematous wound without drainage or fluctuance; treat with antibiotics typically active against gram-positive and gram-negative organisms.
3. Wound infections associated with drainage or fluctuance should be opened; drainage and dressing changes are usually all the treatment that is needed, and antibiotics are used only if there is a component of cellulitis or systemic evidence of infection.
4. Infection over vascular grafts require expert care; graft removal may be required and the operating surgeon should be notified immediately.

D. Line Sepsis
1. Indwelling IV catheters should be changed every 3 to 4 days to avoid line sepsis.
2. Fever workups should first include routine examinations and tests.
3. If no other source can be found, the catheter should be checked for infection by drawing a blood culture through it.
4. A peripheral blood culture is obtained at the same time as the central catheter is cultured; if both are positive, the catheter is left in place and antibiotics are given.
5. If only the central culture is positive, the catheter is removed.

E. Peritonitis
1. Anastomotic failure after intestinal resection
   a. Patients usually have the picture of an ileus, hypovolemia, and free air.
   b. Free air can normally be seen in patients after abdominal exploration for up to a week postoperatively.
   c. A fistula may become evident by enteric contents draining from the wound; small bowel fistulas may resolve without operation.
   d. Intraabdominal abscesses usually present with localized tenderness and spiking fevers.
   e. A CT scan is the study of choice to evaluate the possibility of an abscess, which may be drained either percutaneously using CT guidance or operatively.
   f. Broad-spectrum antibiotics are indicated.
2. A bile leak after biliary surgery will also present as

peritonitis and is usually associated with nausea and vomiting; ultrasound may reveal a fluid collection.

3. A postoperative patient can develop an abdominal process not directly related to the procedure.
   a. Perforated ulcer
   b. Acalculous cholecystitis
   c. Pancreatitis
   d. Appendicitis
   e. Intestinal ischemia

F.   Meningitis

1. Meningitis should be excluded as a cause of postoperative fever.
2. Meningeal signs are usually evident on physical examination.
3. A lumbar puncture is performed when meningitis is suspected.

G.   Endocarditis

1. Endocarditis may be a cause of persistent fever.
2. Endocarditis most often occurs in patients with a history of valvular disease.
3. Echocardiography should be performed to search for vegetations.
4. Antibiotic prophylaxis should be given to all patients at risk (e.g., valvular heart disease, prosthetic valves) who are undergoing instrumentation of the oral, respiratory, GI, and urinary tracts.

H.   Sinusitis

1. Sinusitis is commonly seen in patients with prolonged nasal intubations (ET or NG tubes).
2. Diagnosis is made by sinus films.
3. Treatment is with drainage, antibiotics, and nasal vasoconstrictors.

I.   Soft Tissue Infections

1. Infection associated with soft tissue inflammation usually requires surgical intervention.
2. The patient often presents with fever, leukocytosis, and a specific area of inflammation; the site should be examined for inflammatory reaction, fluctuance, crepitus, and tissue necrosis.
   a. The presence of erythema without fluctuance or drainage with no devitalized tissue is most likely cellulitis.

    b. An area of erythema occurring over a vein associated with a palpable cord may be suppurative thrombophlebitis.

    c. Linear red streaks proximal to an inflammatory reaction of a distal limb represent lymphangitic spread.

3. Treatment includes warm soaks, elevation, and antibiotics; usual antibiotics are either penicillin G or penicillinase-resistant penicillin (nafcillin, methicillin, dicloxacillin).

4. Failure to improve rapidly should lead one to suspect a resistant organism or abscess.

5. Deep inflammation is characterized by the presence of local inflammation associated with fluctuance, drainage, or sinus tracts.

    a. Needle aspiration with a large-bore needle and a small syringe may be helpful to determine if an undrained collection is present.

    b. If there is no collection, an abscess may not have formed yet, or an unconsidered diagnosis may exist.

    c. If a collection is present, surgical drainage is required, since an abscess is resistant to the action of antibiotics.

6. The presence of devascularized skin, deep necrosis, and crepitus indicates the possibility of a more serious soft tissue infection.

    a. A history of crush injury with devitalized tissue, foreign body, systemic signs of toxemia, muscle necrosis, and gram-positive rods are signs of clostridial myositis (gas gangrene).

    b. Extensive debridement is necessary and often requires limb amputation.

    c. Aggressive circulatory support is needed to maintain tissue perfusion.

    d. Penicillin G 20 to 24 million U/day IV is given.

    e. Hyperbaric O_2 may be helpful; however, treatment by debridement has priority over transfer to hyperbaric O_2 chamber.

7. The presence of a rapidly spreading infection, mixed organisms on Gram's stain, necrotic fascia, and thrombosis and obliteration of subcutaneous vessels are signs of necrotizing fasciitis; gram-negative synergistic necrotizing cellulitis is part of a spectrum of necrotizing infections which may present as a necrotizing infection of the abdominal wall.

a. Extensive debridement of necrotic fascia is necessary, but limbs can usually be salvaged.

b. High-dose, broad-spectrum antibiotics are given.

c. Circulatory support is necessary to maintain perfusion.

VII.   INFECTION IN THE IMMUNOCOMPROMISED HOST

A.   The Immunocompromised Host

1. The immunocompromised host is any patient with impaired host defenses who is at increased risk of developing infection; such infections are likely to be of greater severity than in the normal host.

2. The increasing prevalence of immunocompromised patients is due to the following:

   a. Advances in cancer chemotherapy

   b. Organ transplantation

   c. Immunosuppressive therapy of nonmalignant disease

   d. Increasing prevalence of AIDS

3. In the immunocompromised host, infection is the most common immediate cause of death.

4. Infection is likely to be due to opportunistic pathogens; since the host's ability to mount an inflammatory response is impaired, signs of serious systemic infection may be nonspecific or absent.

B.   Defects in the Immune Response

1. Granulocytopenia

   a. Absolute granulocyte count $< 500/\mu L$ or defect in phagocytosis; incidence or severity of infection related to absolute granulocyte count and rapidity of onset of granulocytopenia

   b. Etiology includes the following:

      (1) Leukemia, lymphoma, collagen-vascular disease

      (2) Cytotoxic chemotherapy or radiation therapy for malignant disease

      (3) Immunosuppressive therapy for autoimmune disease and posttransplantation (corticosteroids, azathioprine)

   c. Common pathogens include the following:

      (1) Gram-positive: *S. aureus, S. epidermidis*

      (2) Gram-negative: *E. coli, K. pneumoniae, P. aeruginosa*

  (3) Fungal: *C. albicans, Aspergillus* and *Mucor* organisms
  (4) Viral: Herpes viruses, especially CMV
2. Cellular immune dysfunction
  a. Etiology
    (1) Lymphoma
    (2) AIDS
    (3) Autoimmune disease
    (4) Organ transplant recipients (corticosteroids, immunosuppressive therapy)
  b. Common pathogens
    (1) Bacterial: *Listeria monocytogenes, Salmonella* organisms, *Nocardia asteroides, Legionella* organisms, mycobacteria
    (2) Fungal: *Cryptococcus neoformans, Candida* organisms, *Histoplasma capsulatum, Coccidioides immitis*
    (3) Viral: VZV, CMV, HSV
    (4) Parasitic: *P. carinii, Toxoplasma gondii, Giardia lamblia, E. histolytica, Cryptosporidium enteritis, Strongyloides stercoralis*
3. Humoral immune dysfunction
  a. Etiology
    (1) Multiple myeloma, chronic lymphocytic leukemia, sickle cell disease
    (2) Chemotherapy
  b. Common pathogens
    (1) *Streptococcus pneumoniae*
    (2) *H. influenzae*
C. **Evaluation of the Immunocompromised Patient**
  1. Evaluation of potential infection in the immunocompromised host is similar to evaluation in the normal patient, with some exceptions.
    a. The subtle and atypical nature of symptoms and signs demands a high index of clinical suspicion, willingness to intervene early and persistence in search for potential causative organisms by rigorous and repeated septic workups.
    b. Minimal symptoms demand complete evaluation.
  2. Nonspecific signs (clinical deterioration leukocytosis, leukopenia, hypothermia, hypotension, glucose intolerance, low-grade pyrexia) may require full septic workup.

3. Identification of infectious agent must be prompt and precise.

4. Consider early use of invasive diagnostic procedures (transbronchial or open-lung biopsy).

D.   Therapy

1. Required information for therapeutic intervention

   a. Presence of immunologic deficiencies in the compromised host

   b. Infections the patient is susceptible to on basis of impaired host defenses

2. General principles

   a. Drainage or debridement of localized collections of infected material

   b. Specific antibiotics

   c. Reconstruction of deficient antimicrobial defenses (FFP for complement deficiencies, immune serum globulin for IgG deficiency, reduction or cessation of immunosuppressive therapy, colony-stimulating factor, WBC transfusion)

3. Empiric antibiotic therapy

   a. Broad-spectrum regimen against potential major gram-positive and gram-negative pathogens

   b. Use of synergistic antibiotic combinations rather than single-agent or nonsynergistic combinations reduces morbidity and mortality (e.g., vancomycin + ticarcillin + amikacin, ceftazidime + amikacin)

   c. Amphotericin B for a febrile, neutropenic patient who is unresponsive to antibacterial treatment

4. Prevention of infection

   a. Avoid damage to physical barriers (repeated venipuncture, indwelling venous or urinary catheters, prolonged intubation).

   b. Bolster host defenses (immune serum globulin, hyperimmune varicella-zoster immune globulin, vaccination against *Pneumococcus, Haemophilus,* and *Meningococcus* organisms)

   c. Maintain optimal nutritional status.

   d. Avoid acquisition of new potential pathogens (sterility, isolation).

   e. Use prophylaxis for specific infections with high incidence in certain populations (trimethoprim-sulfamethoxazole and aerosolized pentamidine for protection against *Pneumocystis carinii* pneumonia in patients with AIDS)

VIII. ANTIBIOTICS
A. Principles of Antimicrobial Therapy
1. Mechanisms of action
   a. Bacteriostatic: Prevention of growth and multiplication of bacteria (bacteria not killed); infection cleared by host defenses
   b. Bactericidal: Bacterial killing; mandatory in immuno-compromised host
2. Use of multiple antibiotics
   a. Possible or proven multiple organisms (e.g., gram-negative septicemia)
   b. Prevention of emergence of resistant strains (e.g., *Pseudomonas* organisms, mycobacteria)
3. Antimicrobial synergy
   a. Potentiation at a biochemical level
   b. Assistance to cellular penetration (e.g., action of penicillin at cell wall level interferes with the ability of *S. faecalis* to resist penetration by aminoglycosides)
   c. Protection (e.g., clavulanic acid—broad-spectrum enzyme inhibitor—protects amoxicillin against degradation by β-lactamase)
4. Antibiotic incompatibilities: Interference with action of β-lactam antibiotics on cell wall synthesis by bacteriostatic agents (tetracyclines)
5. Monitoring of serum levels
   a. Guide to drug dosage (ensure therapeutic levels, minimize complications)
   b. Mandatory if renal function impaired
   c. Most accurate dosing regimen provided by individualized pharmokinetics: steady-state levels achieved after fifth dose
      (1) Peak levels measured 1 hour after IV or IM administration
      (2) Trough levels measured immediately prior to next dose
   d. Important for agents with known toxicity, dose-related complications, narrow therapeutic range
      (1) Aminoglycosides
      (2) Vancomycin

(3) Ketoconazole

(4) Chloramphenicol

B. Complications of Antibiotic Therapy

1. Antibiotics: May induce hepatic enzyme activity, which increases metabolism of concurrently administered drugs

2. Hypersensitivity reactions

   a. Most frequently seen with β-lactam agents

   b. 6% cross-sensitivity with cephalosporins

3. Suppression of normal flora and superinfection

   a. Candidiasis or other fungal infection

   b. *C. difficile* (pseudomembranous) enterocolitis

4. Neurotoxicity: Aminoglycosides

5. Encephalitic reactions: High-dose penicillin, cephalosporins, nalidixic acid

6. Peripheral neuropathy: Isoniazid, chloramphenicol, metronidazole, nitrofurantoin

7. Neuromuscular blockade: Aminoglycosides

8. Marrow toxicity

   a. Sulfonamides

   b. Chloramphenicol: Aplastic anemia (non–dose-dependent with 50% mortality)

   c. Penicillins: Hemolytic anemia, granulocytopenia

C. Specific Agents

1. Aminoglycosides

   a. Activity

      (1) Bactericidal against most aerobic and facultative anaerobic gram-negative bacilli

      (2) Moderate activity against gram-positive cocci

      (3) No activity against anaerobes

   b. Adverse reactions

      (1) There is a narrow therapeutic margin, and monitoring of serum levels is required.

      (2) Nephrotoxicity is rare on initial administration; adjustment of dosage intervals allows use in established renal failure.

      (3) Ototoxicity is a vestibular or auditory dysfunction resulting from seventh cranial nerve injury.

      (4) A neuromuscular blockade is an anticholinesterase effect.

   c. Drug interactions

       (1) Cephalosporins: Synergistic nephrotoxicity

       (2) Diuretics: May potentiate ototoxicity and nephrotoxicity as a result of volume contraction

       (3) Penicillin: Inactivation of aminoglycosides (clinical significance unknown)

  d. Specific agents

       (1) Gentamycin, tobramycin: Similar spectrum; gentamycin slightly more nephrotoxic

       (2) Amikacin: Active against many strains which are resistant to gentamycin or tobramycin

       (3) Netilmicin: Less nephrotoxic and ototoxic, but may cause hepatic toxicity

2. Penicillins

  a. Bactericidal against majority of the following:

       (1) Gram-positive cocci

       (2) Gram-negative cocci

       (3) Gram-positive bacilli

  b. Adverse reactions

       (1) Hypersensitivity: Fever, rash, serum sickness, anaphylaxis

       (2) Neurotoxicity: Convulsions, encephalitis, encephalopathy

       (3) Nephrotoxicity: Interstitial nephritis

       (4) Hematologic: Display of Coombs'-positive hemolytic anemia

       (5) Hypercalcemia: Following high dosage with renal insufficiency

  c. Drug interactions

       (1) Aminoglycosides are inactivated by penicillin.

       (2) Probenecid, aspirin, indomethacin may block renal tubular secretion of penicillin and lead to high serum levels.

  d. Specific agents

       (1) Penicillin G: Most active against streptococci

       (2) Ampicillin: Enterococcus organisms, *H. influenzae*

       (3) Methicillin: Penicillinase-resistant; may be associated with interstitial nephritis

       (4) Nafcillin: Penicillinase-resistant; less nephrotoxic than methicillin; may be associated with neutropenia, phlebitis

(5) Oxacillin: Penicillinase-resistant; may be associated with hepatotoxicity

(6) Azlocillin, mezlocillin, piperacillin (uriedopenicillin): Broad spectrum against gram-negative organisms; activity against *E. coli, Proteus* and *Enterobacter* organisms, and many strains of *Pseudomonas* organisms mezlocillin and piperacillin also active against some strains of *Klebsiella* and *Serratia* organisms

(7) Carbenicillin, ticarcillin (carboxypenicillin): Highly active against gram-negative organisms, including *Pseudomonas;* may be associated with hepatitis, hypokalemia, and decreased platelet aggregation

3. Cephalosporins
   a. First generation: Effective against gram-positive and some gram-negative bacteria
   b. Second generation: Increased gram-negative but less gram-positive activity
   c. Third generation: Main effect on gram-negative bacteria
   d. Adverse reactions: Large safety margin and high therapeutic margin
      (1) Hypersensitivity: Cross-sensitivity in penicillin-allergic patients is 6% to 9%; use avoided in patients with history of anaphylactic penicillin hypersensitivity
      (2) Nephrotoxicity: Interstitial nephritis
      (3) Neurotoxicity: Convulsions, confusion
      (4) Hematologic: Coombs'-positive anemia, thrombophlebitis, inhibition of platelet aggregation, suppression of vitamin K-dependent clotting factors

4. Vancomycin
   a. Activity: Bactericidal against all gram-positive bacteria, including methicillin-resistant staphylococci and *Clostridium* (pseudomembranous colitis) organisms
   b. Adverse reactions
      (1) Ototoxicity: Associated with high serum levels
      (2) Nephrotoxicity: Infrequent

        (3) Hypotension: Associated with rapid infusion

        (4) Hypersensitivity

    c. Dose: 20 to 30 mg/kg/24 hr (1 g IV q12h)

    d. Monitored serum levels

        (1) Peak: 35 µg/ml

        (2) Trough: 10 µg/ml

5. Metronidazole

    a. Activity against anaerobic bacteria, *Trichomonas* and *Giardia* organisms, and *E. histolytica*

    b. Adverse reactions

        (1) Nausea, vomiting

        (2) Headache, ataxia, vertigo, neuropathy, seizures

    c. Dose: 30 mg/kg/24 hr (500 mg IV q6h)

6. Clindamycin

    a. Activity: Gram-positive bacteria and gram-negative anaerobes

    b. Adverse reactions

        (1) Diarrhea in 20% to 30%

        (2) Hepatotoxic

        (3) Pseudomembranous colitis

    c. Dose: 30 to 40 mg/kg/24 hr (600 to 900 mg IV q8h)

7. Chloramphenicol

    a. Activity: Gram-negative bacteria, including species resistant to conventional agents (rickettsial disease, psittacosis, lymphogranuloma venereum)

    b. Adverse reactions: Bone marrow suppression (aplastic anemia)

    c. Dose: 0.25 to 1 g PO q6h (500 mg); 0.5 to 1.0 g IV q6h

    d. Monitored serum levels

        (1) Peak: 20 µg/ml

        (2) Trough: 2 µg/ml

8. Erythromycin

    a. Activity: Bacteriostatic (bactericidal in high doses) against gram-positive bacteria; good substitute for penicillin in allergic patient

    b. Adverse reactions

        (1) Nausea, vomiting, epigastric discomfort, diarrhea

        (2) Cholestatic jaundice (>10-day course, repeated courses)

        (3) Thrombophlebitis

    c. Dose: 0.25 to 1 g PO or IV q6h

9. Imipenem-cilastatin
   a. Broad spectrum of activity against *Pseudomonas, Serratia,* and *Enterobacter* organisms; enterococcus; anaerobes
   b. May cause seizures, nausea, vomiting
   c. Dose: 0.5 to 1 g IV q6-8h
10. Quinolones
    a. Active against most aerobic gram-positive and gram-negative bacteria, mycobacteria, *Mycoplasma* organisms, chlamydia
    b. Useful for UTI, enteric infection
    c. May cause nausea, vomiting, dizziness, seizures
    d. Dose
       (1) Norfloxacin 400 mg PO q12h
       (2) Ciprofloxacin 200 to 300 mg IV q12h; 750 mg PO q8-12h
11. Trimethoprim-sulfamethoxazole (TMP-SMX)
    a. Active against *Pneumocystis* and *Shigella* organisms, and gram-negative bacilli except *Pseudomonas* organisms
    b. May cause nausea, vomiting, blood dyscrasias
    c. Dose: 10 to 20 mg/kg/24 hr in 2 to 4 divided doses (based on trimethoprim component)
    d. Available for injection: TMP 80 mg and SMX 400 mg/5ml
12. Aztreonam
    a. Bactericidal against gram-negative aerobes, including *Pseudomonas* organisms
    b. May cause nausea, vomiting, phlebitis
    c. Dose: 1 to 2 g IV q6-8h
13. Tetracyclines
    a. Bacteriostatic against a variety of gram-positive and gram-negative bacteria, rickettsia, *Mycoplasma* organisms, chlamydia
    b. High incidence of bacterial resistance limits use
    c. May cause hepatotoxicity, GI upset, thrombophlebitis
    d. Dose: 250 to 500 mg PO q6h; 500 mg IV q12h (5 mg/ml infusion; 2 ml/hr)
14. Amphotericin B
    a. Active against most fungi, including *Histoplasma, Coccidioides, Candida, Aspergillus, Blastomyces,*

Cryptococcus, Sporotrichum, and *Phycomycetes* organisms

b. Adverse reactions

   (1) Nephrotoxicity is dose-related; most patients experience a 30% decrease in GFR with standard treatment; volume loading reduces renal toxicity.

   (2) Chills, fever, headache, anorexia, weight loss, nausea, vomiting (50% to 80%)

   (3) Thrombophlebitis, anemia, hypersensitivity

   (4) Arachnoiditis, auditory neurotoxicity

c. Systemic: Total dose of amphotericin B usually 6 mg/kg; should not usually exceed 8 mg/kg (total dose of 3 to 5 g prescribed for more severe or persistent infections)

   (1) Dilution in D_5W to concentration of 10 mg/dL; stable for 24 hours

   (2) Slow IV infusion over 6 hours, monitoring BP, pulse, respiratory rate, and temperature q30min during treatment

   (3) Test dose (1 mg) given over 30 minutes with observation for 1 hour, monitoring for fever, hypotension, tachycardia

   (4) First day: 0.25 mg/kg IV over 6 hours; increase dose by 0.1 mg/kg/day to dose of 0.5 to 0.7 mg/kg/day

   (5) Discontinuation of treatment or dose reduction if temperature > 38.9°C; systolic BP < 100 mm Hg, fall in systolic BP of > 30 mm Hg; pulse > 130

   (6) May ameliorate febrile or hypotensive reaction by premedicating with 125 mg hydrocortisone IV 30 minutes before treatment; may also be beneficial to use diphenhydramine and acetaminophen

d. Amphotericin B bladder irrigation

   (1) Amphotericin B 50 mg in 1 L NS infused through Foley catheter over 8 hours as continuous bladder irrigation

   (2) Irrigation is usually continued for 7 to 10 days

   (3) Following cessation of bladder irrigation, urine is cultured for fungal culture

15. Flucytosine

   a. Active against *Candida* and *Cryptococcus* organisms

    b. May cause diarrhea, colitis, allergic rash, neutropenia, thrombocytopenia, hepatotoxicity

    c. High incidence of resistance when used as single agent; used in combination with amphotericin B to reduce dose of latter

    d. Dose

       (1) Amphotericin B reduced to 0.3 mg/kg/day IV

       (2) Flucytosine 375 mg/kg q6h PO

16. Fluconazole

    a. Indications: Oral, pharyngeal, and esophageal candidiasis, cryptococcosis, and coccidioidal meningitis

    b. Adverse reactions: Hepatic toxicity; monitoring of liver function tests recommended

    c. Recommended dose for oral pharyngeal candidiasis: 200 mg PO loading dose followed by 100 mg PO q6h

    d. Doses of up to 400 mg/day for severe esophageal candidiasis or cryptococcal meningitis

    e. Parenteral administration (doses per PO administration) is by IV infusion: maximum rate 200 mg/hr

17. Nystatin

    a. For use in oral candidiasis

    b. Dose: Nystatin liquid 5 ml PO q6h (swish and swallow); nystatin tablets one or two PO q6h

18. Ketoconazole

    a. Active against *Candida, Coccidioides, Histoplasma, Blastomyces,* and *Paracoccidioides* organisms, dermatophytes

    b. May cause hepatotoxicity, hepatic necrosis, pruritus, dizziness, somnolence

    c. Dose: 400 mg/day PO

19. Acyclovir

    a. Active against HSV-1, HSV-2, VZV, EBV, inactive against human CMV

    b. Dose

       (1) IV: 5 to 10 mg/kg q8h

       (2) PO: 50 to 200 mg PO q4-8h (suppression therapy)

       (3) Topical: 5% ointment, four to six applications per day

20. Ganciclovir

    a. Activity against CMV

b. Dose: 5 mg/kg q12h IV × 14 to 21 days, then 5 mg/kg/day maintenance

SUGGESTED READING

Balkwill FR, Burke F: The cytokine network, *Immunol Today* 10:299, 1989.

Bone R et al: Definitions of sepsis and organ failure and guidelines for use of innovative therapies in sepsis, *Chest* 101:1644, 1992.

Brengelmann GL: *Body temperature regulation.* In Patton, editor: *Textbook of physiology,* vol 2, *Circulation, respiration, body fluids, metabolism and endocrinology,* ed 21, Philadelphia, 1989, WB Saunders.

Feld R: The compromised host, *Eur J Cancer Clin Oncol* 25(suppl 2):1, 1989.

Keighley MRB, Giles GR: *The investigation and treatment of surgical infections.* In Cuschieri A, Giles GR, and Moossa AR, editors: *Essential surgical practice,* ed 2, Bristol, England, 1988, John Wright.

Rubin RH, Young LA, editors: *Clinical approach to infection in the compromised host,* ed 2, New York, 1988, Plenum Medical Book.

VENTILATOR MANAGEMENT

21

Stanley A. Gall, Jr.

I. **INDICATIONS FOR VENTILATORY SUPPORT**
A. **Conditions Which Require Ventilatory Support**
   1. Level of consciousness compromising ventilation or inadequate to protect airway
   2. Secretions in excess of patient's capacity to clear
   3. Inadequate muscle strength
   4. Excessive work of breathing
   5. Upper airway obstruction
   6. Inadequate oxygenation
   7. Atelectasis or consolidation unresponsive to more conservative therapy
B. **Partial Ventilatory Support**
   1. May be adequate for patients exhibiting spontaneous ventilation
   2. Advantages over total ventilatory support
      a. Periodic normalization of pleural pressure
         (1) Allows greater venous return
         (2) May improve cardiac performance
      b. Limits disuse atrophy and discoordination of respiratory musculature
      c. Less sedation and analgesia required to control patient anxiety
      d. Ventilation better distributed to dependent portions of lung
      e. Partial support always needed to overcome the obligatory resistance of the breathing circuit
C. **Indications for Endotracheal Intubation**
   1. Failure of airway adjuncts
      a. Oral airways
      b. Positioning
      c. Reversal of sedation

2. Inadequate bag-mask-valve ventilation
3. Required prolonged ventilatory support
4. Patients with compromised airways
   a. Maxillofacial fractures
   b. Massive hemoptysis
   c. Supraglottic obstruction
   d. Airway protection when high risk for aspiration
      (1) Excessive secretions
      (2) Massive upper GI bleeding
5. Elective intubation under controlled circumstances preferable to waiting for respiratory failure requiring emergent intubation

D. Mandatory Equipment at Bedside for Intubation
   1. Laryngoscope
   2. Endotracheal tube, stylet, and syringe
   3. Oxygen with bag-valve-mask
   4. Suction apparatus
   5. Intravenous access
   6. Medications: Epinephrine, lidocaine, atropine
   7. Monitoring: BP, ECG
   8. Magill forceps
   9. Stethoscope

II. TRACHEOSTOMY
A. Indications for Tracheostomy
   1. Upper respiratory obstruction
   2. Secretions from upper respiratory tract not controlled
   3. Inadequate pulmonary toilet of lower respiratory tract, although otherwise able to ventilate
   4. Inadequate strength or vital capacity (neurologic or obstructive)
   5. Anticipated mechanical ventilatory support in excess of 3 weeks

B. Advantages of Tracheostomy Over Translaryngeal Intubation
   1. Upper airway obstruction bypassed
   2. Reduction of ventilatory dead space (V_D)
   3. Reduction of work of breathing
   4. Improved access to lower respiratory tract for pulmonary toilet
   5. More secure airway

C. **Disadvantages of Tracheostomy Compared to Translaryngeal Intubation**
   1. Requires operative procedure
   2. Increased exposure of lower respiratory tract to colonization with pathological organisms
D. **Complications of Tracheostomy**
   1. 1.5% mortality rate
   2. 5.9% morbidity rate
      a. Early complications
         (1) Displacement of tracheostomy tube
         (2) Infection
         (3) Perioperative hemorrhage
      b. Late complications
         (1) Erosion into mediastinal vessels; tracheo-innominate artery fistula
         (2) Dysphagia
         (3) Subglottic stenosis
         (4) Tracheoesophageal fistula

III. **TYPES OF VENTILATORS**
A. **Volume-Cycled Ventilation**
   1. The ventilator delivers a preset, constant V_T.
   2. Pressure limits are set to avoid excessive inspiratory pressures.
   3. The ventilator provides more constant ventilation under conditions of changing compliance.
   4. Part of V_T is lost to the compliance of the breathing circuit (usually 3 to 4 ml/cm H_2O), especially at lower V_T and higher inspiratory pressures.
   5. It is difficult to compensate for delivered volume lost to air leaks.
B. **Pressure-Cycled Ventilation**
   1. Inspiration is terminated by preset peak pressure.
   2. Delivered volume is dependent on total compliance and applied pressure.
   3. Incomplete exhalation limits subsequent ventilatory volume.
      a. Respiratory rate increases to compensate
      b. May result in pathologically high mean airway pressure
   4. Airway leaks are well compensated.
   5. It is primarily used in infants and small children.
      a. Compliance is more constant in these patients.

      b. Appropriate endotracheal tube size selection mandates a small leak.

C. **Time-Cycled, Pressure-Limited Ventilation**
  1. This type of ventilation is similar to pressure-cycled ventilation.
    a. Addition of an inspiratory pause maintains airway pressure at the preset maximum for a predetermined time.
    b. Delivered volume is dependent on applied pressure, compliance, and degree of equilibration between airway and alveolar pressures.
  2. Alveolar units with diminished compliance and lengthened ventilation time constants will equilibrate when inspiratory pause time is lengthened.
  3. If airway-alveolar pressure equilibration does not occur, V_T will be unpredictable.

IV. **VENTILATOR MODES**
A. **Controlled Mandatory Ventilation (CMV)**
  1. The ventilator delivers calculated minute-ventilation.
    a. Determined by the preset V_T and rate
    b. Independent of patient's breathing
  2. No air flow is provided between ventilator breaths.
  3. CMV is appropriate when the patient is unable to initiate breaths.
    a. Paralyzing agents
    b. Anesthesia
    c. Neurologic disease

B. **Assisted Ventilation**
  1. Assist/control ventilation
    a. The ventilator delivers preset V_T when triggered by the patient's negative inspiratory pressure.
    b. A full breath is delivered each cycle; no partial breaths are possible.
    c. A minimum mandatory rate may be set.
    d. Anxious or hyperpneic patients are at risk for hyperventilation.
    e. Triggering sensitivity must be set at critical level.
      (1) Should avoid respiratory alkalosis (too sensitive)
      (2) Wasted inspiratory effort (too insensitive)
    f. Respiratory muscles are at risk for further atrophy.

2. Pressure support
  a. The ventilator provides a constant pressure during patient-triggered inspiration.
    (1) Augments patient's own inspiratory effort
    (2) May be used in conjunction with other ventilator modes
    (3) May be used alone
      (a) Synchronized
      (b) Requires spontaneous ventilatory effort
      (c) Does not guarantee a minimum minute ventilation
  b. May be weaned independently from decreases in intermittent mandatory ventilation rate
  c. Preserves respiratory muscle coordination
  d. Limits disuse atrophy when adjusted to provide the minimally effective augmentation of inspiration

C. **Intermittent Mandatory Ventilation (IMV) and Synchronized Intermittent Mandatory Ventilation (SIMV)**
  1. Machine delivered rate and V_T are set.
  2. Air flow is provided so the patient may breathe spontaneously, although unassisted, between breaths.
  3. V_T and rate settings may be adjusted to provide tapering support as a weaning mode.
  4. SIMV allows ventilator breaths to be synchronized with patient-initiated breaths to improve patient comfort.
  5. In absence of patient initiation, IMV/SIMV provides the same ventilation as CMV.
  6. Advantages over AC or CMV modes include the following:
    a. Less sedation is required.
    b. Less disuse atrophy of respiratory muscles occurs.
  7. Some patients may be unable to synchronize with the ventilator.
    a. Evaluation for hypoxia
    b. May require ventilation in an alternate mode
    c. May require sedation or paralysis

D. **High-Frequency Jet Ventilation**
  1. Provides ventilation at reduced peak airway pressures
    a. Lower incidence of pulmonary barotrauma
    b. Less decrease in cardiac output
    c. Less of an increase ICP

2. Methods
    a. Jet injector lumen endotracheal tube
    b. 14-gauge needle injector
    c. Sliding venturi, which provides the greatest V_T
3. Setup of ventilator
    a. Frequency of 50 to 300 cycles/min
    b. Duty cycle of 20% to 30%
    c. Drive pressure of 5 to 50 psig
    d. V_T of 3 to 4 ml/kg
        (1) May be adjusted by altering duty cycle
        (2) May be adjusted by changing the drive pressure
4. Tip of endotracheal tube positioned 10 cm proximal to the carina to prevent preferential single lung ventilation
5. Established indications
    a. Bronchopleural fistula
        (1) PIP must be less than opening pressure of bronchopleural fistula
        (2) Will limit air leak and allow healing
    b. Bronchoscopy or laryngoscopy
    c. Infants who are hypoxic on standard ventilatory modalities
    d. Excessive PIP on standard ventilator modes (relative indications)
6. Complications
    a. Inadequate minute ventilation
    b. Inadequate humidification
    c. Tracheal mucosal injury secondary to high shear forces

V. STANDARD VENTILATOR SETTINGS
A. Rate
1. Frequency of respirator cycling, usually set at 10 to 15 breaths/min
2. Adjusted in tandem with inspiratory flow rate (IFR) to provide for appropriate I:E ratio
3. Exhalation time shortened by increased rate at a constant IFR

B. Tidal Volume
1. Volume-cycled ventilators: Set directly (10 to 15 ml/kg)
2. Pressure-cycled ventilators: The product of inspiratory pressure, rate, and IFR
3. For jet ventilation: V_T is 3 to 4 ml/kg

C. **Inspiratory Flow Rate**
   1. Increases in IFR
      a. Shortens the period of inspiration
      b. Provides a longer period for exhalation
   2. Importance of lung compliance
      a. Lungs with normal compliance are relatively insensitive to IFR.
      b. When compliance is diminished, high IFR results in excessive PIP.
   3. Normal I : E ratio is 1 : 2 to 1 : 3

D. **Peak Inspiratory Pressure**
   1. Pressure-cycled ventilator: Determines airway pressure and V_T at which inspiration will be terminated
   2. Volume-cycled ventilator: Overpressure alarm
   3. Combined with an inspiratory pause
      a. The airway pressure is allowed to plateau at PIP.
      b. Ventilation is a pressure-limited time-cycled mode.
   4. Adequate PIP delivery
      a. Good breath sounds bilaterally
      b. Visible chest movement
      c. Sufficient V_T delivery to maintain a normal $Paco_2$

E. **Fio_2**
   1. Fio_2 is the fraction of oxygen in inspired air (room air = 0.21).
   2. Adjust Fio_2 to provide for Pao_2 of 60 to 90 mm Hg and $Sao_2 > 90\%$.
   3. Fio_2 may be directly and safely reduced using $Pao_2 : Fio_2$ ratio.

$$\text{Desired } Fio_2 = [(\text{Actual } Fio_2/(\text{Actual } Pao_2))]$$
$$\times \text{ Desired } Pao_2$$

   4. An Fio_2 in excess of 0.5 subjects the patient to the risk of oxygen toxicity.

F. **Positive End-Expiratory Pressure**
   1. PEEP maintains positive airway pressure at end expiration.
      a. Counterbalances airway closing forces
      b. Increases functional residual capacity (FRC)
      c. Maintains small airway patency at end expiration
   2. A PEEP of 5 cm H_2O is comparable to physiologic PEEP provided by glottic closure.

   3. RV performance is limited by excessive PEEP.
      a. The RV must eject against a higher afterload with a limited preload.
         (1) Airway pressure increases pulmonary vascular resistance.
         (2) Capacitance volume shifts out of the thorax limiting preload to the RV.
      b. LV performance is also reduced by preload limitation.
      c. This functional hypovolemia may be ameliorated by increasing intravascular volume.
   4. PEEP levels above 10 cm H_2O mandate invasive monitoring of intravascular volume.
   5. High levels of PEEP narrow the delivered pressure amplitude, limiting V_T.
   6. PEEP may be critical to adequate ventilation and oxygenation.
      a. Optimal PEEP may vary depending on delivered V_T.
      b. Institute PEEP to recruit alveolar units and reduce Fio_2 below toxic levels.
      c. Optimize by maximizing compliance without limiting Do_2.

G. Pressure Support
   1. Allows inspiratory support of patient initiated breaths
   2. Stepwise reduction allows gradual strengthening of respiratory muscles in deconditioned patients

H. Continuous Positive Airway Pressure (CPAP)
   1. Physiologically equivalent to PEEP plus pressure support
   2. Maintains small airway patency by improving FRC
   3. May be contraindicated in patients with a normal FRC
      a. Possibility of lung overexpansion
      b. Decreased compliance
      c. Increased work of breathing
      d. Diminished gas exchange
   4. Used postoperatively to hasten return of FRC to preoperative levels

I. Sensitivity
   1. Inspiratory force the patient must generate to trigger an inspiratory cycle
   2. If too high (excessively insensitive), may waste energy attempting to initiate breaths

3. If set too low (too sensitive), may trigger breaths too easily and result in hyperventilation

VI. TROUBLESHOOTING
A. Hypercarbia

1. Ventilator malfunction
   a. Causes
      (1) Disconnection
      (2) Inadequate V_T because of circuit capacitance or air leak
   b. Solutions
      (1) Reconnect patient to ventilator.
      (2) Review ventilator and alarm settings.
      (3) Eliminate air leaks.
2. Inadequate V_T
   a. Causes
      (1) Bronchospasm
      (2) Mucus plugging
      (3) Atelectasis
      (4) Tension pneumothorax
      (5) Incorrect ventilator settings
      (6) Inadequate compensation for dead space
   b. Solutions
      (1) Treat bronchospasm and mucus plugging.
      (2) Increase V_T or PEEP to improve compliance and recruit alveoli.
      (3) Exclude pneumothorax.
3. Increased physiologic dead space
   a. Causes
      (1) PE
      (2) Diminished cardiac output with inadequate perfusion
   b. Solutions
      (1) Exclude or treat PE.
      (2) Improve cardiovascular dynamics.
4. Increased CO_2 production
   a. Causes
      (1) Fever
      (2) Shivering
      (3) Rewarming
      (4) Hypermetabolic state

        (5) Sepsis

        (6) Excessive carbohydrate to fat caloric ratio

    b. Solutions

        (1) Treat and correct the underlying problem.

        (2) Consider muscle paralysis to control shivering until postoperative rewarming is complete.

B. **Hypoxia and Sudden Respiratory Decompensation**

  1. Patient disconnected from the ventilator and hand ventilated with 100% Fio_2

  2. Physical examination

    a. Evaluate for adequate bilateral ventilation.

    b. Evaluate hemodynamic status.

  3. Laboratory evaluation

    a. Obtain ABG and mixed venous blood gas.

    b. Obtain CXR.

        (1) Check endotracheal tube position.

        (2) Exclude pneumothorax.

        (3) Assess lung fields for edema, consolidation, or Westermark's sign.

  4. Treatment

    a. Low resistance to manual ventilation

        (1) Hemodynamically stable

            (a) Exclude ventilator malfunction

            (b) Consider PE, subjective dyspnea, shortness of breath

            (c) Correct subjective dyspnea by increasing V_T.

            (d) Exclude pathologic processes before increasing sedation.

        (2) Hemodynamically unstable

            (a) Exclude pneumothorax.

            (b) Consider PE, sepsis, and relative hypovolemia.

    b. High resistance to manual ventilation

        (1) Obstructed endotracheal tube

            (a) Differentiate between kinked tube and mucus or thrombus plug.

            (b) Endotracheal suctioning excludes obstructed endotracheal tube.

        (2) If no obstruction, should consider one of the following:

            (a) Malpositioned tube; CXR obtained for tube position

      (b) Mucus or thrombus plugging in trachea distal to endotracheal tube

      (c) Bronchospasm or pulmonary edema

C. **Alarms**

  1. Low pressure (disconnect alarm)

    a. Senses absence of positive pressure in circuit

    b. Excellent monitoring of disconnection

    c. Most common failure due to failure to reactivate after endotracheal suctioning

  2. Low exhaled volume

    a. If the exhaled V_T does not match the inhaled V_T, an air leak or disconnection exists.

    b. The alarm may be set at 90% to 100% of the V_T to account for the portion of delivered volume lost to circuit capacitance.

  3. Maximum PIP

    a. Alarm set 15% above PIP

    b. Triggering of alarm

      (1) Lack of synchronization with the patient's breathing

      (2) Inadequate exhalation time resulting in breath-stacking

      (3) Malpositioned endotracheal tube

  4. O_2 concentration of inspired gases

    a. Set at Fio_2, plus or minus 0.10.

    b. Alarm signals ventilator failure or failure of oxygen source.

  5. End-tidal CO_2

    a. The gold standard for verifying tracheal intubation

    b. Low end-tidal CO_2

      (1) Disconnection

      (2) Extubation

      (3) Esophageal intubation

    c. On-line assessment of Pco_2 given by measurement

      (1) It is usually 4 to 6 mm Hg lower than measured $PaCO_2$.

      (2) Values may be 10 to 12 mm Hg lower when large Vd.

VII. WEANING FROM MECHANICAL VENTILATION

A. **Methodology**

  1. Most patients are ventilated in the SIMV mode.

    a. Progressive decreases in rate allow the patient to perform an increasing fraction of ventilation.

    b. Add pressure support.

        (1) Will compensate for resistance of ventilator

        (2) Will assist spontaneous breaths

        (3) Weaned independently of IMV rate

2. Reduce sedation to optimize respiratory drive.

3. Patients on long-term mechanical ventilation will have a loss of endurance. Rest patient with increased support each night to allow a recovery period between daytime weaning trials.

B. Criteria

1. Ability to oxygenate: $Po_2 > 60$ to 80 mm Hg with $Fio_2 \leq 0.50$

2. Patient alert

    a. Responsive to commands

    b. Sustained head lift (>5 seconds)

    c. Bilateral hand grip

    d. Ability to cough (intact gag reflex)

3. Adequate muscular strength

    a. Muscular paralysis is reversed.

    b. A V_T of 4 ml/kg indicates inadequate strength to sustain ventilation.

    c. Rapid, shallow breathing is an adaptation to compensate for inadequate muscular strength or endurance.

4. Predictors for successful extubation

    a. $V_T > 4$ ml/kg

    b. F (respiratory rate) = 8 to 25 breaths/min

    c. F/V_T ratio < 100 breaths/min

    d. Negative inspiratory force maximum < −25 cm H_2O

5. Ventilator support compatible with extubation

    a. IMV < 8

    b. PEEP ≤ 5 cm H_2O

    c. Pressure support ≤ 8 cm H_2O

    d. $Fio_2 < 0.50$

C. Difficult to Wean Patients

1. Patient factors

    a. Correct or treat underlying pulmonary diseases.

    b. A degree of acidosis (pH near 7.3) may be required to effect adequate respiratory drive.

    c. Reduce excessive ventilation demands by holding carbohydrates to <33% of caloric intake.

d. Theophylline increases diaphragmatic contractility.
e. Use CPAP to maintain FRC off ventilator.
f. Excess Fio_2 results in resorption atelectasis.
   (1) Reduce Fio_2.
   (2) Keep $Pao_2 \geq 60$ mm Hg.
g. Respiratory rates > 30 indicate fatigue; this requires increased ventilator support or better synchronization.

2. Ventilator factors
   a. Partial ventilator support, and therefore weaning, may not be possible on some ventilators because of excessive resistance of circuit and valves.
   b. A PEEP of 5 cm H_2O and pressure support of 3 to 5 cm H_2O may be required during mechanical ventilation to overcome ventilator impedance and provide a physiologic PEEP.

3. Airway factors
   a. Excessive work required by small endotracheal tubes
   b. Functional internal diameter limited by partial obstruction of the endotracheal tube
   c. Excessive V_D
      (1) Tracheostomy reduces V_D by 100 to 150 ml.
      (2) This will favorably improve V_D/V_T.

VIII. EXTUBATION

A. Preparation

1. Review respiratory mechanics, last ABG, and physical examination to insure that extubation is appropriate.
2. Explain the process to the patient to minimize anxiety.
3. Utilize endotracheal suctioning.

B. Removal of Endotracheal Tube

1. Perform expeditiously with all equipment for reintubation immediately available.
2. Deflate the balloon; if the patient can ventilate around the ET tube, laryngeal edema is not significant.
3. Give a large bagged breath and remove the endotracheal tube on exhalation.
4. Encourage the patient to cough.
5. Apply supplemental O_2 via the facemask.
   a. Administer Fio_2 that is 0.10 to 0.15 above Fio_2 on the ventilator.
   b. Obtain ABG after 10 to 15 minutes.

6. Monitor the respiratory rate, pulse oximetry, and hemo-dynamics for signs of decompensation.

IX. MECHANICAL VENTILATION COMPLICATIONS
A. Disconnection
1. The most frequent mechanical complication of mechanical ventilation
2. Easily diagnosed by appropriate alarms and settings if they have not been disabled

B. Infection
1. Intubation inhibits normal airway defenses.
   a. Mucociliary elevator
   b. Macrophage killing
   c. Nasotracheal filtering/humidification
2. Colonization of the normally sterile trachea with gram-negative rods proceeds rapidly after intubation (<72 hours).
3. Hypoxia, hyperoxia, and acidosis of critical illness further impede host resistance.
4. Sinusitis occurs in 2% to 5% of patients with nasotracheal intubation.
   a. Physical signs
      (1) Fever
      (2) Purulent exudate
   b. Radiologic evaluation
      (1) Sinus films
      (2) May require CT for adequate visualization
   c. Treatment
      (1) Change route of intubation.
      (2) Administer antibiotics based on culture and sensitivity.
      (3) Drain sinuses in resistant cases.
5. Pneumonia
   a. Risk raised 20-fold by mechanical ventilation
   b. Usually due to enteric, gram-negative rods
   c. Sources of pathogens
      (1) Orophyarngeal colonization
      (2) Aspiration
      (3) Inhalation from contaminated ventilatory circuitry
      (4) Hematogenous spread
   d. Treatment
      (1) Adequate pulmonary toilet
      (2) Antibiotics based on culture and sensitivity

C. **Barotrauma**
   1. A function of PIP
      a. Distended alveoli at increased risk
      b. Hyperventilation of normal tissue in presence of large regions of low compliance
         (1) Atelectasis
         (2) Contusion
         (3) Pneumonia
      c. High-risk conditions
         (1) COPD
         (2) Mucus plugging
         (3) Bronchoscopy
         (4) CPR
   2. Results in alveolar rupture
      a. Air dissecting along perivascular tissue planes
         (1) Pneumomediastinum
         (2) Subcutaneous emphysema
      b. Results in pneumothorax from disruption of parietal pleura
   3. Solutions
      a. Spontaneous assisted ventilation will result in lowest peak airway pressures.
      b. Muscular paralysis will improve the chest wall compliance portion of total lung compliance.
      c. Jet ventilation will allow adequate gas exchange at a lower PIP.

D. **Tracheal and Laryngeal Stenosis**
   1. Endotracheal tubes cause mucosal ulceration and chronic inflammation.
   2. Resultant problems include the following:
      a. Fibrosis
      b. Tracheomalacia
      c. Stenosis
      d. Tracheoesophageal fistulae
   3. Solutions include the following:
      a. Use thin-walled, low-pressure, high-volume cuffs.
      b. Maintain a cuff pressure of < 20 to 25 mm Hg.

E. **Disuse Atrophy and Respiratory Muscle Discoordination**
   1. Minimize by using partial ventilator support, allowing spontaneous ventilatory effort.
   2. After prolonged periods of ventilatory support, gradual

reductions in support over the course of several days may be necessary.

3. Maintain a positive nitrogen balance to avoid catabolism of respiratory muscles.

SUGGESTED READING

Kirby RR, Banner MJ, and Downs JB, editors: *Clinical applications of ventilatory support,* New York, 1990, Churchill Livingstone.

Pepe PE: Acute post-traumatic respiratory physiology and insufficiency, *Surg Clin North Am* 69:157, 1989.

Yang KL, Tobin MJ: A prospective study of indexes predicting the outcome of trials of weaning from mechanical ventilation, *N Engl J Med* 324:1445, 1991.

NUTRITION   **22**

Bradley H. Collins

I.   NUTRITIONAL ASSESSMENT
A.   Patients at Risk for Malnutrition
1. Malnutrition present at the time of admission
   a. Decreased oral intake
   b. Malignancy
   c. Chronic disease (hepatic, renal, or cardiac failure)
2. Malabsorption
   a. Short bowel syndrome
   b. Intestinal fistula
   c. Inflammatory bowel disease
   d. Pancreatic exocrine insufficiency
3. Inadequate oral intake secondary to disease process
   a. GI obstruction
   b. Pancreatitis
   c. Peptic ulcer disease
   d. Superior mesenteric artery syndrome
4. Prolonged fasting
   a. Prolonged preoperative/postoperative NPO status
   b. Protracted postoperative ileus
5. Increased energy expenditure resulting from hypermetabolic state
   a. Sepsis
   b. Multiple trauma or major burns
   c. Extensive surgery

B.   Nutritional Assessment of the Surgical Patient
1. History
   a. Dietary habits
   b. Unintentional weight loss
   c. Presence of chronic illness
2. Physical signs of malnutrition
   a. Fat and muscle wasting
   b. Peripheral edema, ascites

  c. Excessive hair loss
  d. Neuropathy, dementia
  e. Hepatomegaly
3. Anthropometric measurements to evaluate body fat and skeletal protein mass
  a. Triceps skinfold thickness
   (1) Measured with skinfold calipers
   (2) Useful in the assessment of fat reserves
   (3) Increased accuracy if measured at more than one anatomic location
  b. Arm circumference
   (1) Indicative of skeletal muscle mass
   (2) Taken at the midportion of the upper arm
4. Laboratory findings
  a. Total lymphocyte count
   (1) Total lymphocyte count equal to 1200 to 2000 cells/mm^3 indicates mild protein malnutrition.
   (2) Total lymphocyte count equal to 800 to 1200 cells/mm^3 indicates moderate deficiency.
   (3) Total lymphocyte count less than 800 cells/mm^3 indicates severe deficiency.
  b. Serum albumin
   (1) Most widely used serum indicator of malnutrition
   (2) Half-life of approximately 20 days; therefore it does not accurately reflect early protein malnutrition
   (3) Decreased albumin also associated with other conditions
    (a) Overhydration
    (b) Liver disease
    (c) Open wounds
   (4) Interpretation of levels
    (a) Normal > 3.4 g/dL
    (b) Mild visceral protein deficiency = 2.9 to 3.3 g/dL
    (c) Moderate deficiency = 2.2 to 2.8 g/dL
    (d) Severe deficiency < 2.2 g/dL
  c. Serum transferrin
   (1) Serum concentration less affected by state of hydration than albumin
   (2) Half-life of approximately 9 days
    (a) Better indicator of early visceral protein malnutrition

       (b) More indicative of the effects of feeding
     (3) Interpretation of levels
       (a) Normal = 250 to 300 mg/dL
       (b) Mild visceral protein deficiency = 150 to 200 mg/dL
       (c) Moderate deficiency = 100 to 150 mg/dL
       (d) Severe deficiency < 100 mg/dL

  d. Other serum proteins that are more sensitive indicators of acute changes in visceral proteins
    (1) Retinol-binding protein ($t_{1/2}$ = 10 hours)
    (2) Prealbumin ($t_{1/2}$ = 24 hours)

C. Classification of Malnutrition

1. Marasmus
  a. Malnutrition resulting from insufficient protein and caloric intake as compared to energy expenditure
  b. Usually occurs over an extended period of starvation
  c. Anthropometric measurements diminished due to muscle and fat wasting
  d. Visceral organs usually spared, thus biochemical parameters within normal limits

2. Kwashiorkor
  a. Occurs in the setting of sufficient caloric intake in association with inadequate protein
  b. Normal skeletal muscle and body fat stores (anthropometric parameters normal)
  c. Pathophysiology largely due to the effects of insulin
    (1) Carbohydrate intake stimulates insulin release.
    (2) Insulin enhances lipogenesis, reduces lipolysis, and stimulates protein synthesis.
    (3) Visceral organs are not subject to the anabolic effects of insulin.
      (a) The protein deficit is compensated for by proteolysis of the viscera.
      (b) Patients exhibit edema, low albumin and transferrin levels, and defects in cell-mediated immunity

3. Protein-energy malnutrition
  a. Also known as mixed malnutrition
  b. Represents a combination of marasmus and kwashiorkor

D. Metabolism

1. Estimation of the energy expenditure of patients
  a. No stress/minimal activity: 28 kcal/kg/day

    b. Mild stress: 30 kcal/kg/day

    c. Moderate stress: 35 kcal/kg/day

    d. Severe stress: 40 kcal/kg/day

2. Basal energy expenditure (BEE)

    a. BEE is the energy required to maintain necessary bodily functions, such as the circulation, respiration, and body temperature

    b. The Harris-Benedict formula provides an estimate of BEE utilizing age (years), height (cm), and weight (kg).

       (1) Females

$$BEE \text{ (kcal/kg/day)} = 665 + (9.6 \times weight) + (1.8 \times height) - (4.7 \times age)$$

       (2) Males

$$BEE \text{ (kcal/kg/day)} = 66 + (13.7 \times weight) + (5.0 \times height) - (6.8 \times age)$$

3. Actual energy expenditure (AEE)

    a. Takes into account both the BEE and the energy associated with clinical stressors

    b. AEE (kcal/kg/day) = BEE × (Activity factor) × (Stress factor)

       (1) Activity factors

          (a) Ventilator-dependent: 1.10

          (b) Bed rest: 1.15

          (c) Normal activity: 1.25

       (2) Stress factors

          (a) Elective surgery: 1.24

          (b) Skeletal trauma: 1.32

          (c) Blunt trauma: 1.37

          (d) Trauma: 1.61

          (e) Sepsis: 1.79

          (f) Burns: 2.32

4. Approximate caloric values of these metabolic fuel sources

    a. Fat = 9 kcal/g

    b. Carbohydrate

       (1) 4 kcal/g enterally

       (2) 3.4 kcal/g intravenously

    c. Protein = 4 to 5 kcal/g

5. Respiratory quotient (RQ)

a. Ratio of carbon dioxide production to oxygen consumption

$$RQ = V_{CO_2}/V_{O_2}$$

b. Gives an indication of the balance of fuel substrates being metabolized
   (1) Values for various fuels
       (a) Fat = 0.7
       (b) Protein = 0.8
       (c) Carbohydrate = 1
   (2) Clinical interpretation
       (a) RQ approaching 0.7 indicates fat oxidation (prolonged starvation).
       (b) RQ approaching 1.0 indicate glucose oxidation.
       (c) RQ > 1.0 signifies fat synthesis.
6. Nitrogen balance
   a. Indicator of protein status
   b. Calculated by subtracting nitrogen excretion from nitrogen intake
      (1) Normally nitrogen intake and excretion are equal.
      (2) A negative nitrogen balance indicates loss of lean body mass.
          (a) Starvation
          (b) Catabolic state associated with stress (injury, sepsis, burns)
      (3) A positive nitrogen balance indicates the following:
          (a) Implies gains in lean body mass
          (b) Associated with refeeding after starvation

II. ENTERAL ALIMENTATION
A. Indications
1. Malnutrition or extended hypermetabolic state
2. Severe dysphagia
3. Major burns
4. Trauma
5. Low output enterocutaneous fistulas (if feedings are administered distal to fistula)
B. Contraindications
1. Absolute contraindications
   a. Complete intestinal obstruction
   b. Severe ileus

      c. Shock

      d. Massive GI bleeding

      e. Enteric losses > 600 ml/24 hours

         (1) Severe diarrhea

         (2) High output intestinal fistulas

      f. Aggressive nutritional support not desired by patient

  2. Relative contraindications

      a. Severe pancreatitis (some evidence that tube feeding intrajejunally may not stimulate the exocrine pancreas)

      b. Malabsorption syndromes

      c. Ileus

         (1) Normal gastric propulsive activity returns in 48 to 72 hours.

         (2) Small intestinal activity returns in 12 hours after abdominal surgery.

         (3) Colon activity returns in 72 hours after abdominal surgery.

C. Advantages of Enteral Feeding

  1. Physiologic

      a. Enteral feeding allows maintenance of intestinal structure via trophic effects of intestinal nutrients.

         (1) Intestinal integrity of the intestinal mucosa is preserved.

         (2) Risk of sepsis secondary to bacterial translocation is decreased.

      b. GI hormonal function is generally maintained.

      c. Usual pattern of nutrient absorption into the portal circulation is preserved.

  2. Formulations more nutritionally complete than intravenous options

  3. Less expensive than intravenous hyperalimentation

  4. No specialized personnel required for administration

D. Methods of Delivery for Enteral Nutrition

  1. Stomach

      a. Nasogastric or gastrostomy tube

      b. Advantages

         (1) Tube placement is simple.

         (2) Delivery of food into the stomach simulates normal GI function.

         (3) High osmolar loads are tolerated.

         (4) Bolus feeding is tolerated.

      c. Disadvantages

   (1) The infusion of food into the stomach increases the
       risk of aspiration.
       (a) Patients must be alert.
       (b) Patients must have an intact gag reflex.
   (2) Standard nasogastric tubes are stiff and large caliber.
       (a) Patient discomfort
       (b) Gastroesophageal reflux/aspiration
       (c) Erosion of nasal cartilage and septum
   (3) Frequent measurement of gastric residuals is man-
       datory.
2. Small intestine
   a. Nasoduodenal or jejunostomy tube
   b. Advantages
      (1) Significantly reduced risk of aspiration
      (2) Enables use of enteral nutrition in patients who are
          not candidates for gastric feeding
          (a) Patients with altered mental status, including co-
              matose patients
          (b) Patients with gastroparesis
          (c) Patients with proximal enterocutaneous fistulas
              (tube placed distal to fistula)
   c. Disadvantages
      (1) Continuous feeding is necessary; bolus feeding to the
          small intestine is tolerated poorly.
      (2) Nasoduodenal tubes are difficult to place.
      (3) Nasoduodenal and needle jejunostomy tubes are
          prone to obstruction.
      (4) Nasoduodenal tubes are prone to dislodgment.

E. Enteral Formulas

1. Carbohydrate
   a. Starch (fruit, vegetables, cereals)
   b. Glucose polymers
   c. Monosaccharides (glucose, fructose)
   d. Disaccharides (sucrose, lactose, maltose)
   e. Polysaccharides
2. Fat
   a. Vegetable oils
   b. Medium-chain triglycerides
      (1) Transported directly into the portal system
      (2) Do not require elaborate digestive and absorptive
          steps

   (3) Indicated in patients with fat absorption abnormalities
   c. Milk butterfat
3. Protein
   a. Intact protein
   b. Partially hydrolyzed protein (dipeptides, tripeptides, and oligopeptides)
   c. Amino acids
4. Vitamins and minerals
   a. Vitamins and minerals are present in nutritional formulations in adequate quantities so that daily requirements are satisfied when caloric support is complete.
   b. Care must be taken to determine vitamin and mineral intake if diluted formulas are utilized or total caloric intake is insufficient.
   c. Vitamin and mineral supplements are available and may be added to enteral feedings as indicated.
5. Fiber (occasionally referred to as residue)
   a. Fiber is thought to be clinically beneficial.
   b. Content varies among enteral formulations (residue-free, low-residue, and fiber-supplemented diets).
6. Glutamine
   a. Primary fuel source of a number of rapidly dividing cells
      (1) Enterocytes and colonocytes
      (2) Lymphocytes
   b. Increased uptake and metabolism during stress
   c. Experimental evidence that absence from the diet results in progressive intestinal atrophy with the following:
      (1) Breakdown of the mucosal barrier
      (2) Bacterial translocation
      (3) Sepsis
   d. Generally present in only small quantities in most enteral formulations
      (1) The instability of glutamine in solution precludes its routine addition to most enteral formulas.
      (2) Glutamine supplements are available in the form of L-glutamine powder; the recommended daily dose is 6 to 8 g/day.
7. Osmolality
   a. Reflects the protein, carbohydrate, amino acid, electrolyte, and mineral content of the solution

b. Generally ranges from 200 to 900 mOsm/kg in commercial formulas
c. Side effects of high osmolality (hypertonic) feeding solutions
   (1) Delayed gastric emptying
   (2) Diarrhea
   (3) Dehydration
   (4) Electrolyte abnormalities

8. Formula selection
   a. Determine the actual energy requirement of the patient.
   b. Determine protein requirements.
      (1) Daily protein requirements vary for a number of clinical conditions.
         (a) Recommended daily allowance: 0.8-1 g/kg
         (b) Low stress—maintenance: 1.0-1.2 g/kg
         (c) Low stress—anabolic: 1.3-1.7 g/kg
         (d) Hypermetabolic (trauma, sepsis): 1.5-2.5 g/kg
         (e) Severe burns: 2-3 g/kg
         (f) Liver failure: 0.5-1.5 g/kg
         (g) Renal failure—without dialysis: 0.5-0.6 g/kg
         (h) Renal failure—hemodialysis: 1.2-1.4 g/kg
         (i) Renal transplant: 1.3-1.5 g/kg
      (2) Calculation of daily protein requirement is the following:

         Protein requirement in g
            = (patient's weight in kg)
            × (protein requirement for illness in g/kg)

   c. Determine nonprotein caloric requirements.
      (1) Calories required from nonprotein sources = (total required calories) − (required protein calories)
      (2) Fat
         (a) Efficient source of energy
         (b) Provides essential fatty acids
         (c) Should be approximately 20% to 30% of the calories obtained from nonprotein sources
         (d) Exercise caution in hyperlipidemic patients
      (3) Carbohydrate
         (a) The remaining 70% to 80% of nonprotein calories are obtained from carbohydrates.

        (b) Closely monitor blood sugar levels of glucose intolerant patients.

   d. Calorie to nitrogen ratio

     (1) Nitrogen constitutes approximately 16% of protein (6.25 g of protein = 1 g of nitrogen).

     (2) A calorie to nitrogen ratio of 100 to 150:1 is desirable in the postoperative setting.

        (a) A patient requiring and receiving 100 g of protein will receive 16 g of nitrogen.

        (b) Utilizing the calorie to nitrogen ratio, the appropriate nonprotein calories would range from 1600 to 2400 kcal/day.

F. Administration of Enteral Nutrition

  1. Stomach

   a. Intermittent (bolus) feeding

     (1) Begin with approximately 100 ml of half-strength hyperosmolar formula or 100 ml of full-strength isotonic formula administered q4h.

     (2) If tolerated for the first 3 or 4 feedings, hyperosmolar formulas may be advanced to three fourths and full strength at 8 to 12 hour intervals.

     (3) Once full-strength feedings are tolerated, then the volume should be advanced by 50 to 100 ml every 8 to 12 hours as tolerated, until full support is achieved.

     (4) Gastric residuals must be checked prior to each intermittent feeding.

     (5) The tube must be flushed with 25 to 50 ml of water after each feeding.

   b. Continuous infusion

     (1) Initiate with half-strength hyperosmolar or full-strength isotonic formula

        (a) Begin at rate of 50 ml/hr.

        (b) Increase rate by 25 ml/hr every 8 hours as tolerated until appropriate rate achieved.

     (2) Hyperosmolar formulas are increased to three fourths and then full strength at 8 hour intervals.

     (3) Residuals should be assessed every 4 hours.

     (4) The tube should be flushed regularly with water.

  2. Small intestine

   a. Route most likely to be utilized in the critically ill

   b. Must administer infusions continuously, not intermittently
      (1) Initiate feedings with half-strength hyperosmolar or full-strength isotonic formula, approximately 50 ml/hour.
      (2) Increase rate by 25 ml/hour every 8 hours as tolerated until the appropriate rate is achieved.
      (3) Hyperosmolar formulas should be increased to three fourths and then full strength at 8 hour intervals.
      (4) Frequent flushing with water is imperative (small bore tube clogs easily).

G. Monitoring
1. Physical examination
   a. General
      (1) Progression or reversal of fat and muscle wasting
      (2) Alteration in severity of ascites and peripheral edema
      (3) Change in anthropometric measures
   b. Abdominal examination for distention
   c. Daily weights
2. Accurate recording of total input and output
3. Laboratory studies
   a. Potassium
      (1) Hypokalemia is the most common electrolyte abnormality associated with tube feeding.
      (2) Hyperkalemia may also occur.
   b. Glucose
      (1) Causes of hyperglycemia
         (a) High carbohydrate levels in enteral formulas
         (b) Diabetes
         (c) Glucose intolerance associated with major illness or sepsis
      (2) Treatment of hyperglycemia
         (a) Treat underlying condition.
         (b) Utilize insulin as necessary.

H. Complications of Enteral Feeding
1. Diarrhea
   a. Occurs in 60% to 70% of critically ill patients receiving enteral alimentation.
   b. Etiology in this subset of patients is variable.
      (1) Rate of infusion too rapid
      (2) Excessive osmolality
      (3) Bacterial contamination of the formula

      (4) Underlying disease process

  c. Treatment includes the following:

      (1) Search for the etiology.

      (2) Treat the underlying conditions.

      (3) Diet-related causes may be managed by decreasing the infusion rate or osmolality.

2. Aspiration pneumonia

3. Tube misplacement

4. Tube dislodgment

I. Comorbid Conditions Influencing Enteral Nutrition

1. Renal failure

  a. Dialysis judiciously employed to correct abnormalities

  b. Limited ability to handle nitrogenous waste

      (1) Adjust the daily protein provision.

        (a) Renal failure without dialysis: 0.5 to 0.6 g/kg/day

        (b) Renal failure with hemodialysis: 1.2 to 1.4 g/kg/day

        (c) Renal failure with peritoneal dialysis: 1.2 to 1.6 g/kg/day

      (2) Catabolic illness in any patient produces an increased demand for nitrogen.

      (3) Adequate supplementation must be provided to achieve positive nitrogen balance.

      (4) Frequent dialysis is usually necessary to remove nitrogenous wastes.

  c. Electrolytes: Estimates of the daily electrolyte supplementation for critically ill renal failure patients with normal electrolyte levels

      (1) Potassium: 40 to 60 mEq/day

      (2) Sodium: 40 to 50 mEq/L

      (3) Phosphorus: 200 to 400 mg/day

      (4) Calcium: 800 mg/day

      (5) Magnesium: 100 mg/day

2. Hepatic failure

  a. Hepatic encephalopathy: Protein intolerance reflected by worsening encephalopathy

  b. Management

      (1) Protein restriction

      (2) Intravenous glucose to limit protein catabolism until encephalopathy resolves

      (3) Protein administered enterally as tolerated once encephalopathy resolves

3. Cardiac failure
    a. Etiology of malnourishment with severe cardiac disease
        (1) Chronic malnutrition
        (2) Hypercatabolism associated with severe illness
    b. Management
        (1) Fluid restriction is usually necessary.
        (2) Formulas that have high caloric density (1.5 to 2 kcal/ml) are useful.
        (3) Advance enteral diets by increasing the concentration before the rate is increased (limits fluid).
4. Glucose intolerance
    a. Alterations in glucose metabolism in critically ill patients
        (1) Increased hepatic glucose production
        (2) Insensitivity of organs and tissues to the effects of insulin
    b. Clinical approach
        (1) Determine the etiology of the glucose intolerance.
            (a) Rule out sepsis.
            (b) Treat the underlying cause.
        (2) Consider limiting the carbohydrate content of enteral alimentation.

III. PARENTERAL NUTRITION
A. Indications
1. Massive small bowel resection (short bowel syndrome)
2. Impaired intestinal motility
3. High-output enterocutaneous fistulas not amenable to enteral feeding
4. Radiation enteritis
5. Complicated inflammatory bowel disease
6. Moderate to severe acute pancreatitis
7. Intensive chemotherapy
8. Anticipated inability to utilize the intestinal tract within 7 to 10 days

B. Contraindications
1. Functional GI tract
2. TPN required for less than 7 to 10 days
3. Aggressive nutritional support not desired by patient
4. Risks of TPN exceed possible benefits

C. Advantages
1. Provides satisfactory nutrition for patients with nonfunctioning or absent intestinal tracts

    2. Can be tailored to meet the specific needs of patients with a variety of disorders

    3. Allows infusion of hyperosmolar solutions

       a. High caloric density tolerated

       b. May allow fluid restriction while maintaining adequate nutritional support

D. Disadvantages

    1. Development of disuse atrophy of the intestinal tract

    2. Not a physiologic method of nutrient delivery

    3. Necessary cannulation of a large vein

    4. Expense

    5. Electrolyte abnormalities

    6. Metabolic complications

    7. Liver enzyme elevations

       a. Elevated transaminase most common

       b. Usually peak at 10 to 15 days, then resolve

E. Components of TPN Solutions

    1. Fluid requirement

       a. Patients receiving TPN require an additional 500 to 800 ml/day of fluid in excess of maintenance fluid requirements.

         (1) Decreased endogenous water production associated with anabolism

         (2) Endogenous water generated in catabolic patients by proteolysis and the oxidation of fat

       b. Ongoing fluid losses include the following:

         (1) Measurable losses: Wound drainage, diarrhea

         (2) Immeasurable losses: Third-space losses

         (3) Ventilated patients: Loss of fluid through the ventilator circuit

         (4) Elevated body temperature: Additional 350 to 400 ml fluid loss per day for each degree elevated

    2. Caloric requirements

       a. Calculation of energy requirements

       b. Energy sources

         (1) Carbohydrate

            (a) The most common source in TPN is dextrose (caloric value = 3.4 kcal/g).

            (b) The dextrose concentration of commercially available solutions ranges from 2.5% to 70%.

            (c) Dextrose usually constitutes 50% to 80% of the caloric content.

    (2) Fat
        (a) Efficient source of calories
        (b) Provides essential fatty acids (2% to 4% of nonprotein calories in the form of fat necessary to prevent essential fatty acid deficiency)
        (c) Fat emulsions available in concentrations of 10% (1.1 kcal/ml) and 20% (2.2 kcal/ml)
        (d) Usually constitutes 20% to 50% of daily caloric requirements
        (e) May facilitate weaning ventilator-dependent patients by reducing carbohydrate and increasing fat effecting a decrease in the respiratory quotient
    (3) Protein
        (a) Determine the protein requirement (usually 1 to 2 g/kg/day).
        (b) Maintain calorie to nitrogen ratio of 135 to 200:1.
        (c) Administered as amino acids.
        (d) Protein facilitates anabolism, specifically protein synthesis.
        (e) Patients with severe catabolic stress utilize protein as an energy source.
  c. Electrolytes
    (1) Approximate daily requirements are the following:
        (a) Sodium: 1 to 2 mEq/kg/day
        (b) Potassium: 1 to 2 mEq/kg/day
        (c) Chloride: 1 to 2 mEq/kg/day
        (d) Calcium: 0.2 to 0.3 mEq/kg/day
        (e) Magnesium: 0.25 to 0.35 mEq/kg/day
        (f) Phosphate: 7 to 9 mmol/1000 kcal/day
    (2) The electrolyte content of amino acid solutions should be taken into account prior to supplementation.
  d. Vitamins
    (1) Fat- and water-soluble vitamin supplements must be added to TPN solutions.
    (2) Formulations for adults do not contain vitamin K. Add vitamin K directly to TPN solution, 1 to 2 mg/day, or administer SQ or IM 5 to 10 mg/week.
  e. Trace element recommended daily supplementation: Zinc, copper, manganese, chromium, selenium

f. Other additives
   (1) Albumin: 25 g/day in TPN solution until appropriate serum levels achieved
   (2) Heparin (1000 U/L): To decrease the risk of catheter thrombosis
   (3) Insulin: For patients with glucose intolerance
g. Glutamine
   (1) Presently not in TPN solutions
      (a) Glutamic acid has been added to some solutions.
      (b) Lability of glutamine has precluded its addition to solutions.
   (2) May be added to TPN in future

F. Monitoring
1. Accurate assessment of daily input and output
2. Daily weights
3. Physical examination
   a. Decreased fat and muscle wasting
   b. Decreased ascites and peripheral edema
   c. Improved anthropometric measures
4. Laboratory studies
   a. Daily
      (1) Serum electrolytes and BUN
      (2) Serum glucose
   b. Twice weekly
      (1) Serum electrolytes (Ca, P, and Mg)
      (2) Blood studies (Hb, hct, WBC)
      (3) Urine glucose, ketones, and specific gravity
   c. Weekly
      (1) Liver function tests (transaminases, bilirubin, and alkaline phosphatase)
      (2) Visceral protein indicators (albumin, transferrin and prealbumin)
      (3) Triglyceride level (provides indication of patient's ability to tolerate lipid infusion)
      (4) Nitrogen balance (indicative of adequacy of nutritional support)

G. Discontinuing TPN
1. TPN infusion is associated with increased serum insulin levels.
   a. Sudden cessation of TPN is occasionally associated with hypoglycemia.

b. Hypoglycemia can occur in as few as 15 minutes.
2. Methods of tapering TPN include the following:
   a. Elective taper
      (1) If patient receiving > 500 g of glucose per day, decrease glucose by 250 g per day to 500 g per day.
      (2) When 500 g/day of glucose is attained, discontinue TPN and administer 5% dextrose at 75 to 125 ml/hour for 6 to 8 hours.
      (3) Remove TPN catheter.
   b. Emergent taper
      (1) Indications
         (a) Catheter sepsis
         (b) Emergency surgery
      (2) Procedure
         (a) Administer 5% dextrose (with ¼ or ½ NS and potassium) at the same rate TPN was infused prior to cessation.
         (b) Restart TPN when appropriate.

H. Comorbid Conditions Influencing Parenteral Nutrition

1. Renal failure
   a. Concentrated solutions of carbohydrate, fat, and amino acids may be utilized so that total volume of infusion is decreased.
   b. Dialysis should be utilized liberally so full nutritional support may be maintained.
2. Hepatic failure
   a. Patients with mild liver failure are capable of tolerating TPN solutions.
   b. Patients with moderately severe hepatic dysfunction have depressed levels of branched-chain amino acids and may benefit from formulas with increased levels.
   c. Patients with fulminant hepatic failure may be difficult to manage.
      (1) Continuous infusion of glucose is necessary to limit CNS damage.
      (2) Amino acids (especially branched-chain) are required to serve as substrates for liver regeneration.
3. Cardiac failure
   a. Patients are unable to tolerate large volume loads.
   b. Use concentrated solutions of carbohydrate, fat, and amino acids.
4. Pulmonary failure

   a. Patients with respiratory muscle weakness or acute pulmonary parenchymal disease should receive standard TPN solutions.
   b. Patients with chronic obstructive lung disease would probably benefit from decreased respiratory quotient and increase fat and decrease carbohydrate calories.
5. Glucose intolerance
   a. Blood glucose levels must be under control prior to the initiation of TPN.
   b. TPN should be advanced slowly in these patients over a period of a few days.
   c. Blood glucose levels must be monitored closely.
   d. Administer insulin.
      (1) One half of the patient's daily maintenance insulin dose should be placed in the initial TPN solution bag and then adjusted as necessary in subsequent bags.
      (2) Some patients may require separate TPN and insulin drips so that blood glucose may be managed more precisely.

SUGGESTED READING

Deitel M: *Nutrition in clinical surgery,* ed 2, Baltimore, 1985, Williams and Wilkins.

Grant JP: *Handbook of total parenteral nutrition,* ed 2, Philadelphia, 1992, WB Saunders.

Rombeau, JL, Caldwell, MD: *Clinical nutrition: enteral and tube feeding,* ed 2, Philadelphia, 1990, WB Saunders.

Rombeau JL, Caldwell MD: *Clinical nutrition: parenteral nutrition,* ed 2, Philadelphia, 1993, WB Saunders.

Wilmore DW: *The metabolic management of the critically ill,* New York, 1977, Plenum Medical Book.

ANESTHESIA 23

Clarence H. Owen

I. **GOALS OF ANESTHETIC ADMINISTRATION**
A. **Safety During Surgical Procedures and Intensive Care Monitoring**
   1. Minimize or eliminate patient motion.
   2. Facilitate placement/maintenance of monitoring systems.
   3. Ensure adequate oxygenation, ventilation, circulation at all times.
B. **Homeostasis of Body Functions**
   1. Optimize conditions for maintenance of respiratory and circulatory functions.
   2. Minimize fluctuations in function caused by stress and anesthetic agents.
C. **Optimization of the Patient's Experience**
   1. Provide insensibility during invasive procedures.
   2. Provide relief of pain and anxiety.
D. **Anesthesia**
   1. General anesthesia: The state of unconsciousness brought about by irregular descending depression of the central nervous system; divided into four well-defined clinical stages:
      a. Stage I: Induction period—gradually increasing amnesia, analgesia
      b. Stage II: Onset of unconsciousness—unpredictable reactions, involuntary movements, irregular respirations, persistence of reflexes, loss of all volitional responses
      c. Stage III: Surgical anesthesia—progressive obtundation, gradual loss of protective reflexes, progressive hypoventilation and generalized paralysis
      d. Stage IV: Medullary paralysis—respiratory arrest, myocardial depression, obtundation of catecholamine release, flaccid paralysis

2. Regional anesthesia: Insensibility of an anatomic portion of the body produced by interruption of the sensory nerve conductivity of that region

3. Balanced anesthesia: Utilization of a combination of anesthetic agents to provide the desired effect while minimizing the potential undesirable effects of any given agent

II. INDUCTION AGENTS

Induction agents produce a state of unconsciousness via progressive depression of the CNS.

A. Barbiturates

Thiopental, thiamylal, methohexital

1. Indications and mode of action
   a. Ultrashort onset of action (30 seconds), excellent for induction
   b. Depress reticular activating system, augment inhibitory tone of CNS GABA pathways, depress release of CNS excitatory neurotransmitters
   c. Produce no analgesia
2. Pharmacology
   a. Early reawakening (5 to 10 minutes) as a result of tissue redistribution, high lipid solubility
   b. Metabolized to inactive products by the liver, excreted by the kidneys
   c. Long elimination half-life a result of redistribution
3. Side effects
   a. Dose-dependent decrease in BP, myocardial contractility; minimal effect on HR
   b. Dose-dependent decrease in respiratory rate, tidal volume; occasionally apnea
4. Dosage and administration (induction): 3 to 4 mg/kg thiopental, 0.7 to 1 mg/kg methohexital

B. Ketamine

1. Indications and mode of action
   a. Usually used for induction
   b. Produces analgesia, amnesia, "dissociative" anesthesia (eyes open, normal muscle tone)
   c. Useful for short, painful procedures in ICU setting
2. Pharmacology: An arylcyclohexylamine, similar to phencyclidine
3. Side effects

      a. Mildly depresses respiration, with minimal effect on responsiveness to hypercarbia; less likely to produce apnea than barbiturates

      b. Activates the sympathetic nervous system, causing increased HR, BP; ideal for hypovolemic patients; contraindicated in patients with CAD

      c. Causes cerebral vasodilation and increased intracranial pressure; contraindicated in patients with increased intracranial pressure or space-occupying lesions

      d. Stimulates oral secretions necessitating pretreatment with an antisialogogue (glycopyrrolate 0.1 to 0.2 mg IM/IV or atropine 0.2 mg IM/IV)

      e. Often associated with restlessness, agitation, hallucinations during emergence from anesthesia, which may be treated/prevented with benzodiazepines

   4. Dosage and administration

      a. Induction: 1 to 2 mg/kg IV or 5 to 10 mg/kg IM

      b. Sedation: 0.2 mg/kg IV (titrated to effect)

C. Etomidate

   1. Indications and mode of action

      a. Ultrashort onset of action (30 seconds); often used for induction

      b. Appears to augment inhibitory tone of GABA pathways in the CNS

   2. Pharmacology

      a. An imidazole-containing hypnotic, unrelated to other anesthetic agents

      b. Early reawakening (3 to 5 minutes) as a result of tissue redistribution

   3. Side effects

      a. Minimal effects on BP, HR, myocardial contractility; ideal for compromised patients

      b. Dose-dependent depression of respiratory rate, tidal volume (less than barbiturates)

      c. Reduces cerebral blood flow and metabolism; ideal for patients with increased ICP, but may activate seizure foci, precipitate myoclonus

      d. Occasionally associated with postoperative nausea and vomiting

      e. May suppress adrenal corticosteroid synthesis, particularly after prolonged infusion

   4. Dosage and administration (induction): 0.3 mg/kg IV

D. **Propofol**
1. Indications and usage
   a. Unknown mode of action
   b. Useful as induction agent, for continuous anesthesia or sedation
   c. Produces no analgesia
2. Pharmacology
   a. Rapid onset of action (30 to 45 seconds); conscious sedation with low dosages
   b. Early reawakening as a result of tissue redistribution
3. Side effects
   a. Dose-dependent decrease in respiratory rate, tidal volume; occasionally apnea
   b. Dose-dependent decrease in BP, myocardial contractility; minimal effect on HR
4. Dosage and administration
   a. Induction: 2 to 2.5 mg/kg IV
   b. Continuous infusion for maintenance of anesthesia: 0.1 to 0.2 mg/kg/min
   c. Continuous infusion for sedation: 3 to 4 mg/kg/hr
   d. 1% isotonic oil-in-water emulsion containing egg lecithin, glycerol and soybean oil; high associated venous irritation; caution with use in patients with lipid disorders, pancreatitis, or history of allergy to egg products

III. **INHALATION ANESTHETIC AGENTS**
A. **Indications and Mode of Action**
1. Typically used for maintenance of general anesthesia rather than induction, although often used as induction agents in pediatric patients
2. Generally not used in the ICU setting, but effects must be considered in postoperative patients
3. Interaction with cellular membranes in CNS
B. **Pharmacology**
1. The rate of absorption/elimination is a function of the agent's solubility in blood; decreased solubility leads to increased rates of absorption/elimination.
2. Elimination is predominantly via exhalation, although hepatic metabolism contributes for the more blood-soluble agents (especially halothane, up to 15%)
3. Dosages are expressed as minimal alveolar concentration

or the percent atmospheric pressure at which movement in response to skin incision is inhibited in 50% of patients.

C. **Specific Agents**

1. Nitrous oxide
    a. Relatively low solubility, high rate of absorption/ elimination
    b. Dose-dependent analgesia, but high minimal alveolar concentration precludes ability to obtain surgical anesthesia
    c. Often used in combination with other inhalational agents, increasing alveolar concentration of second gas at lower total inspired volumes
    d. Causes mild myocardial and respiratory depression, sympathetic activation
    e. May increase pulmonary vascular resistance in adults
    f. May limit Fio_2 during administration and cause diffusion hypoxia following cessation of administration due to rapid diffusion from blood into alveoli
    g. Should be avoided in the presence of closed gas-containing spaces (pneumothorax, obstructed bowel, occluded middle ear, air embolus, etc.) because of expansion caused by diffusion of nitrous oxide into closed spaces in exchange for nitrogen

2. Volatile agents (halothane, enflurane, isoflurane)
    a. Liquids at standard temperature and pressure with potent evaporative vapors
    b. Produce unconsciousness and amnesia at relatively low inspired concentrations
    c. Rate of absorption/elimination inversely proportional to solubility in blood:

       Halothane > enflurane > isoflurane
       > desflurane > sevoflurane

    d. Tend to increase cerebral blood flow and decrease cerebral metabolism
    e. Produce dose-dependent myocardial depression and systemic vasodilation
    f. May sensitize the myocardium to arrhythmogenic effects of catecholamines

      g. Produce dose-dependent respiratory depression (decreased tidal volume)

      h. Tend to cause bronchodilation but may be bronchial irritants/precipitate bronchospasm

      i. Tend to decrease hepatic perfusion; rarely associated with hepatitis (halothane)

      j. Tend to decrease renal perfusion; rarely associated with nephrotoxicity as a result of release of fluoride ions (enflurane and sevoflurane)

IV. NEUROMUSCULAR BLOCKING AGENTS

A. Indications and Mode of Action

    1. Act via interference with normal acetylcholine neuromuscular transmission

    2. Cause generalized paralysis, facilitating endotracheal intubation and/or mechanical ventilation, decreasing systemic Vo_2, and optimizing surgical conditions

    3. Must be used in conjunction with other agents providing analgesic and/or amnestic effects

    4. Necessitate mechanical ventilation

B. Depolarizing Agents

Succinylcholine

    1. Pharmacology

      a. Binds and activates the acetylcholine receptor, leading to normal postjunctional depolarization

      b. Degraded much more slowly than acetylcholine; requires plasma cholinesterase activity

      c. Leads to muscle fasciculation followed by relaxation, absence of posttetanic potentiation, absence of fade following tetanic or train-of-four stimulation

    2. Side effects

      a. May cause transient increases in HR and BP as a result of vagolytic effects

      b. May cause transient increases in intraocular and intragastric pressures (fasciculation)

      c. May cause an elevation of serum potassium levels up to 0.5 mEq/L due to sustained depolarization; should be avoided in patients with renal insufficiency or hyperkalemia

      d. May lead to prolonged neuromuscular blockade in patients with the following:

 (1) Low levels of plasma cholinesterase: Patients with burns, shock, cardiac failure, liver insufficiency, starvation, hypothyroidism, third trimester of pregnancy

 (2) Pharmacologic inhibition of cholinesterase resulting from anticholinesterases, echothiophate eye drops, phenelzine (monoamine oxidase inhibitor), organophosphate compounds

 (3) Atypical plasma cholinesterase—4% of population heterozygous, 1/2800 homozygous

C.   **Nondepolarizing Agents**

 Pancuronium, vecuronium, atracurium

 1. Competitive inhibition with acetylcholine (bind receptor, no postjunctional depolarization)

 2. Action terminated by redistribution and subsequent metabolism of agent

 3. Two pharmacologic classes—steroid derivatives and benzylisoquinolines

 4. Leads to relaxation without fasciculation, posttetanic potentiation, and the presence of fade following tetanic or train-of-four stimulation

 5. Vary on rate of onset, duration of action, cardiovascular side effects, and metabolism

D.   **Dosage and Administration (Table 23-1)**

TABLE 23-1.

Neuromuscular Blocking Agents

Agent	Dose (mg/kg)	Onset (min)	Duration (min)	Elimination
Depolarizing				
Succincylcholine	0.5-1	1	5-10	Plasma cholinesterase
Nondepolarizing				
Pancuronium*	0.05-0.10	2-5	45-60	80% renal
Vecuronium†	0.05-0.10	2-3	25-30	80% hepatic
Atracurium‡	0.4-0.5	2-3	25-30	Hofmann elimination
Anticholinesterases				
Edrophonium	0.5-1	1	40-65	70% renal, 30% hepatic
Neostigmine	0.03-0.06	7	55-75	50% renal, 50% hepatic
Pyridostigmine	0.25	10-13	80-130	75% renal, 25% hepatic

*Repeat doses of 20%-25% initial dose may be given every 45-60 min to maintain relaxation

†Vecuronium dose for continuous infusion = 1 g/kg/min

‡Atracurium dose for continuous infusion = 6-8 g/kg/min

E. **Reversal of Neuromuscular Blockade**

1. Recovery following administration of succinylcholine cannot be reversed pharmacologically but typically occurs within 10 to 15 minutes (except situations noted above).

2. Action of nondepolarizing agents may be reversed by administration of anticholinesterases which cause a transient increase in acetylcholine available for competition at neuromuscular junction.

3. Anticholinesterase administration causes peripheral side effects (bradycardia, salivation) resulting from effects of acetylcholine on muscarinic receptors (may be attenuated with atropine or glycopyrrolate)

V. **BENZODIAZEPINES**

Diazepam, midazolam, lorazepam

A. **Indications and Mode of Action**

1. Produce dose-dependent sedative, amnestic, muscle relaxant, and anticonvulsant effects

2. Produce no analgesia, often used in combination with opioids for effects ranging from control of mild postoperative pain/anxiety to maintenance of general anesthesia

3. Bind to specific receptors in the CNS, seem to enhance inhibitory tone of GABA pathways

B. **Pharmacology**

1. Metabolized in the liver; activity prolonged in elderly or patients with hepatic insufficiency

2. Rapid conversion of midazolam to inactive metabolites in the liver (relatively short duration)

3. Conversion of diazepam and lorazepam to active metabolites (longer duration of action)

C. **Side Effects**

1. Produce mild depression in BP and cardiac output; may be more pronounced when given rapidly or with a narcotic, particularly in hemodynamically compromised patients

2. Produce mild, dose-dependent depression in respiratory rate and tidal volume; may be more pronounced in elderly or debilitated patients, particularly if administered with a narcotic

3. Associated with variable response between patients; requires careful monitoring

4. Associated with birth defects when administered during pregnancy, especially first trimester

5. Should be avoided in patients receiving valproate; may precipitate psychotic episode

D. **Dosage and Administration** (Table 23-2)

E. **Benzodiazepine Reversal**

Flumazenil

1. Competitive antagonist
2. Should be used cautiously in patients on long-term therapy or patients treated for seizures
3. Dosage: 0.3 mg IV bolus, repeated q30-60sec up to 5 mg

VI. NARCOTICS

Morphine, meperidine, fentanyl

A. **Indications and Mode of Action**

1. Dose-dependent analgesia and sedation; anesthesia in high-dose administration
2. Act at specific opioid (endorphin) receptors in the brain and spinal cord

B. **Pharmacology**

Primarily metabolized by the liver, excreted by the kidneys

C. **Side Effects**

1. Minimal cardiovascular effects, although may cause bradycardia (central vagal stimulation) and/or peripheral vasodilation (sympathetic depression and/or histamine release)
2. Dose-dependent respiratory depression, particularly decreased respiratory rate and diminished response to hypercarbia; apnea with large doses
3. Smooth muscle stimulation resulting in increased GI secretions and decreased motility, precipitating gastric retention, biliary colic, constipation, urinary retention
4. Nausea and vomiting due to direct stimulation of the chemoreceptor trigger zone

TABLE 23-2.

Intravenous Benzodiazepines

Agent	Induction Dose (mg/kg)	Sedation Dose (mg)	Onset (min)	Elimination $t_{1/2}$ (hr)
Midazolam	0.15-0.35	0.5-1	1-2	2-4
Diazepam	0.3-0.4	2.5-5	4-8	20
Lorazepam	0.04-0.06	0.5	20-40	15

5. Dose-dependent muscle rigidity, particularly of thoracic and abdominal musculature

6. Dose-dependent pupillary constriction (miosis), often useful for monitoring effect of agent

D.   Dosage and Administration

1. Intravenous dosages of commonly used agents are summarized in Table 23-3.

2. Patient-controlled anesthesia is a popular method of postoperative pain control in which individual bolus administration of narcotics is provided upon demand by the patient via an intravenous pump system, incorporating preset incremental dosage amounts and maximum numbers of doses per unit time. The initial "loading" dose often facilitates delivery of adequate analgesia, and dosage parameters are titrated based upon utilization and symptomatology.

E.   Narcotic Reversal

Naloxone

1. Competitive antagonist to narcotics at opioid receptors

2. Dose-dependent reversal of narcotic effects

3. Peak CNS effects within 1 to 2 minutes; diminished effects within 30 minutes

4. May precipitate abrupt onset of pain with associated hypertension, tachycardia

5. Dosage: 0.04 mg IV bolus repeated q2-3min to reach desired effect; may be given IM

6. Crosses the placenta; may decrease neonatal respiratory depression caused by narcotics

VII.   NONNARCOTIC ANALGESIC AGENTS

Ketorolac

TABLE 23-3.

Intravenous Narcotics

Agent	Relative Potency	Analgesic Dose (mg/kg)	PCA Dose (mg)*	Elimination $t_{1/2}$ (hr)
Morphine	1	0.05-0.20	0.5-3	3-4
Meperidine	0.1	0.5-2	5-30	3-4
Fentanyl	100	0.001-0.002	0.01-0.08	4-7

*PCA: Patient-controlled analgesia

A. **Indications and Mode of Action**
1. Parenteral NSAID recently approved in U.S.
2. Adjunct to narcotic agents for management of acute pain
3. Inhibition of cyclooxygenase; decreased prostaglandin synthesis

B. **Pharmacology**
1. Onset of action approximately 10 minutes, duration 4 to 8 hours
2. Metabolized in the liver; excreted by the liver and kidneys
3. Dosage: 30 to 60 mg, followed by 15 to 30 mg q6hr (IV, IM, or PO)

C. **Side Effects**
Similar to other NSAIDs
1. Gastric irritation and ulceration
2. Renal dysfunction
3. Platelet dysfunction

VIII. LOCAL ANESTHETIC AGENTS

A. **Indications and Mode of Action**
1. Temporary local or regional anesthesia
2. Blockade of local nerve action potential propagation via specific interaction of ionized moiety with receptors on intracellular portion of axonal Na^+ channels, inhibiting Na^+ ion influx

B. **Pharmacology**
1. Composed of aromatic ring (hydrophobic) and a tertiary amine (hydrophilic) connected by either ester or amide linkage
2. All weak bases; degree of ionization relevant to lipid solubility and ability to cross axonal membrane (directly correlates with potency, rate of onset)
3. Duration of effect related to degree of protein binding, mechanism of metabolism
4. Esters rapidly degraded by plasma cholinesterase to inactive products including p-aminobenzoic acid (may cause allergic reactions)
5. Amides degraded by n-dealkylation and hydrolysis, primarily in the liver—toxicity possibly more likely in patients with hepatic insufficiency
6. Adjuvant agents
   a. Epinephrine: Prolongs duration of anesthesia, decreases systemic toxicity and bleeding, increases

    intensity of nerve block; must be avoided in areas with poor collateral blood flow (nose, digits, penis)

    b. Sodium bicarbonate: Raises the pH, increasing concentration of nonionized base; increases rate of onset of blockade and decreases pain associated with local infiltration

C. Side Effects

1. Allergic reactions: Rare; must be differentiated from common responses (syncope, vasovagal)
2. Systemic reactions: Usually due to accidental intravascular injection or overdose
3. CNS toxicity: Restlessness, lightheadedness, tinnitus, metallic taste, circumoral numbness, muscle twitching, loss of consciousness, generalized seizure, apnea, coma

    a. Treatment consists of stopping administration of the drug and ventilation with 100% O_2. Utilize anticonvulsant therapy as indicated with diazepam or thiopental.

    b. Intubation and neuromuscular blockade may be necessary when other therapies fail.

4. Cardiovascular toxicity: Decreased conduction, depressed contractility, loss of peripheral vasomotor tone, cardiovascular collapse

    a. Treat with 100% O_2, volume replacement, and inotropic agents as needed.

    b. Intravascular injection of bupivacaine is particularly toxic and may require prolonged CPR until effects of the drug have subsided.

IX. TECHNIQUES OF REGIONAL ANESTHESIA

A. Spinal (Subarachnoid) Anesthesia

1. Indications and mode of action

    a. Surgical anesthesia (either used alone or in combination with general anesthesia) is occasionally useful for postoperative pain management.

    b. The effect of a direct blockade of spinal nerves is greater on smaller fibers (pain) than on larger fibers (motor, proprioception).

2. Pharmacology

    a. Agents most commonly utilized include lidocaine, bupivacaine, tetracaine (with or without epinephrine), either as isobaric, hyperbaric, or hypobaric solutions

       b. May use morphine or fentanyl for postoperative pain control

   3. Side effects

       a. Hypotension: Related to degree of sympathetic blockade

       b. Dyspnea: Caused by proprioceptive blockade or apnea with direct C3-C5 blockade; delayed respiratory depression occasionally following narcotic administration

       c. Nausea and vomiting: Caused by hypotension or unopposed vagal stimulation

       d. Headache: Usually 24 to 48 hours postoperatively as a result of continued CSF leak; usually managed conservatively, occasionally requiring "blood patch"

       e. Urinary retention: Sacral blockade with atonic bladder

       f. Infection: Rare

   4. Dosage and administration (Table 23-4)

B. Epidural Anesthesia

   1. Indications and mode of action

       a. Surgical anesthesia and/or postoperative pain control

       b. Administered as single dose, multiple injections, or continuous infusion

       c. Catheter may be left in place for several days

TABLE 23-4.

Neuroaxial Local Anesthetics and Narcotics

Agent	Epidural		Subarachnoid	
	Dose (mg)	Duration (hr)	Dose (mg)	Duration (hr)
Local Anesthetics				
Procaine	—	—	120	0.5-1
Chloroprocaine	80	0.5	—	—
Tetracaine	—	—	12	1.5-2
Tetracaine/ epinephrine	—	—	12	3-5
Lidocaine	50	0.75-1.5	60	0.5-1
Bupivacaine	20-25	2-4	9	1.5-2
Narcotics				
Morphine	1-10	6-24	0.1-0.5	8-24
Meperidine	200-200	6-8	10-30	10-30
Fentanyl	0.025-0.15	4-6	0.025	3-6

      d. Acts at spinal nerve roots located laterally in epidural space

      e. Caudal blocks: Administration of anesthesia into caudal space, the direct extension of the epidural space below the sacral hiatus

  2. Pharmacology

      a. Chlorprocaine and bupivacaine are used most commonly.

      b. Narcotics are often used for postoperative pain control.

  3. Side effects

      a. Similar to subarachnoid anesthesia

      b. Epidural hematoma: Uncommon, but may require urgent laminectomy when severe; epidural anesthesia relatively contraindicated in patients requiring systemic anticoagulation

      c. Dural puncture: Can be managed by conversion to spinal anesthesia or replacement at higher level; may result in inadvertent total spinal anesthesia if unrecognized

      d. Direct spinal cord injury, nerve root trauma, anterior spinal cord ischemia (uncommon)

  4. Dosage and administration: Summarized in Table 23-4

C. Regional Nerve Blocks

  1. Useful for surgical anesthesia and/or postoperative pain control

  2. Require accurate identification of peripheral nerve anatomy and infiltration with local agent

D. Local Infiltration

  1. Surgical anesthesia for localized procedures

  2. Most effective when administered according to anatomic distribution of cutaneous nerves

SUGGESTED READING

Collins, VJ, editor: *Principles of anesthesiology,* ed 3, Philadelphia, 1993, Lea and Febiger.

Davidson JK, Eckhardt WF, Perese DA, editors: *Clinical anesthesia procedures of the Massachusetts General Hospital,* ed 4, Boston, 1993, Little, Brown.

Stoelting RK, Miller RD: *Basics of anesthesia,* ed 2, New York, 1989, Churchill Livingstone.

MEDICATIONS

24

Scott K. Pruitt

Drug*	Use	Form	Dosage
Acebutolol (Sectral)	Antihypertensive; β-antagonist	Cap: 200, 400 mg	200-600 mg PO bid
Acetaminophen (Tylenol)	Antipyretic	Cap: 325 mg; Elix: 100 mg/ml, 160 mg/5 ml; Supp. 125, 325, 650	650 mg PO/PR q3-4h, prn
Acetaminophen with codeine (Tylenol #3 or #4)	Analgesic	Tab #3: 300 mg acetaminophen/30 mg codeine Tab #4: 300 mg acetaminophen/60 mg codeine Elix: 120 mg acetaminophen/12 mg codeine/5 ml	1-2 PO q3-4h, prn; 15 ml PO q3-4h, prn
Acetaminophen with oxycodone (Percocet)	Analgesic	Tab: 325 mg acetaminophen/5 mg oxycodone; Cap: 500 mg/5 mg	1-2 PO q3-4h, prn
Acetazolamide (Diamox)	Diuretic; carbonic anhydrase inhibitor; HCO_3 excretion	Inj: 500 mg/5 ml; Tab: 125, 250 mg/Sustained release tab: 500 mg	250-375 mg PO qd; 250-500 mg IV q8h × 3 doses
Acyclovir (Zovirax)	Antiviral	Inj: 500 mg/10 ml	5-10 mg/kg IV over 1 hr q8h × 7 days
Adenosine (Adenocard)	Antiarrhythmic	Inj: 3 mg/ml (2 ml), 25 mg/ml (10 ml)	6 mg IV bolus, then 12 mg IV if needed
Albuterol (Proventil, Ventolin)	Bronchodilator; β₂-agonist	Inhaler: 90 µg/dose; Tab: 2, 4 mg; Susp: 2 mg/5 ml	1-2 puffs q4-6h; 2-4 mg PO tid-qid

*Trade name given in parentheses

Continued.

Drug*	Use	Form	Dosage
Allopurinol (Zyloprim)	Xanthine oxidase inhibitor	Tab: 100, 300 mg	200–600 mg PO qd
Alprazolam (Xanax)	Benzodiazepine, antianxiety	Tab: 0.25, 0.5, 1, 2 mg	0.25–3 mg PO tid
Alteplase (Activase, TPA)	Tissue plasminogen activator	Inj: 1 mg/ml	100 mg IV over 2 hr (then start heparin)
Amiloride (Midamor)	Potassium-sparing diuretic	Tab: 5 mg	5–20 mg PO qd
Aminocaproic acid (Amicar)	Inhibitor of fibrinolysis	Inj: 250 mg/ml	Load: 4–5 g in 250 ml D_5W over 1 hr Infusion: 1 g/50 ml/1 hr for 8 hr
Aminophylline	Bronchodilator	Inj: 1, 2, 25 mg/ml; Tab: 100, 200 mg	See theophylline
Amiodarone (Cordarone)	Antiarrhythmic	Tab: 200 mg	Load: 800–1600 mg PO qd Maintenance: 400–800 mg PO qd
Amitriptyline (Elavil)	Antidepressant	Inj: 10 mg/ml; Tab: 10, 25, 50, 75, 100, 150 mg	25–50 mg PO tid; 20–30 mg IM qid
Amphotericin B (Fungizone)	Antifungal	Inj: 5 mg/10 ml (dilute 1:50 in D_5W before use)	Systemic: 0.3–1 mg/kg/day IV; Bladder irrigation: 50 mg/L D_5W/day
Amrinone (Inocor)	Inotrope	Inj: 5 mg/ml (20 ml)	Load: 0.75 mg/kg; Infusion: 5–10 µg/kg/min
Aspirin (ASA)	Analgesic; antipyretic; antiinflammatory; antiplatelet activity	Cap: 325 mg; Enteric coated: 325 mg; Supp: 125, 325, 650 mg; Tab: 325 mg	650 mg PO/PR q-3-4h, prn
Atenolol (Tenormin)	Antihypertensive; β-antagonist	Tab: 25, 50, 100 mg	50–100 mg PO qd
Atracurium (Tracrium)	Nondepolarizing neuromuscular blocking agent	Inj: 1, 2 mg/ml	0.3–0.5 mg/kg IV

Atropine	Anticholinergic	Inj: 0.05, 0.1, 0.3, 0.4, 0.5, 0.8, 1 mg/ml
Azathioprine (Imuran)	Immunosuppressive	Inj: 10, 100 mg/ml; Tab: 50 mg
		Initial: 3-5 mg/kg qd; Maintenance: 1-3 mg/kg qd
Beclomethasone (Vanceril)	Antiasthmatic; corticosteroid	Inhaler: 42 µg/dose
		2 puffs q3-4h
Benazepril (Lotensin)	Antihypertensive; ACE inhibitor	Tab: 5, 10, 20, 40 mg
		10-40 mg PO qd
Bretylium tosylate (Bretylol)	Antiarrhythmic	Inj: 50 mg/ml (10 ml)
		Load: 5-10 mg/kg; Infusion: 1-2 mg/min
Bumetanide (Bumex)	Diuretic	Inj: 0.25 mg/ml; Tab: 0.5, 1.0 mg
		0.5-2 mg/day PO; 0.5-1 mg IV q4h up to 10 mg/day
Calcitriol (Rocaltrol)	Vitamin D supplement in CRF	Cap: 0.25, 0.5 µg/ Inj: 1, 2 µg/ml
		0.25-1 µg/day
Calcium chloride	Calcium supplement	Inj: 100 mg/ml (10 ml); 13.6 mEq (272 mg) Ca/g of CaCl$_2$ as 10% solution
		For CPR: 0.5-1 g IV; For Ca supp: 0.5-1 g IV q1-3d
Calcium gluconate	Calcium supplement	Inj: 100 mg/ml (10 ml); 4.5 mEq (90 mg) ca/g of Ca gluconate (Neocalglucon) 155 mg Ca/5 ml
		For Ca: 0.5-2 g IV; 15-30 ml PO tid (Neocalglucon)
Captopril (Capoten)	Antihypertensive; ACE inhibitor	Tab: 12.5, 25, 50, 100 mg
		25-150 mg PO bid or tid
Chloral hydrate	Sedative; hypnotic	Cap: 250, 500 mg; Supp: 500 mg; Susp: 50, 100 mg/ml
		50-1000 mg PO/PR qhs, prm
Chlorpromazine (Thorazine)	Antipsychotic; tranquilizer	Inj: 25 mg/ml; Supp: 25, 100 mg; Tab: 10, 25, 50, 100, 200 mg; Cap: 30, 75, 150, 200, 300 mg; Susp: 30, 100 mg/ml
		Acute psychosis: 25 mg IM, then 25-400 mg IM q4-6h; Control of nausea/vomiting: 10-25 mg PO/PR/IM tid

*Trade name given in parentheses

Continued.

Drug*	Use	Form	Dosage
Cimetidine (Tagamet)	Antiulcer; H_2 antagonist	Inj: 6, 150 mg/ml; Tab: 200, 300, 400, 800 mg; Liq: 60 mg/ml	300 mg PO/IV q6h; 37.5-50 mg/hr IV continuous infusion
Cisapride (Propulsid)	GI prokinetic agent	Tab: 10 mg	10-20 mg PO qid
Clonidine (Catapres)	Antihypertensive	Tab: 0.1, 0.2, 0.3 mg; Transdermal patch: 2.5, 5, 7.5 mg	0.1-1.2 mg PO bid; Topical: q7d
Codeine	Narcotic; analgesic; antitussive	Inj: 15, 30, 60 mg/ml; Tab: 15, 30, 60 mg	30-60 mg PO/IM q3-4 pm
Colchicine	Gout therapy	Inj: 0.5 mg/ml; Tab: 0.5, 0.6, 0.65 mg	Initial 2 mg IV/PO, then 0.5 mg PO/IV q6h
Cyclosporine (Sandimmune)	Immunosuppressive	Inj: 50 mg/ml; Liq: 20 mg/ml; Cap: 25, 100 mg	Initial: 10-14 mg/kg/day; Maintenance: 3-10 mg/kg/day
Cytomegalovirus immune globulin (Cytogam)	Antiviral	Inj: 250 mg/ml (10 ml)	50-150 mg/kg over 6 hr, q2 wks
Dantrolene (Dantrium)	Malignant hyperthermia therapy	Inj: 20 mg/60 ml	1 mg/kg IV bolus; repeat until symptoms resolve or total dose of 10 mg/kg
Darvocet-N-100	Analgesic	Tab: 100 mg propoxyphene/ 650 mg acetominophen	1-2 PO q3-4h, pm
Deferoxamine (Desferal)	Iron-chelating agent	Inj: 500 mg/2 ml	1 g IV followed by 500 mg IV q4-12h (total not > 6 g/24h)
Desmopressin acetate (DDAVP)	Diabetes insipidus; bleeding in hemophilia A and von Willebrand's	Inj: 4 µg/ml	DI: 1-2 µg IV/SQ q12h; Bleeding: 0.3 µg/kg IV single dose

Dexamethasone (Decadron)	Corticosteroid	Inj: 4, 8, 10, 20, 24, 40 mg/ml; Tab: 0.25, 0.5, 0.75, 1, 1.5, 2, 4, 6 mg; Elix: 0.1, 0.5, 1 mg/ml	10 mg IV q6h
Diazepam (Valium)	Antianxiety; tranquilizer	Inj: 5 mg/ml; Tab: 2, 5, 10 mg	2-10 mg PO bid-qid, prn; 2-10 mg IV/IM q3-4h prn; Seizure: 5-10 mg IV q10-15 min, prn
Diazoxide (Hyperstat)	Antihypertensive	Inj: 15 mg/ml (20 ml)	1-3 mg/kg IV q5-15 min until dBP < 100 mm Hg
Digoxin (Lanoxin)	Cardiac glycoside	Inj: 0.1, 0.25, 0.5 mg/ml; Elix: 0.05 mg/ml; Tab: 0.125, 0.25, 0.5 mg; Cap: 0.05, 0.1, 0.2 mg	Load: 0.4-0.6 mg IV bolus, then 0.1-0.3 mg q4-8h; Maintenance: 0.125-0.5 mg qd
Dihydrotachysterol (Hytakerol)	Vitamin D analogue	Cap: 0.125 mg; Tab: 0.125, 0.2, 0.4 mg; Solution: 0.2 mg/ml	Load: 0.8-2.4 mg PO qd; Maintenance: 0.2-1.0 mg PO qd
Diltiazem (Cardizem)	Antianginal; calcium channel blocker	Inj: 5 mg/ml; Tab: 30, 60, 90, 120 mg; Cap: 60, 90, 120, 180, 240, 300 mg	0.25-0.35 mg IV bolus (may be repeated), then 5-15 mg/hr IV continuous infusion; Maintenance: 120-480 mg PO qd (divided by 4 for tabs, 2 for sustained release, 1 for once daily capsules)
Diphenhydramine (Benadryl)	Antihistamine	Inj: 10, 50 mg/ml; Cap: 25, 50 mg; Elix: 2.5 mg/ml	25-50 mg PO/IV q4-6h, prn

*Trade name given in parentheses

Continued.

Drug*	Use	Form	Dosage
Diphenoxylate (Lomotil)	Antidiarrheal	Tab, Solution: 2.5 mg diphen-oxylate 0.025 mg atropine per tab or 5 ml	1-2 tab PO qid, prn
Dipyridamole (Persantine)	Antiplatelet aggregation	Tab: 25, 50, 75 mg; Inj: 5 mg/ml	75-100 mg PO qid
Disopyramide (Norpace)	Antiarrhythmic	Cap: 100, 150 mg; Controlled release: 100, 150 mg	100-200 mg PO q6-8h; 200-400 mg PO q12h
Dobutamine (Dobutrex)	Inotrope, β-agonist	Inj: 12.5 mg/ml (5 ml)	2-20 μg/kg/min
Docusate sodium (Colace)	Stool softener	Cap: 50, 100, 250 mg; Tab: 50, 100 mg; Syrup: 60 mg; Liq 10 mg/ml	100 mg PO bid
Dopamine (Intropin)	Dopamine receptor agonist, β₁-agonist, α-agonist	Inj: 40, 80, 160 mg/ml (15 ml)	0.5-2 μg/kg/min (stimulates dopamine receptors); 2-10 μg/kg/min (β₁ stimulator); 10-20 μg/kg/min (α stimulator)
Edrophonium (Tensilon)	Cholinergic; curare antagonist	Inj: 10 mg/ml	10 mg IV over 30-45 sec, re-peat as necessary to total of 40 mg
Enalapril (Vasotec)	Antihypertensive; ACE inhibitor	Inj: 1.25 mg/ml; Tab: 2.5, 5, 10, 20 mg	5-40 mg PO qd; 1.25-5 mg IV q6h
Enoxaprin	Low molecular weight heparin; DVT prophylaxis	Inj: 30 mg/0.3 ml	30 mg SQ bid
Epinephrine (Adrenalin)	Inotrope; pressor; broncho-dilator	Inj: 0.1 (1:10,000), 0.3, 0.5, 1 (1:1,000) mg/ml	0.01-0.15 μg/kg/min

Esmolol (Brevibloc)	Antiarrhythmic; β-antagonist	Inj: 10, 250 mg/ml	Load: 500 µg/kg over 1 min; Infusion: 50-200 µg/kg/min
Ethacrynic acid (Edecrin)	Loop diuretic	Inj: 1 mg/ml; Tab: 25; 50 mg	25-100 mg PO qd; 0.5-1 mg/kg IV
Etomidate (Amidate)	Induction agent	Inj: 2 mg/ml	0.2-0.6 mg/kg IV
Famotidine (Pepcid)	H$_2$-antagonist	Inj: 10 mg/ml; Tab: 20, 40 mg	20 mg PO/IV q12h; 40 mg PO qhs
Fentanyl (Sublimaze)	Analgesic	Inj: 0.05 mg/ml	0.002-0.05 mg/kg IV
Flecainide (Tambocor)	Antiarrhythmic	Tab: 50, 100, 150 mg	50-200 mg PO bid
Fluconazole (Diflucan)	Antifungal	Inj: 2 mg/ml; Tab: 50, 100, 200 mg	200-400 mg PO/IV qd × 1, then 100-200 mg PO/IV qd
Flucytosine (Ancobon)	Antifungal	Cap: 250, 500 mg	12.5-37.5 mg/kg PO q6h
Flurazepam (Dalmane)	Hypnotic	Cap: 15, 30 mg	15-30 mg PO qhs, pm
Fosinopril (Monopril)	Antihypertensive; ACE inhibitor	Tab: 10, 20 mg	10-80 mg PO qd
Furosemide (Lasix)	Diuretic	Inj: 10 mg/ml; Tab: 20, 40, 80 mg; Solution: 10 mg/ml	10-40 mg PO bid for hypertension; 20-80 mg IV/PO q6h pm for pulmonary edema/fluid overload
Ganciclovir (Cytovene)	Antiviral	Inj: 50 mg/ml	5 mg/kg IV q12h × 14-21 days
Glipizide (Glucotrol)	Oral hypoglycemic	Tab: 5, 10 mg	2.5-40 mg PO qd
Glucagon	Hypoglycemia treatment	Inj: 1 U/ml	0.5-1 U/IM/SQ
Glyburide (Micronase)	Oral hypoglycemic	Tab: 1.25, 2.5, 5 mg	2.5-20 mg PO qd
Glycopyrrolate (Robinul)	Anticholinergic	Inj: 0.2 mg/ml; Tab: 1, 2 mg	To reverse neuromuscular blocking agent: 0.2 mg IV for each 1 mg neostigmine

*Trade name given in parentheses

Continued.

Drug*	Use	Form	Dosage
Guanethidine (Ismelin)	Antihypertensive	Tab: 10, 25 mg	10-50 mg PO qd
Haloperidol (Haldol)	Antipsychotic; sedative/hypnotic	Inj: 5 mg/ml; Solution: 2 mg/ml; Tab: 0.5, 1, 2, 5, 10, 20 mg	0.5-5 mg PO/IM bid-tid; 2-5 mg IV/IM q30-60 min, prn
Heparin sodium	Anticoagulant	Multiple formulations	Load: 5000 U IV; Continuous IV infusion: 20,000-40,000 U/24 hr in 1000 ml NaCl 0.9%
Hydralazine (Apresoline)	Antihypertensive; vasodilator	Inj: 20 mg/ml; Tab: 10, 25, 50, 100 mg	10-50 mg PO qid; 10-40 mg IM q1-2h prn; 10-40 mg IV, prn
Hydrochlorothiazide	Diuretic (thiazide)	Tab: 25, 50, 100 mg; Solution: 10 mg/ml	25-100 mg PO qd
Hydrocortisone (Solu-Cortef)	Corticosteroid	Inj: 100, 250, 500, 1000 mg/vial	100-500 mg IV q2-6h, prn
Hydromorphone (Dilaudid)	Analgesic	Inj: 1, 2, 3, 4, mg/10 ml; Tab: 2, 3, 4 mg; Supp: 3 mg	2-4 mg PO/IM q4-6h, prn; 3 mg PR q6-8h prn
Hydroxyzine (Atarax, Vistaril)	Antianxiety	Inj: 25, 50 mg/ml; Syrup: 2 mg/ml; Tab: 10, 25, 50, 100 mg	25-100 mg PO/IM qid
Ibuprofen	Antiinflammatory; analgesic	Tab: 300, 400, 600, 800 mg; Susp: 20 mg/ml	300-800 mg PO tid-qid
Imipramine (Tofranil)	Antidepressant	Inj: 25 mg/vial; Cap: 75; 100; 125; 150 mg; Tab: 10, 25, 50 mg	25-50 mg PO/IM qid
Indomethacin (Indocin)	Antiinflammatory	Cap: 25, 50 mg; Supp: 50 mg; Susp: 25 mg/5 ml	25-50 mg PO/PR bd-tid

Drug (Trade name)	Action	Formulations	Dosing
Ipratropium bromide (Atrovent)	Anticholinergic bronchodilator	Inhaler: 18 µg/dose, 0.03%	2 puffs qid + prn
Isoproterenol (Isuprel)	β-Agonist	Inj: 0.2 mg/ml (5 ml)	0.1–1.0 µg/kg/min
Ketamine (Ketalar)	Induction; short acting anesthetic	Inj: 10, 50, 100 mg/ml	1.0–4.5 mg/kg IV
Ketoconazole (Nizoral)	Antifungal	Tab: 200 mg; Susp: 100 mg/5 ml	200–400 mg PO qd
Ketorolac (Toradol)	Analgesic; antiinflammatory	Inj: 15, 30, 60 mg/ml	Load 30–60 mg IM, then 15–30 mg IM q6h, prn
Labetalol (Trandate)	Antihypertensive; adrenergic antagonist	Inj: 5 mg/ml; Tab: 100, 200, 300 mg	100–400 mg PO bid; Load: 20 mg IV, Infusion: 0.5–2 mg/min IV
Lactulose (Cephulac)	Hepatic encephalopathy	Syrup: 10 g/15 ml (67%)	15–50 ml PO tid; 300 ml in 700 ml NS PR for 30–60 min q4-6h
Levothyroxine (Synthroid)	Synthetic thyroid hormone	Inj: 200, 500 µg/vial; Tab: 50, 75, 88, 100, 112, 125, 137, 150, 175, 200, 300 µg	25–300 µg PO/IM qd; 200–500 µg IV for myxedema
Lidocaine	Antiarrhythmic	Inj: 10, 15, 20, 25, 40, 100, 200 mg/ml	50–100 mg IV bolus, repeat if necessary after 5 min, then 1–4 mg/min IV infusion
Lisinopril (Zestril)	Antihypertensive; ACE inhibitor	Tab: 5, 10, 20, 40 mg	10–40 mg PO qd
Loperamide (Imodium)	Antidiarrheal	Cap: 2 mg	Load: 4 mg PO; 2 mg PO after each stool up to 16 mg/day
Lorazepam (Ativan)	Anxiolytic; sedative	Inj: 2, 4 mg/ml; Tab: 0.5, 1, 2 mg	2–3 mg/day PO/IM given bid-tid; 2–4 mg IV, prn

*Trade name given in parentheses

Continued.

Drug*	Use	Form	Dosage
Mannitol	Osmotic diuretic	Inj: 5, 10, 15, 20, 25% solutions	50-150 g IV, prn
Meperidine (Demerol)	Analgesic	Inj: 25, 50, 75, 100 mg/ml; Elixer: 10 mg/ml; Tab: 50 mg	0.5-2.0 mg/kg IV q2-3h; 50-150 mg PO/IM/SQ q3-4 h, prn
Metaproterenol (Alupent)	Bronchodilator; β-agonist	Inhalation solution: 0.4, 0.6, 5%; Susp: 2 mg/ml; Tab: 10, 20 mg	20 mg PO tid-qid; Nebulization: 1 vial q4h, prn
Metaraminol (Aramine)	Sympathomimetic; therapy for hypotension with spinal anesthesia	Inj: 10 mg/ml	2-10 mg SQ/IM; Infusion: 15-100 mg in 500 ml NS IV prn
Methohexital (Brevital)	Induction agent	Inj: 10 mg/ml	0.7-1.5 mg/kg IV
Methyldopa (Aldomet)	Antihypertensive	Inj: 50 mg/ml; Tab: 125, 250, 500 mg; Susp: 250 mg/ml	250-500 mg PO bid-tid; 250-500 mg IV q6-8h
Methylprednisolone (Solu-Medrol)	Corticosteroid	Inj: 40, 125, 500, 1000, 2000 mg/vial; Tab: 2, 4, 8, 16, 24, 32 mg	30 mg/mg IV q4-6h × 48-72 hr
Metoclopramide (Reglan)	Gastric motility stimulant	Inj: 5 mg/ml; Tab: 5, 10 mg; Syrup: 1 mg/ml	10-15 mg PO/IV qid or q6h
Metolazone (Zaroxolyn)	Diuretic	Tab: 2.5, 5, 10 mg	5-20 mg PO qd
Metoprolol (Lopressor)	Antihypertensive, β₁-antagonist	Inj: 1 mg/ml; Tab: 50, 100 mg	50-200 mg PO bid; 5 mg IV q2min, prn
Mexiletine (Mexitil)	Antiarrhythmic	Tab: 150, 200, 250 mg	200-400 mg PO q8h
Midazolam (Versed)	Antianxiety; sedation; induction	Inj: 1, 5 mg/ml	0.15-0.35 mg/kg IV

Monooctanoin (Moctanin)	Dissolves gallstones	Solution: 120 mg/bottle	3-5 ml/hr perfused into bile duct
Morphine	Analgesic	Inj: 0.2, 2, 3, 4, 5, 8, 10, 15, 25, 50 mg/ml	0.05-0.2 mg/kg IV q1h; 2-10 mg IM q3-4h
Nadolol (Corgard)	Antihypertensive, β-antagonist	Tab: 20, 40, 80, 120, 160 mg	40-80 mg PO qd
Naloxone (Narcan)	Narcotic antagonist	Inj: 0.02, 0.4, 1 mg/ml	0.4-2 mg IV q2-3min, pm (up to 10 mg total)
Neostigmine	Anticholinesterase; reversal or neuromuscular block	Inj: 1 mg/ml (1:1000), 0.5 mg/ml (1:2000)	0.5-2 mg IV, repeat pm up to 5 mg total
Nifedipine (Procardia)	Antihypertensive; calcium channel blocker	Cap: 10, 20 mg	10-30 mg PO tid; 10 mg sublingual pm
Nitroglycerin	Vasodilator	Inj: 0.5, 0.8, 5, 10 mg/ml; Tab: 0.15, 0.3, 0.4, 0.6 mg; Ointment: 2% (1 inch = 15 mg)	0.3-0.6 mg sublingually q5min, pm; 0.5-4 in topically q4-8h; 0.1-2 µg/kg/min
Nitroprusside (Nipride)	Antihypertensive; vasodilator	Inj: 10, 25 mg/ml	0.3-10 µ/kg/min
Norepinephrine (Levophed)	Rx of hypotension; vasopressor	Inj: 1 mg/ml (4 ml)	0.01-0.02 µg/kg/min
Ocetreotide acetate (Sandostatin)	Somatostatin analog	Inj: 0.05, 0.1, 0.5, 1 mg/ml	50-100 µg SQ q8-12h
OKT3	Immunosuppressive	Inj: 1 mg/ml	
Omeprazole (Prilosec)	Proton pump inhibitor	Cap: 20 mg	20 mg PO qd
Oxazepam (Serax)	Antianxiety; tranquilizer	Cap: 10, 15, 30 mg; Tab: 15 mg	10-30 mg PO tid-qid
Oxycodone (Percodan)	Analgesic	Tab: 325 mg aspirin/0.38 oxycodone terephthalate/4.5 mg oxycodone HCl	1-2 PO q4h, pm

*Trade name given in parentheses

Continued.

Drug*	Use	Form	Dosage
Pancreatin	Pancreatic enzyme replacement	Tab: (pancreatin, 325 mg; lipase, 650 U; protease, 8,125 U; amylase 8,125 U	1-3 PO with meals
Pancrelipase (Cotazym, Viokinase)	Pancreatic enzyme replacement	Cotazym Cap: lipase, 8,000 U; protease, 30,000 U; calcium carbonate, 25 mg; Viokinase Tab: lipase, 8,000 U; protease, 30,000 U; amylase 30,000 U	1-3 tab/cap PO before meals
Pancuronium (Pavulon)	Neuromuscular blockade	Inj: 1, 2 mg/ml	0.04-0.1 mg/kg IV, prn
Paregoric	Antidiarrheal	Liq: 2 mg/5 ml (0.04% MSO₄)	5-10 ml PO qid, prn
Pentazocine (Talwin)	Analgesic	Inj: 30 mg/ml	30 mg IV/IM/SQ q3-4h, prn
Phenobarbital	Anticonvulsant	Inj: 30, 60, 130 mg/ml; Tab: 8, 16, 32, 65, 100 mg; Elix: 4 mg/ml	1-5 mg/kg/day PO/IV
Phenoxybenazmine (Dibenzyline)	α-Adrenergic antagonist	Tab: 10 mg	10-40 mg PO q8-12h
Phentalamine (Regitine)	α-Adrenergic antagonist	Inj: 5 mg/vial	5 mg IM/IV/IV
Phenylephrine (Neo-Synephrine)	Vasopressor	Inj: 10 mg/ml (1 ml)	0.6-5 µg/kg/min
Phenytoin (Dilantin)	Anticonvulsant; antiarrhythmic	Inj: 50 mg/ml; Cap: 30, 100 mg; Susp: 30, 125 mg/5 ml	100-30 mg PO tid; Load: 10-15 mg/kg IV; Maintenance: 4-8 mg/kg/day
Prazosin (Minipress)	Antihypertensive	Cap: 1, 2, 5 mg	1-5 mg PO tid

Prednisone	Corticosteroid	Tab: 1, 2.5, 5, 20, 50 mg; Solution: 5 mg/5 ml	5-6 mg PO qd
Procainamide (Pronestyl)	Antiarrhythmic	Inj: 100, 500 mg/ml; Cap: 250, 375, 500 mg; Sustained release: 250, 500, 750, 1000 mg	Load: 750-1000 mg IV; Infusion: 2-6 mg/min IV; Maintenance: 250-500 mg PO q4h or 500-1000 mg PO q6h
Prochlorperazine (Compazine)	Antiemetic	Inj: 5 mg/ml; Tab: 5, 10, 25 mg; Supp: 2.5, 5, 25 mg	5-10 mg PO/IM q4-6h, prn; 25 mg PR bid, prn
Promethazine (Phenergan)	Antiemetic	Inj: 25, 50 mg/ml; Tab: 12.5, 25, 50 mg; Supp: 12.5, 25, 50 mg	12.5-25 mg PO/IM q4-6h, prn; 25 mg PR tid-qid, prn
Propofol (Diprivan)	Anesthesia; sedation	Inj: 10 mg/ml	1.5-3 mg/kg IV for induction; 25-150 µg/kg/min IV continuous infusion
Propranolol (Inderal)	Antiarrhythmic, β-adrenergic antagonist, antihypertensive	Inj: 1 mg/ml; Tab: 10, 20, 40, 60, 80, 90 mg; Sustained release cap: 60, 80, 120, 160 mg	1-3 mg IV q20min up to total of 0.15 mg/kg; 10-60 mg PO q6h
Protamine sulfate	Heparin antagonist	Inj: 10 mg/ml	1 mg IV to reverse 90 U bovine heparin, 100 U porcine heparin (Ca²⁺), 115 U porcine heparin (Na⁺)
Quinapril (Accupril)	Antihypertensive; ACE inhibitor	Tab: 5, 10, 20, 40 mg	10-80 mg PO qd
Quinidine sulfate (Quinidex)	Antiarrhythmic	Tab: 100, 200, 300 mg	400-600 mg PO q2-3 h until PSVT terminated; Maintenance: 200-300 mg PO tid-qid

Continued.

*Trade name given in parentheses

Drug*	Use	Form	Dosage
Ranitidine (Zantac)	H$_2$-antagonist; antiulcer	Inj: 1, 25 mg/ml; Tab 150, 300 mg; Susp: 15, 16.8 mg/ml	150 mg PO q12h; 50 mg IV q6-8h; 6.25 mg/hr IV continuous infusion
Sodium bicarbonate	Alkalinizing agent	Amp: 50 mEq/50 ml	Adjusted for acid-base status
Spironolactone (Aldactone)	Diuretic; antialdosterone	Tab: 25, 50, 100 mg	25-200 mg PO qd
Streptokinase	Plasminogen activator; thrombolytic	Inj: 250,000; 750,000; 1,500,000 U/vial	For thrombotic events: 250,000 U IV load over 30 min, then 100,000 U/hr × 72 hr
Succinylcholine	Depolarizing neuromuscular blocking agent	Inj: 20 mg/ml	0.6-2 mg/kg IV
Sucralfate (Carafate)	Antiulcer; cytoprotective	Tab: 1g; Solution: 1 g/10 ml	1 g PO/via NG q6h
Tacrolimus (Prograf, FK506)	Immunosuppressant	Cap: 1, 5 mg; Inj: 5 mg/ml	0.05-0.1 mg/kg/day IV continuous infusion; 0.075-0.15 mg/kg PO q12h
Terbutaline (Brethine)	β-Agonist; bronchodilator	Inhaler: 200 µg/dose; Inj: 1 mg/ml; Tab: 2.5, 5 mg	1-2 puffs q4-6h; 0.25-0.5 mg SC q4h; 5 mg PO q6h
Theophylline	Bronchodilator	Inj (aminophylline): 25 mg/ml; Solution: 80, 150 mg/15 ml; Tab: 100, 200, 300, 400 mg	Load: 6 mg/kg IV; Infusion: 0.6-0.9 mg/kg/hr; 5-8 mg/kg PO q6-8h
Thiopental	Anesthetic (short acting)	Inj: 20 mg/ml	50-75 mg IV, prn
Thioridazine (Mellaril)	Antipsychotic	Tab: 10, 15, 25, 50, 100, 150, 200 mg; Susp: 25, 30, 100 mg/ml	50-250 mg PO tid
Timolol (Blocadren)	Antihypertensive; β-antagonist	Tab: 5, 10, 20 mg	10-20 mg PO bid

Drug (Trade name)	Category/Use	Formulation	Dosing
Tocainide (Tonocard)	Antiarrhythmic	Tab: 400, 600 mg	400–800 mg PO q8h
Tolazamide (Tolinase)	Oral hypoglycemic	Tab: 100, 250, 500 mg	100–500 mg PO qd-bid
Triazolam (Halcion)	Hypnotic	Tab: 0.125, 0.25, 0.5 mg	0.125–0.5 mg PO qhs, prn
Trimethaphan (Arfonad)	Antihypertensive	Inj: 50 mg/ml	3–4 mg/min IV continuous infusion
Vasopressin (Pitressin)	Rx of diabetes insipidus	Inj: 20 U/ml	5–10 U IV bid-tid, prn
Vecuronium (Norcuron)	Nondepolarizing neuromuscular blocking agent; induction agent	Inj: 1 mg/ml	0.08–0.1 mg/kg IV
Verapamil (Isoptin, Calan)	Antiarrhythmic; calcium channel blocker	Inj: 2.5 mg/ml; Tab: 40, 80, 120 mg; Sustained release: 240 mg	Load: 0.75–0.15 µg/kg; Infusion: 5 µg/kg/min; 40–120 mg PO q8h
Warfarin (Coumadin)	Oral anticoagulant; vitamin K antagonist	Tab: 2, 2.5, 5, 7.5, 10 mg	5–15 mg PO qd (monitor PT)

*Trade name given in parentheses

INDEX

Page numbers in italics indicate illustrations; *t* indicates tables.